Humanistic Approaches to Medical Practice

Humanistic Approaches to Medical Practice

Editors

Beatrice Gabriela Ioan
Magdalena Iorga

MDPI • Basel • Beijing • Wuhan • Barcelona • Belgrade • Manchester • Tokyo • Cluj • Tianjin

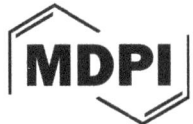

Editors
Beatrice Gabriela Ioan
Legal Medicine Department
Grigore T. Popa University of
Medicine and Pharmacy
Iasi
Romania

Magdalena Iorga
Behavioral Sciences
Department
Grigore T. Popa University of
Medicine and Pharmacy
Iasi
Romania

Editorial Office
MDPI
St. Alban-Anlage 66
4052 Basel, Switzerland

This is a reprint of articles from the Special Issue published online in the open access journal *Medicina* (ISSN 1648-9144) (available at: www.mdpi.com/journal/medicina/special_issues/humanistic_medical).

For citation purposes, cite each article independently as indicated on the article page online and as indicated below:

LastName, A.A.; LastName, B.B.; LastName, C.C. Article Title. *Journal Name* **Year**, *Volume Number*, Page Range.

ISBN 978-3-0365-5564-5 (Hbk)
ISBN 978-3-0365-5563-8 (PDF)

© 2022 by the authors. Articles in this book are Open Access and distributed under the Creative Commons Attribution (CC BY) license, which allows users to download, copy and build upon published articles, as long as the author and publisher are properly credited, which ensures maximum dissemination and a wider impact of our publications.

The book as a whole is distributed by MDPI under the terms and conditions of the Creative Commons license CC BY-NC-ND.

Contents

About the Editors vii

Preface to "Humanistic Approaches to Medical Practice" ix

Sana Loue
Teaching and Practicing Humanism and Empathy through Embodied Engagement
Reprinted from: *Medicina* **2022**, *58*, 330, doi:10.3390/medicina58030330 1

Bianca Hanganu, Magdalena Iorga, Lavinia Maria Pop and Beatrice Gabriela Ioan
Socio-Demographic, Professional and Institutional Characteristics That Make Romanian Doctors More Prone to Malpractice Complaints
Reprinted from: *Medicina* **2022**, *58*, 287, doi:10.3390/medicina58020287 9

Sînziana Călina Silișteanu, Maria Totan, Oana Raluca Antonescu, Lavinia Duică, Elisabeta Antonescu and Andrei Emanuel Silișteanu
The Impact of COVID-19 on Behavior and Physical and Mental Health of Romanian College Students
Reprinted from: *Medicina* **2022**, *58*, 246, doi:10.3390/medicina58020246 25

Lavinia Duică, Elisabeta Antonescu, Maria Totan, Gabriela Boța and Sînziana Călina Silișteanu
Borderline Personality Disorder "Discouraged Type": A Case Report
Reprinted from: *Medicina* **2022**, *58*, 162, doi:10.3390/medicina58020162 35

Marta Rzadkiewicz, Gorill Haugan and Dorota Włodarczyk
Mature Adults at the GP: Length of Visit and Patient Satisfaction—Associations with Patient, Doctor, and Facility Characteristics
Reprinted from: *Medicina* **2022**, *58*, 159, doi:10.3390/medicina58020159 43

Dragos Bumbacea, Carmen Panaitescu and Roxana Silvia Bumbacea
Patient and Physician Perspectives on Asthma and Its Therapy in Romania: Results of a Multicenter Survey
Reprinted from: *Medicina* **2021**, *57*, 1089, doi:10.3390/medicina57101089 57

Vlad Ioan Covrig, Diana Elena Lazăr, Victor Vlad Costan, Roxana Postolică and Beatrice Gabriela Ioan
The Psychosocial Role of Body Image in the Quality of Life of Head and Neck Cancer Patients. What Does the Future Hold?—A Review of the Literature
Reprinted from: *Medicina* **2021**, *57*, 1078, doi:10.3390/medicina57101078 69

Magdalena Iorga, Lavinia-Maria Pop, Nicoleta Gimiga, Luminița Păduraru and Smaranda Diaconescu
Assessing the Opinion of Mothers about School-Based Sexual Education in Romania, the Country with the Highest Rate of Teenage Pregnancy in Europe
Reprinted from: *Medicina* **2021**, *57*, 841, doi:10.3390/medicina57080841 83

Oana-Maria Isailă, Sorin Hostiuc and George-Cristian Curcă
Perspectives and Values of Dental Medicine Students Regarding Domestic Violence
Reprinted from: *Medicina* **2021**, *57*, 780, doi:10.3390/medicina57080780 97

Lavinia-Maria Pop, Magdalena Iorga, Lucian-Roman Șipoș and Raluca Iurcov
Gender Differences in Healthy Lifestyle, Body Consciousness, and the Use of Social Networks among Medical Students
Reprinted from: *Medicina* **2021**, *57*, 648, doi:10.3390/medicina57070648 . . . . **105**

Win-Long Lu, Yuan-Ti Lee and Gwo-Tarng Sheu
Metabolic Syndrome Prevalence and Cardiovascular Risk Assessment in HIV-Positive Men with and without Antiretroviral Therapy
Reprinted from: *Medicina* **2021**, *57*, 578, doi:10.3390/medicina57060578 . . . . **121**

Magdalena Iorga, Camelia Soponaru, Răzvan-Vladimir Socolov, Alexandru Cărăuleanu and Demetra-Gabriela Socolov
How the SARS-CoV-2 Pandemic Period Influenced the Health Status and Determined Changes in Professional Practice among Obstetrics and Gynecology Doctors in Romania
Reprinted from: *Medicina* **2021**, *57*, 325, doi:10.3390/medicina57040325 . . . . **131**

Israel Macías-Toronjo, José L. Sánchez-Ramos, María J. Rojas-Ocaña and Esperanza Begoña García-Navarro
Fear-Avoidance Behavior and Sickness Absence in Patients with Work-Related Musculoskeletal Disorders
Reprinted from: *Medicina* **2020**, *56*, 646, doi:10.3390/medicina56120646 . . . . **151**

About the Editors

Beatrice Gabriela Ioan

Beatrice Gabriela Ioan is a Professor of Legal Medicine and Bioethics at "Grigore T. Popa"University of Medicine and Pharmacy and a physician at the Institute of Legal Medicine of Iași, Romania. She graduated from the Faculty of Medicine in 1993 and received her PhD in 2003. She also graduated from the Faculty of Psychology in 2002 and from the Law Faculty in 2012. In 2004, she completed the Master of Art Program in Bioethics at Case Western Reserve University, USA, and in 2013 the Master du Droit et Gestion de la Santé at Institut Catholique de Rennes, France. She is member of the Steering Committee for Human Rights in the Fields of Biomedicine and Health of the Council of Europe and its former Chair. Since 2016 she has been a member of the International Bioethics Committee of UNESCO. She is also the Chair of the Bioethics Commission and member of the Superior Discipline Commission of the Romanian College of Physicians. She has authored many scientific articles, books and book chapters on Bioethics and Legal Medicine. Her main areas of interest are: bioethics, medical communication and medical liability.

Magdalena Iorga

Magdalena IORGA is a PhD Associate Professor at "Grigore T. Popa"Faculty of Medicine at the University of Medicine and Pharmacy from Iași, Romania. She also works as a PhD supervisor in the field of Psychology at the Faculty of Psychology and Education Sciences at "Alexandru Ioan Cuza"University of Iași. In 2001, she completed the Master in Intercultural Education. She has published five books and more than 100 scientific research articles in ISI databases, including more than 80 articles in BDI journals. She has coordinated research grants and national and international projects in the field of medical psychology and behavioral sciences. Her main areas of interests are applied psychology in the medical field, ethics, higher education and child psychology.

Preface to "Humanistic Approaches to Medical Practice"

Medical practice is a mixture of science and art, technique and humanism. The importance of human beings is more obvious in medicine than in any other field. The patient is at the center of medical care and the relationship between the patient and the doctor/medical staff is the foundation of the entire medical system.

The doctor–patient relationship is built on trust; i.e., the patient trusts the doctor's professional ability to cure the disease he/she is suffering from and, equally, expects the doctor to exhibit humanistic behavior [1].

Overspecialization is a big component of modern medicine, with professionals working in increasingly narrow fields, which makes patients routinely treated by multidisciplinary teams. This draws attention to the importance of appropriate relationships between members of the medical team for the success of the therapy. Thus, interactions between healthcare professionals, as well as those between them and their patients, must be filtered through the rigors of humanistic values and behaviors [2, 3].

Humanism in medicine is based on internal values, such as integrity, honesty, care and compassion, altruism, empathy, respect for oneself, patients and colleagues [1, 2]. This "way of being" is patient-centered and recognizes that the cognitive, psychological, emotional, social, and spiritual dimensions of clinical interactions affect both patients and healthcare professionals [4]. Humanistic values applied in medical practice characterize humanistic behaviors [2].

Medical professionalism is reflected in the way the doctor treats the patient and correctly applies, on the one hand, their clinical knowledge and skills and, on the other hand, a humanistic approach to their patients [1]. In this way, humanism is a central feature of professionalism [1] and a core competency of doctors [2]. Therefore, focusing only on the technical aspects and ignoring the humanistic and moral aspects of the medical profession can seriously damage the professionalism of doctors, decrease the quality of medical services provided to patients and deteriorate the doctor–patient relationship [5].

Montgomery et al. proposed a developmental model of medical humanism, centered on the interaction between "heart" and "head", which captures the indissoluble link between humanism and professionalism. In this model, the "heart" represents the emotional aspects of humanism (such as altruism, empathy, and care), and the "head" signifies its cognitive aspects (knowledge, attitudes, and ethics), the latter being attributes of professionalism [6].

Humanistic medicine views the patient as a person, from a holistic perspective, not just the disease from which he/she suffers [7], promoting bio-psycho-social-spiritual models of care [1, 4]. Medical practice that reflects the humanistic values of the profession involves doctor–patient interactions in which the patient is approached as a unique human being who must be treated with dignity and respect [2].

Lee Roze des Ordons et al. identified five defining attitudes and behaviors of humanism in medicine: the holistic care of the patient, considering their emotional, social and spiritual dimensions; respect for the intrinsic value of each person; taking into account other people's perspectives and understanding the experiences of patients and their families related to the disease; the recognition of the universality/the common elements of the human condition, which allows for the identification of common ground for the doctor and patient and overcoming professional boundaries; and focusing on the multiple relationships that are established between the actors of the medical act (healthcare professionals, patients, their families, and students) [4].

In addition to understanding physical diseases on a scientific basis, healthcare professionals must focus on the suffering of the patient, on the life changes, dilemmas and stress caused by the disease. So, a much more comprehensive paradigm opens up to the healthcare professionals, i.e., suffering-based medicine (SBM). SBM differs from evidence-based medicine (EBM). While EBM is defined as "the conscientious explicit and judicious use of current best evidence in helping individual patients make decisions about their care in the light of their personal values and beliefs"[8], SBM focuses on "all nonphysical personal aspects of the illness experience not amenable to being solved by finding the best evidence"[9]. SBM is not a substitute for scientific medicine but helps the patient to improve clinically. The experience of illness determines the perception of loss of wholeness, loss of certainty and control, loss of freedom to act, and loss of the familiar world [10]. So, healthcare professionals must guide the patient through the process of changing to the new life brought by the illness and to deal with the suffering. Suffering is determined by an individual's cultural background, religious beliefs, and socio-economic constraints, and must be taken into account by the specialist. For patients that are not familiarized with being ill, and for chronically ill patients or end-life patients, medical care must be adjusted. Maybe the healthcare professionals were happy to use new technology in order to better care for the patient but neglecting their psychological aspects or suffering is surely a mistake. In order to adjust themselves to various kinds of patients, medical professionals must collect a comprehensive anamnesis and also clinically relevant data needed for both a diagnosis and a therapeutic plan without eliminating any possible medical type of intervention.

Practicing humanistic medicine has benefits for both patients and healthcare professionals. In the study by Lee Roze des Ordons et al., humanism was identified as a basic principle of patient care and the physician's well-being [4].

Humanistic behaviors help doctors to favorably solve communication problems with patients, to ensure adequate information is provided, understand their perspectives and respect their rights. Trust and mutual understanding facilitate cooperation between doctors and patients, reporting of symptoms and sharing of information—including patients' life experiences, which play a critical role in the diagnosis and acceptance of treatment [5].

Focusing healthcare around the needs and preferences of patients and their active involvement in the decision-making process (which characterizes the so-called patient-centered care) are prerequisites for improving clinical outcomes, quality of care and patients'satisfaction, while reducing healthcare costs and health disparities [11].

In the study carried out by Hirpa et al., which aimed to evaluate patients' priorities in obtaining medical care, the humanistic qualities of doctors and shared decision making were among the most important aspects outlined by the participants, with the study concluding that providing effective, quality healthcare requires understanding what matters most to patients [11].

Higuita-Gutiérrez et al. investigated the preferences of cancer patients regarding healthcare and showed that one of the problems most frequently reported by the participants was the dehumanization of the interaction between the patient and the doctor, which represents a burden for the patient in addition to the one imposed by the disease from which he/she suffers. Participants emphasized a preference for doctors who use their professional knowledge and skills to better know their patients and their individuality—including from the perspectives of their daily lives, finding out the truth, being aware of their own limits, and being open to communication and to shared decision making [12].

Humanistic medical practice helps doctors both in their careers and in their lives. In a study conducted by Chou et al., in 2014 [13], it was shown that doctors believed that treating their patients humanistically serves to prevent burnout in themselves. Doctors who empathized with their patients have higher job satisfaction, are less prone to occupational burnout and made fewer errors which lead to complaints [5, 14].

The humanistic behaviors of medical professionals are also beneficial in the process of training students, teaching professionalism and instilling the humanistic values of the profession, which are essential for future medical professionals [1, 7]. The models of humanistic behavior offered by teachers during the clinical training of students have a major role, given that students learn not only from the explanations provided but, above all, from observing the daily actions and behaviors of their teachers, included in the so-called hidden curriculum [1, 5, 7]. Dealing with diseases means connecting with patients and their families. This is why teaching medical students and medical professionals how to adopt humanistic approaches during medical processes is mandatory. During their medical formation, medical students must be helped to gain awareness and sensitivity to many physical and psychological components of people's reaction to restrictions, health, illness, and hospitalization and death anxiety. Thus, many of the medical faculties adopted new curricula in order to adjust students to the new world of medical services. For example, in 2011, The Korean Accreditation Board of Nursing revised nursing college accreditation criteria, and decided that 40% of the curriculum must be composed of subjects related to the humanities and social sciences [15].

Despite the major benefits and positive impact of humanistic medical practice, contemporary medicine is characterized by realities that limit the premises of such an approach.

Dehumanization began to make its presence felt in medicine in the early 19th century with the development of new methods of clinical investigation, and continued with scientific advances in medicine over the next two centuries. Medicine has undergone, in a relatively short time, major changes that have largely determined the reconfiguration of the doctor–patient relationship and the way in which medical care is provided [1].

Current medical practice is dominated by so-called scientific medicine, which originates in the traditional view of natural sciences and focuses on diseases of different parts of the body, offering a "materialistic, reductionist and mechanistic" perspective [7]. From this perspective, the patient is approached as a static and passive object, a set of interacting parts that must be understood, studied and treated by focusing on the diseased parts [4, 7, 12].

The introduction of new technologies and artificial intelligence into medical practice is considered the main reason for the dehumanization of medicine. New technologies for diagnosis have made doctors dependent on technology, while psychological, moral and social aspects have been ignored in diagnosing, treating and ensuring the well-being of patients [1, 5]. Advanced technologies have changed the relationship between doctors and patients, in the sense that doctors tend to pay more attention to the use of technologies than to their interactions with the patient. Added to this is the use in medical practice of technologies that interact with the patient without or with little involvement of the doctor [1]. At the same time, the online environment abounds with information, more or less correct, about diseases, being accessed more and more frequently by patients, so that doctors are no longer the only source of information for them [1].

Researchers identified the dehumanization of medicine in the process of robotizing the medical act. However, science talks about "humanistic robots" and "humanistic care robots"—robots designed "for use in home, hospital, or other settings to assist in, support, or provide care for sick, disabled, young, elderly, or otherwise vulnerable persons"—focusing on the robot caregiving, design, and also on the ethics of robot care [16], highlighting the efficiency of the humanistic medical approach.

The realities of practicing the medical profession today are added to the negative impact of new technologies on the doctor–patient relationship. Doctors are obliged to consult more and more patients in order to be productive, have increasingly busy work schedules, are pressured to solve bureaucratic problems (for example, filling out administrative documents) [1]. The burden of these responsibilities can lead to occupational burnout and weakens the doctors' adherence to the humanistic values of their profession [2, 5].

In the medical climate dominated by technological progress and the new circumstances of practicing medicine, the need to relate to the humanistic values of the medical profession becomes increasingly clear. At the same time, medical professionals must acknowledge the complexity of the medical act in which technical aspects are intertwined with cultural, ethical, legal, psychological, and sociological issues in order to provide the best care to their patients.

This Special Issue is dedicated to the humanistic values of medical practice. It includes articles that approach various aspects of the so-called humanistic medicine, drawing a picture of what contemporary medicine should strive for.

References

1. Mustika, R.; Soemantri, D. Unveiling the Hurdles in Cultivating Humanistic Physicians in the Clinical Setting: An Exploratory Study. The Malaysian Journal of Medical Sciences: MJMS. 2020, 27(3), 117.

2. Cohen, L. G., & Sherif, Y. A. Twelve tips on teaching and learning humanism in medical education. Medical Teacher. 2014, 36(8), 680-684.

3. Weissmann, P., Branch, W., Gracey, C., Haidet, P. & Frankel, R. Role modeling humanistic behavior: Learning bedside manner from the experts. Acad Med. 2006, 81:661–667.

4. Lee Roze des Ordons, A., de Groot, J.M., Rosenal, T., Viceer, N., Nixon, L. How clinicians integrate humanism in their clinical workplace-'Just trying to put myself in their human being shoes'. Perspect Med Educ. 2018, Oct 7(5), 318-324.

5. Hazrati, H., Bigdeli, S., Gavgani, V. Z., Soltani Arabshahi, S. K., Behshid, M., & Sohrabi, Z. Humanism in clinical education: a mixed methods study on the experiences of clinical instructors in Iran. Philosophy, Ethics, and Humanities in Medicine. 2020, 15(1), 1-10.

6. Montgomery, L., Loue, S., Stange, K.C. Linking the Heart and the Head: Humanism and Professionalism in Medical Education and Practice. Fam Med. 2017, May 49(5), 378-383.

7. Vogt, H., Ulvestad, E., Eriksen, T. E., & Getz, L. Getting personal: can systems medicine integrate scientific and humanistic conceptions of the patient? Journal of Evaluation in Clinical Practice. 2014, 20(6), 942-952.

8. Sackett, D.L., Rosenberg W.M. The need for evidence-based medicine. Journal of the Royal Society of Medicine. 1995, 88(11), 620–624.

9. Del Giglio, A. Suffering-based medicine: practicing scientific medicine with a humanistic approach. Medicine, Health Care and Philosophy. 2020, 23(2), 215-219.

10. Toombs, S.K. Meaning of illness: A phenomenological approach to the patient-physician relationship. The Journal of Medicine and Philosophy. 1987, 12 (3), 219–240.

11. Hirpa, M., Woreta, T., Addis, H., Kebede, S. What matters to patients? A timely question for value-based care. PLoS One. 2020, Jul 9;15(7), e0227845.

12. Higuita-Gutiérrez, L.F., Estrada-Mesa, D.A., Cardona-Arias, J.A. Preferences in a Group of Patients with Cancer: A Grounded Theory. Patient Prefer Adherence. 2021, Oct 15, 2313-2326.

13. Chou, C.M., Kellom, K., Shea, J.A. Attitudes and habits of highly humanistic physicians.

Academic medicine. 2014, 89(9), 1252-1528.

14. Derksen, F., Bensing, J., Kuiper, S., van Meerendonk, M., Lagro-Janssen, A. Empathy: what does it mean for GPs? A qualitative study, Family Practice. 2015, 32(1), 94–100.

15. Jo, K.H., An, G.J. Effect of end-of-life care education using humanistic approach in Korea. Collegian. 2015. 22(1), 91-97.

16. Vallor, S. Carebots and caregivers: sustaining the ethical ideal of care in the twenty-first century. Philos Technol. 2011, 24, 251.

Beatrice Gabriela Ioan and Magdalena Iorga
Editors

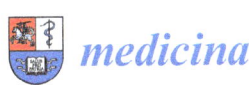

Concept Paper

Teaching and Practicing Humanism and Empathy through Embodied Engagement

Sana Loue

Department of Bioethics, Case Western Reserve University School of Medicine, Cleveland, OH 44106, USA; sana.loue@case.edu

Abstract: Concerns have been raised regarding medicine's dehumanization of patients and providers and regarding the need to include, in the medical school curriculum, components that encourage the development of empathy and humanistic practice. This essay suggests that the development of humanistic practice requires attention to not only the cognitive and affective/emotive aspects of humanism, but also to the nurturing of intersubjectivity between the provider and the patient through strategies designed to promote embodied awareness. Several approaches to the development of embodied awareness are discussed, including puppetry pedagogy, drama, and virtual reality applications.

Keywords: embodiment; empathy; humanism; medical education

Citation: Loue, S. Teaching and Practicing Humanism and Empathy through Embodied Engagement. *Medicina* **2022**, *58*, 330. https://doi.org/10.3390/medicina58030330

Academic Editors: Beatrice Gabriela Ioan and Magdalena Iorga

Received: 30 December 2021
Accepted: 11 February 2022
Published: 22 February 2022

Publisher's Note: MDPI stays neutral with regard to jurisdictional claims in published maps and institutional affiliations.

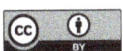

Copyright: © 2022 by the author. Licensee MDPI, Basel, Switzerland. This article is an open access article distributed under the terms and conditions of the Creative Commons Attribution (CC BY) license (https://creativecommons.org/licenses/by/4.0/).

1. Introduction

The extant literature reflects a growing concern with respect to medicine's dehumanization of patients and providers, such that patients are viewed as objectified bodies [1] or body parts [2] biomedicine reduces patients to bodies and body parts [3,4] clinical practice focuses on the organ specifics of disease [5–7] and the nonmaterial components of personhood remain unacknowledged and ignored [7,8]. Additional discussion has focused on the perception of professional competence as comprising solely or primarily the effective application of abstract knowledge [9,10] and technical expertise [11,12]. Emotional competence in the practice of medicine has been depicted as one of emotional distance between the patient and the provider [12], reflecting the longstanding view that it should be one of emotional "toughness" [1], affective neutrality [13], and detached concern [14,15].

More recently, efforts have been made to identify strategies that can be utilized to guide medical students toward a more humanistic, empathetic practice [16–18]. A large body of literature relating to medical education suggests that medical professionalism, comprising humanism's cognitive components of knowledge, attitudes, and ethics [19] may serve as a pathway to the development of a humanistic practice. Montgomery, Loue, and Stange [20] concluded from their review of medical and health professionals education literature that the development of a humanistic practice also requires a focus on the emotive aspects of humanism—altruism, empathy, compassion, and caring [21–24]—and a connection and bidirectional flow between the cognitive (head) and emotive (heart) elements. Their nonlinear model drew from Wilbur's four ways of knowing [25,26]: the interior of an individual; the exterior, referring to knowledge derived from observing individuals' behavior in isolation; the collective interior, i.e., shared norms and values; and the collective exterior, or the observed behavior of a group.

Montgomery and colleagues [20] posited that humanism could be fostered through the creation of a flow between the cognitive and subjective domains within an individual, set into motion through the activation of any one of four levers: personal reflection, action, collective reflection, and system support. This essay builds upon the work of Montgomery and colleagues and others to suggest that the development of humanistic practice also requires the nurturing of intersubjectivity between the provider and the patient through strategies designed to promote embodied awareness. Accordingly, the discussion focuses, first, on defining embodiment and, second, on presenting educational interventions specifically designed to nurture intersubjectivity through embodied awareness.

2. Defining Embodiment

Despite the widespread use of the term "embodiment," there is little consensus about its meaning [27]. In the context of context of medical care, the term has often been used to refer to physicians' qualities and approach to practice: their embodiment of trust [28], of competence, compassion, and kindness [12] and "practicing the professional body" [29]. These understandings suggest that embodiment constitutes the manifestation—or attempted manifestation—of physician characteristics vis-à-vis the patient. Embodiment in this sense is wholly contained within and integrated into the being of the physician, a formulation that essentially assumes but fails to specifically address the intersubjective field that exists between the physician and the patient. The current emphasis on understanding the social determinants of health and the contexts of patients' lives as they relate to their ability to adhere to medical recommendations does little to move away from the view of the Other—the patient—as a being to be acted upon.

In contrast, embodiment may be understood as an intersubjective phenomenon; it is a precondition for intersubjectivity [30]. In writing about body image, Weiss [31] observed, "To describe embodiment as intercorporeality is to emphasize that the experience of being embodied is never a private affair, but is always mediated by our continual interactions with other human and nonhuman bodies." Csordas [32] in describing intersubjectivity as intercorporeality, noted that "because bodies are already situated in relation to one another, intersubjectivity becomes primary." Leder [7] views embodiment as inherently relational, involving relationships between persons and between persons and their environments. Jaye [33] suggested that embodiment is "concerned with the lived experience of one's own body ... ", noting that (i)mplicit within the concept of embodiment is a sense of dynamism or constantly shifting meanings and understandings. Embodiment is experienced within particular historical, cultural, political and societal frames, and these experiences are also shaped by gender and race.

In discussing embodiment in the context of education, Latta and Buck also conceive of embodiment as relational in nature.

(E)mbodied teaching and learning is about building relationships between self, others, and subject matter; living in-between these entities ... neither subject nor otherness are bound entities; they intermingle. Such intertwining makes it necessary to develop a place for the body in teaching and learning that acknowledges the relational intermingling and flux ... a continuous process of reciprocal interaction and modification [34].

"Knowing in any humanly meaningful sense is emergent from and grounded in bodily experience and continuous with the cultural production of meaning" [35]. Research findings lend support to the importance of embodiment. Rizolatti and Craighero [36] have found that because our neural systems recreate what others do and feel, people model others' behavior or mental states as intentional experiences, a phenomenon that has been referred to as "embodied simulation" [37].

Recent nursing literature emphasizes the importance of efforts to understand the Other, an attuned focus that has been termed "engrossment" [38]. There is a difference between curing the body and healing the embodied person, which includes restoring a patient's sense of connectedness, control, and wholeness [39].

The question, therefore, becomes whether can one develop a humanistic practice—compassion, empathy—in the absence of embodiment [40,41] and how an understanding of embodiment may be transmitted in the educational context. Knowledge itself does not lead to caring; empathy suggests connection, connection to be forged through embodiment. Embodied care is a process, "an approach to personal and social morality that shifts ethical considerations to context, relationships, and affective knowledge in a manner that can be fully understood only if care's embodied dimension is recognized. Care is committed to the flourishing and growth of individuals yet acknowledges our interconnectedness and interdependence" [42]. Such care requires movement away from seeing the patient as a body or parts of a body in need of repair to the recognition, acceptance and interaction with the patient as a source of identity and consciousness [43] and the body as a source of meaning [44].

Wisnewski [45] admonished physicians to develop what he termed "sympathetic perception of the patient", a concept similar to what is referred to here as embodiment. He contrasted the patient's concern with "being-in-the-world" with the physician's perception of only a "condition" in front of him or her. In order to convey sympathy, one must perceive sympathetically, "To cultivate sympathetic perception ... is to cultivate an appropriate responsiveness to those situations of need we encounter" [45]. Such an attitude cannot be feigned; "emotional attitudes toward others are conveyed beneath the level of self-consciousness," through inflection and body language [45]; see also [32]. Fuchs [46] recognized the importance of bodily resonance, conceived of as an intuitive understanding of others that occurs in ongoing interactions, often on a pre-reflective level; a process of mutual modifications of bodily and emotional states that takes place as a result of bodily presence [47].

The nonverbal expressions that are revealed through bodily presence constitute a form of knowledge that can be utilized by the health care provider; in essence, the provider "(l)istens within the relationship" with the body [47].

This perspective facilitates the provider's awareness of preconceptions or biases that they may hold, which may be an obstacle to communication and to a full understanding of the patient and their bodily condition, e.g., in situations where the clinician blames the patient for the illness [48]. This knowledge facilitates the development of an ability to feel empathy and sympathy toward the other.

As Merleau-Ponty observed, perception of behavior in other people and the perception of the body itself by a global corporeal schema are two aspects of a single organization that realize the identification of the self with others. Sympathy would emerge from this. Sympathy does not presuppose a genuine distinction between self-consciousness and consciousness of the other, but rather the absence of distinction between the self and the other. It is the simple fact that I live in the facial expressions of the other, as I feel him living in mine [49].

A recent phenomenological study involving 15 physicians lends support for the importance of embodied communication [50]. Physicians reporting on their use of touch during their clinical experiences with patients have indicated that they relied on patients' facial expressions and body language to assess the extent to which touch was welcome and used touch as an embodied form of communication to share emotions and to demonstrate presence and empathy.

3. Developing Embodied Humanistic Practice

Medical students are taught to navigate their way through a professional culture with its own attitudes, behaviors, rituals, specialized knowledge, and institutional hierarchies [51]. As noted above, there exists a core tension between competency and caring [52], such that technical competence appears to often displace caring. Although many physicians do their best to demonstrate compassion and provide support, this often is insufficient. Sometimes doctors must look through the eyes of those for whom they care in order to better serve their needs. By being "on the other side of the stethoscope" and "wearing a gown", providers can learn to better empathize with patients and, ultimately, more effectively ease the pain of living with a disease [53].

Such experiences may lead to better communication, more understanding for patients' difficulties balancing obligations, increased attunement to the emotional aspects of illness, and an understanding of the impact of illness on identity [53]. The question, then, is how this can be achieved without medical students and physicians being patients.

The strategies that are frequently utilized to guide medical students in their development of better communication skills with patients and families and the humanistic practice of medicine are often cognitive in nature, or can be compartmentalized by the learner to be only cognitive, e.g., role playing, journaling. These approaches stand in sharp contrast to the training of osteopaths and homeopaths, which require that they practice skills on each other, requiring that each student feel themselves and the other in their roles as both the provider and the patient.

While we would recognize as ridiculous the suggestion that medical students could be expected to "try out" medication or surgery in themselves, the osteopathy and homeopathy students are expected to experience "being a patient" not only through continued treatment by a qualified practitioner but in the fabric of the organization of training that requires that the students explore their concepts of health and healing and practice their developing skills with each other. During this time, day-to-day absence of the lived body is made visible for the students as they experience new embodied sensations and develop new embodied knowledge. "Playing" the roles of osteopath/homeopath and patient is fundamental to the development of a sense of intersubjectivity and an ability to be reflexive. These new modes of embodied intersubjectivity mean that CAM practitioners are literally and explicitly performing "embodied work". Carrying out "work on yourself" is commonplace language in CAM communities and is required of both patients and practitioners for a successful therapeutic encounter. [54].

Accordingly, mechanisms to develop caring and empathy must resist superficial patient transactions [43] and focus instead on "somatic cultivation," i.e., close attention to body [55]. Similarly, Aoki and Ikemi [56] have suggested that focusing, i.e., an "embodied practice where one attends to a bodily felt sense and uses it in understanding oneself and situations" consists of being aware of a sensation, accepting and acting from the sensation, and finding a comfortable distance from that sensation. This requires that the individual assess whether what they are doing is congruent with what they are feeling. Increases in such focusing have been found to be associated with higher levels of empathy [57].

4. Arts-Based Approaches

It has been suggested that the use of arts-based methods may be critical to the development embodiment because they encourage individuals to challenge their personal assumptions and dominant cultural narratives [58] develop increased insight, and acknowledge emotions [59]. The extent to which specific modalities are effective in inculcating an understanding of embodiment leading to humanistic practice is unclear due to limited details contained in published reports with respect to theoretical framework; program structure, content, and implementation; participants; short- and long-term outcomes; and behavioral assessments [60].

It has been suggested that forms of performance, in particular, may engage the participant and the viewer viscerally, intellectually, physically, and emotionally. As an example of the impact of performance-focused arts-based approaches, Berland described the impact of filming three individuals with wheelchairs equipped with cameras in the production of the movie, Rolling.

"The three participants in this project taught me to see the world in ways I had never imagined. I do not look at a sidewalk or the incline of a hill as I did before. Steps, doors, building entrances, rooms appear different. I now assess manual and power wheelchairs with a critical eye. The impact, however, is broader than that. I listen more carefully. I consider the time and effort it takes for patients to reach my clinic and how long they have waited before coming to see me with a problem" [61].

Tsaplina [62] has recently advocated the use of puppetry pedagogy as an approach to fostering embodiment. She explained, "The art of animating a puppet trains a deep embodied listening that gives voice and form to material and immaterial presences through the imagination" [62]. She recounts her observations of a student who appears unaware of the concept of or need for embodiment:

"I am observing a pre-med student contend with animating a pair of puppet legs that I built and that I purposefully hinged to bend at the knee in opposing directions. He is agitated by these legs. They will not bend to his will, nor how he imagines legs should be. He wants to be a doctor, maybe a psychiatrist. He does not yet understand that his struggle to force these legs to be what they are not is possibly one of the most important things he can learn about the practice of medicine, care and healing" [62].

Without a sense of embodiment, an awareness of breath, of body, of imagination and intersubjectivity, the student is unable to see the puppet as a whole and as it is, but is only able to imagine what he thinks it should be and should do. The puppet challenges the student to be with, rather than do to.

As Tsaplina notes, puppetry practice holds a unique capacity to illuminate how bodies and worlds are interfaces that become each other, continually. This becoming allows for knowledges and articulations to arise by growing our sensitivity and ability to experience and discern diverse phenomena. What is critical to highlight is that the erasure or elimination of this mutual becoming in the name of "unaffected objectivity" is possible only by the application of power by one body over another, thereby rendering bodies silent through force. [62].

Drama also offers the possibility of developing this sense of relational vulnerability or attunement. Acting in a role provides an opportunity for learners to understand the affective components of an interaction, become more self-aware, and develop empathy [63]. A review of literature relating to the effectiveness of arts-based interventions in medical education concluded that of all of the modalities reviewed—mixed arts, poetry, film, prose, visual arts, and performing arts—only performing arts evidence some effect on the development of positive attitudes that include an increase in empathic feelings [60].

Drama must be distinguished from role play and simulations, which are often used in medical education as an opportunity to practice specific skills. In contrast, "the art of drama is used to illuminate some truth about the world" [64]. Drama includes content, theme, substance, subject matter, and curriculum, offering participants an opportunity to learn about themselves and explore situations from multiple perspectives, their own vulnerabilities, and the complexities of human behavior. Theater can present ambiguities, complexities, and contradictions, challenging the students to identify not only such issues, but their potential resolutions as well [65]. Theater is fundamentally a rehearsal for life [66].

The MEET (Medical Education Empowered by Theater) serves as one example of a drama intervention designed to nurture the cognitive, emotional, and volitional components of empathy [65]. The improvisational exercises that comprise the program involve both body and emotions, recognizing that they are critical elements of empathy. Exercises are followed by a debriefing. One scenario that is used involves a pregnant teenage girl who is waiting in the examination room for a prenatal examination with her mother. While she and her mother are arguing, the supervisor enters with five medical students. The supervisor is dismissive of the girl. The five students display different reactions to the supervisor's instructions, with some proceeding to conduct the examination, some remaining silent. Students' narrative evaluations of the program indicated that the course reminded them of the importance of remaining self-aware and to focus on what is happening, rather than accepting situations and events as ordinary and normal.

Scholars have recently noted the underrepresentation in medical education of dance as an approach to the development of embodied awareness [67]. It has been suggested that dance may lead to heightened self-awareness and physical presence and may provide an additional way of knowing.

5. Virtual Reality Training

Li and colleagues have proposed using a virtual reality game application to foster students' close attention to the body [68], noting that this strategy has been used in efforts to foster empathy among medical students [69–72] and facilitate embodiment [73]. They proposed introducing learners to realistic scenarios involving Parkinson's disease and requiring that the learners complete specified tasks under the effects of a simulated tremor. The tasks include using a telephone, picking up and putting down pills in the correct order, turning off an alarm clock, showering, brushing teeth, and preparing a sandwich [68]. At the time of this writing, the application has been tested and was ready for classroom use, but its effectiveness in achieving the desired aims is not yet available.

6. Implications of Embodied Practice

This article has focused on the rationale for the development of a consciously embodied approach among medical students and the need for educational interventions to encourage this development. Teaching strategies designed to bring awareness to and encourage embodied attunement provide opportunities for learners to challenge their personal assumptions and the dominant cultural narratives, and to reframe their perspective such that they are able to encounter the whole person, rather than viewing the patient as a disembodied entity, body part, or condition. As such, it challenges providers' understandings of normality and of viewing differently abled/disabled persons as "others" or as not normal or not healthy [74]. The heightened awareness that comes from an embodied approach is intended to facilitate the development of empathy and humanistic practice. Embodiment as a foundation for humanistic practice necessarily entails authenticity—it is not something that can be manufactured and checked off on a list of qualities to be displayed as a means of encouraging patient adherence or disclosure and giving the illusion of shifting power.

The discussion focused on several strategies commonly utilized in medical education to foster empathy and humanistic practice, e.g., arts-based approaches and virtual reality training. An understanding of the extent to which a specific approach effectuates behavioral change will require additional research and clear descriptions of the underlying theoretical approach; program structure, content, and delivery; and short- and long-term attitudinal and behavioral changes.

Funding: This research received no external funding.

Institutional Review Board Statement: Not applicable.

Informed Consent Statement: Not applicable.

Data Availability Statement: Not applicable.

Acknowledgments: The author gratefully acknowledges the insights contributed by Erin Lamb and Marina Tsaplina in discussions about the nature of embodiment and earlier conceptualizations of this manuscript.

Conflicts of Interest: The author declares no conflict of interest.

References

1. Hafferty, F.W. Cadaver stories and the emotional socialization of medical students. *J. Health Soc. Behav.* **1988**, *29*, 344–356. [CrossRef]
2. Elsey, C.; Challinor, A.; Monrouxe, L.V. Patients embodied and as-a-body within bedside teaching encounters: A videoethnographic study. *Adv. Health Sci. Educ.* **2017**, *22*, 123–146. [CrossRef] [PubMed]
3. Cassell, E. *The Nature of Suffering and the Goals of Medicine*; Oxford University Press: Oxford, UK, 1991.
4. Gordon, D. Tenacious assumptions in Western medicine. In *Biomedicine Examined*; Lock, M., Gordon, D., Eds.; Kluwer Academic Publishers: Dordrecht, The Netherlands, 1988; pp. 19–56.
5. Kirmayer, L. Mind and body as metaphors: Hidden values in biomedicine. In *Biomedicine Examined*; Lock, M., Gordon, D., Eds.; Kluwer Academic Publishers: Dordrecht, The Netherlands, 1988; pp. 57–93.
6. Leder, D. Medicine and paradigms of embodiment. *J. Med. Philos.* **1984**, *9*, 29–43. [CrossRef] [PubMed]
7. Leder, D. A tale of two bodies: The Cartesian corpse and the lived body. In *The body in Medical Thought and Practice*; Leder, D., Ed.; Kluwer Academic Publishers: Dordrecht, The Netherlands, 1992; pp. 17–35.
8. Martensen, R. Alienation and the production of strangers: Western medical epistemology and the architectonics of the body: A historical perspective. *Cult. Med. Psychiatry* **1995**, *19*, 141–182. [CrossRef] [PubMed]
9. Nettleton, S.; Burrows, R.; Watt, I. Regulating medical bodies? The 'modernisation' of the NHS and the disembodiment of clinical knowledge. *Sociol. Health Illn.* **2008**, *30*, 333–348. [CrossRef] [PubMed]

10. Sennett, R. *The Craftsman*; Allen Lane: London, UK, 2008.
11. Bosk, C.L. Professional responsibility and medical error. In *Applications of Social Science and Health Policy*; Aiekn, M.L.H., Mwechanic, D., Eds.; Rutgers University Press: New Brunswick, NJ, USA; pp. 460–477.
12. Connelly, J.E. The other side of professionalism: Doctor-to-doctor. *Camb. Q. Healthc. Ethics* **2003**, *12*, 178–183. [CrossRef] [PubMed]
13. Parsons, T. The sick role and the role of the physician reconsidered. *Milbank Meml. Fund Q. Health Soc.* **1975**, *53*, 257–278. [CrossRef]
14. Fox, R. *Essays in Medical Sociology*; Transaction Publishers: Piscataway, NJ, USA, 1988.
15. Fox, R.C. *Essays in Medical Sociology: Journey into the Field*; Wiley: New York, NY, USA, 1979.
16. Block, S.; Billings, J.A. Nurturing humanism through teaching palliative care. *Acad. Med.* **1998**, *73*, 763–765. [CrossRef]
17. Cohen, J.J. Viewpoint: Linking professionalism to humanism: What it means, why it matters. *Acad. Med.* **2007**, *82*, 1029–1032. [CrossRef]
18. Karnieli-Miller, O.; Frankel, R.M.; Inui, T.S. Cloak of compassion, or evidence of elitism? An empirical analysis of white coat ceremonies. *Med. Educ.* **2013**, *47*, 97–108. [CrossRef]
19. Bickel, J. Proceedings of the AAMC conference on students' and residents' ethical and professional development. October 27–28, 1995. Introduction. *Acad. Med.* **1995**, *71*, 622–623. [CrossRef] [PubMed]
20. Montgomery, L.; Loue, S.; Stange, K.C. Linking the heart and the head: Humanism and professionalism in medical education and practice. *Fam. Med.* **2017**, *49*, 378–383. [PubMed]
21. Bishop, J.P.; Rees, C.E. Hero or has-been: Is there a future for altruism in medical education? *Adv. Health Sci. Educ. Theory Pract.* **2007**, *12*, 391–399. [CrossRef] [PubMed]
22. Marcus, E.R. Empathy, humanism. And the professionalization process of medical education. *Acad. Med.* **1999**, *74*, 1211–1215. [CrossRef] [PubMed]
23. Schoenly, L. Teaching in the affective domain. *J. Contin. Educ. Nurs.* **1994**, *25*, 209–212. [CrossRef] [PubMed]
24. Wear, D.; Zarconi, J. Can compassion be taught? Let's ask our students. *J. Gen. Intern. Med.* **2008**, *33*, 948–953. [CrossRef]
25. Wilbur, K. *A Brief History of Everything*, 1st ed.; Shambhala: Boston, MA, USA, 1996.
26. Wilbur, K. *Sex, Ecology, Spirituality: The Spirit of Evolution*; Shambhala: Boston, MA, USA, 1995.
27. Wilde, M.H. Why embodiment now? *Adv. Nurs. Sci.* **1999**, *22*, 25–38. [CrossRef]
28. Brown, P.R.; Alaszewski, A.; Swift, T.; Nordin, A. Actions speak louder than words: The embodiment of trust by healthcare professionals in gynae-oncology. *Sociol. Health Illn.* **2011**, *33*, 280–295. [CrossRef]
29. Green, B.; Hopwood, N. The body in professional practice, learning and education: A question of corporeality. In *The Body in Professional Practice, Learning and Education; Body/Practice*; Green, B., Hopwood, N., Eds.; Springer International Publishing: Cham, Switzerland, 2015; pp. 15–33.
30. Schultz, A. *The Phenomenology of the Social World*; Heinemann: London, UK, 1972.
31. Weiss, G. *Body Images: Embodiment as Intercorporeality*; Routledge: New York, NY, USA, 1999.
32. Csordas, T.J. Intersubjectivity and intercoreality. *Subjectivity* **2008**, *22*, 110–121. [CrossRef]
33. Jaye, C. Talking around embodiment: The views of GPs following participation in medical anthropology courses. *J. Med. Ethics Med. Humanit.* **2004**, *30*, 41–48. [CrossRef]
34. Latta, M.M.; Buck, G. Enfleshing embodiment: 'Falling into trust' with the body's role in teaching and learning. *Educ. Philos. Theory* **2008**, *40*, 316–329.
35. Bowman, W. Cognition and the body: Perspectives from music education. In *Knowing Bodies, Moving Minds: Towards Embodied Teaching and Learning*; Bresler, L., Ed.; Kluewer Academic Publishers: Boston, MA, USA, 2004; pp. 29–50.
36. Rizzolatti, G.; Craighero, L. The mirror-neuron system. *Annu. Rev. Neurosci.* **2004**, *27*, 169–192. [CrossRef] [PubMed]
37. Gallese, V. Intentional attunement: A neurophysiological perspective on social cognition and its disruption in autism. *Brain Res.* **2006**, *1079*, 15–24. [CrossRef] [PubMed]
38. Noddings, N. *Caring: A Feminine Approach to Ethics and Moral Education*; University of California Press: Berkeley, CA, USA, 1984.
39. Stewart, M.; Brown, J.B.; Weston, W.W.; McWhinney, I.R.; McWilliam, C.L.; Freeman, T.R. *Patient-Centered Medicine: Transforming the Clinical Method*; Sage: London, UK, 1995.
40. Gieser, T. Embodiment, emotion and empathy. *Anthropol. Theory* **2008**, *8*, 299–318. [CrossRef]
41. Schwartz-Franco, O. Touching the challenge: Embodied solutions enabling humanistic moral education. *J. Moral Educ.* **2016**, *45*, 449–464. [CrossRef]
42. Hamington, M. *Embodied Care: Jane Addams, Maurice Merleau-Ponty, and Feminist Ethics*; University of Illinois Press: Urbana, IL, USA, 2004.
43. Hamington, M. Care ethics and corporeal inquiry in patient relations. *Int. J. Fem. Approaches Bioeth.* **2012**, *5*, 52–69. [CrossRef]
44. Merleau-Ponty, M. *Phenomenology of Perception*; Routledge: New York, NY, USA, 1962.
45. Wisnewski, J.J. Perceiving sympathetically: Moral perception, embodiment, and medical ethics. *J. Med. Humanit.* **2015**, *36*, 309–319. [CrossRef]
46. Fuchs, T. Intercorporeality and interaffectivity. *Phenomenol. Mind* **2016**, *11*, 194–209.
47. Engelsrud, G.; Ølen, I.; Nordtug, B. Being present with the patient—A critical investigation of bodily sensitivity and presence in the field of physiotherapy. *Physiother. Theory Pract.* **2019**, *35*, 908–918. [CrossRef]
48. Ekman, E.; Krasner, M. Empathy in medicine: Neuroscience, education and challenges. *Med. Teach.* **2017**, *39*, 164–173. [CrossRef]

49. Merleau-Ponty, M. The Primacy of Perception and Other Essays on Phenomenology, Psychology, the Philosophy of Art, History and Politics. Edie, J.M., Ed.; Northern University Press: Evanston, IL, USA, 1964.
50. Kelly, M.; Svrcek, C.; King, N.; Scherpbier, A.; Dornan, T. Embodying empathy: A phenomenological study of physician touch. *Med. Educ.* **2020**, *54*, 400–407. [CrossRef] [PubMed]
51. Underman, K. Playing doctor: Simulation in medical school as affective practice. *Soc. Sci. Med.* **2015**, *136*, 180–188. [CrossRef] [PubMed]
52. Brosnan, C. Pierre Bourdieu and theory of medical education. In *Handbook of the Sociology of Medical Education*; Brosnan, C., Turner, B.S., Eds.; Routledge: New York, NY, USA, 2009; pp. 51–68.
53. Medical College of Wisconsin. On the Other Side of the Stethoscope: When Doctors Become Patients. Available online: https://www.mcw.edu/mcwknowledge/mcw-stories/on-the-other-side-of-the-stethoscope-when-doctors-become-patients. (accessed on 26 November 2021).
54. Gale, N.K. From body-talk to body-stories: Body work in complementary and alternative medicine. *Sociol. Health Illn.* **2011**, *33*, 237–251. [CrossRef] [PubMed]
55. Shusterman, R. *Body Consciousness: A Philosophy of Mindfulness and Somaesthetics*; Cambridge University Press: New York, NY, USA, 2008.
56. Aoki, T.; Ikemi, A. The Focusing Manner scale: Its validity, research background and its potential as a measure of embodied experiencing. *Pers. Cent. Exp. Psychother.* **2014**, *13*, 31–46. [CrossRef]
57. Nasello, J.A.; Triffaux, J.-M. Focusing: A new challenger for improving the empathy skills of medical students. *Complement. Ther. Med.* **2020**, *53*, 102536. [CrossRef]
58. Gray, J.; Kontos, P. Immersion, embodiment, and imagination: Moving beyond an aesthetic of objectivity in research-informed performance in health. *Forum Qual. Soc. Res.* **2015**, *16*, 29.
59. Haidet, P.; Jarecke, J.; Adams, N.A.; Stuckey, H.L.; Green, M.J.; Shapiro, D.; Wolpaw, D.R. A guiding framework to maximise the power of the arts in medical education: A systematic review and metasynthesis. *Med. Educ.* **2016**, *50*, 320–331. [CrossRef]
60. Perry, M.; Maffulli, N.; Willson, S.; Morrissey, D. The effectiveness of arts-based interventions in medical education: A literature review. *Med. Educ.* **2011**, *45*, 141–148. [CrossRef]
61. Berland, G. The view from the other side—Patients, doctors, and the power of a camera. *N. Engl. J. Med.* **2007**, *357*, 2533–2536. [CrossRef]
62. Tsaplina, M. Bodies speaking: Embodiment, illness and the poetic materiality of puppetry/object practice. *J. Appl. Arts Health* **2020**, *11*, 85–102. [CrossRef]
63. Hobson, W.L.; Hoffman-Longtin, K.; Loue, S.; Love, L.M.; Liu, H.Y.; Power, C.M.; Pollart, S.M. Active learning on center stage: Theater as a tool for medical education. *MedEd Portal* **2019**, *15*, 10801. [CrossRef] [PubMed]
64. Arveklev, S.H.; Wigert, H.; Berg, L.; Burton, B.; Lepp, M. The use and application of drama in nursing education—An interpretive review of the literature. *Nurse Educ. Today* **2015**, *5*, e12–e17. [CrossRef] [PubMed]
65. De Carvalho Filho, M.A.; Ledubino, A.; Frutuoso, L.; da Silva Wanderlei, J.; Jaarsma, D.; Helmich, E.; Strazzacappa, M. Medical education empowered by theater (MEET). *Acad. Med.* **2020**, *95*, 1191–1200. [CrossRef] [PubMed]
66. Boal, A. *The Aesthetics of the Oppressed*; Routledge: New York, NY, USA, 2006.
67. Shevzov-Zebrun, N.; Barchi, E.; Grogran, K. "The spirit thickened": Making the case for dance in the medical humanities. *J. Med. Humanit.* **2020**, *41*, 543–560. [CrossRef]
68. Li, Y.; Ducleroir, C.; Stollman, T.I.; Wood, E. Parkinson's disease simulation in virtual reality for empathy training in medical education. In Proceedings of the 2021 IEEE Conference on Virtual Reality and 3D User Interfaces Abstracts and Workshops, Virtual Conference, 27 March–2 April 2021.
69. Bertrand, P.; Guegan, J.; Robieux, L.; McCall, C.A.; Zenasni, F. Learning empathy through virtual reality: Multiple strategies for training empathy-related abilities using body ownership illusions in embodied virtual reality. *Front. Robot. AI* **2018**, *5*, 26. [CrossRef]
70. Dyer, E.; Swartzlander, B.J.; Gugliucci, M.R. Using virtual reality in medical education to teach empathy. *J. Med. Libr. Assoc.* **2018**, *106*, 498–500. [CrossRef]
71. Louie, A.K.; Coverdale, A.H.; Balon, R.; Beresin, E.V.; Brenner, A.M.; Guerrero, A.P.S.; Roberts, L.W. Enhancing empathy: A role for virtual reality? *Acad. Psychiatry* **2018**, *42*, 747–752. [CrossRef]
72. Swartzlander, B.; Dyer, E.; Gugliucci, M.R. *We Are Alfred: Empathy Learned through a Medical Education Virtual Reality Project. Library Services Faculty Posters*; University of New England: Biddeford, ME, USA, 2017.
73. Bang, E.; Yildirim, C. Virtually empathetic? Examining the effects of virtual reality storytelling on empathy. In *Virtual, Augmented and Mixed Reality: Interaction, Navigation, Visualization, Embodiment, and Simulation*; Chen, J.Y.C., Fragomeni, G., Eds.; Springer International Publishing AG: Cham, Switzerland, 2018; pp. 290–298.
74. Harmon, S.H.E. The invisibility of disability: Using dance to shake from bioethics the idea of 'broken bodies. *Bioethics* **2015**, *29*, 488–498. [CrossRef]

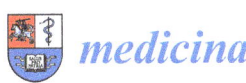

Article

Socio-Demographic, Professional and Institutional Characteristics That Make Romanian Doctors More Prone to Malpractice Complaints

Bianca Hanganu [1], Magdalena Iorga [2,3,*], Lavinia Maria Pop [3] and Beatrice Gabriela Ioan [1]

[1] Legal-Medicine Department, Faculty of Medicine, "Grigore T. Popa" University of Medicine and Pharmacy of Iasi, 700115 Iasi, Romania; bianca-hanganu@umfiasi.ro (B.H.); beatrice.ioan@umfiasi.ro (B.G.I.)
[2] Behavioral Sciences Department, Faculty of Medicine, "Grigore T. Popa" University of Medicine and Pharmacy of Iasi, 700115 Iasi, Romania
[3] Faculty of Psychology and Education Sciences, "Alexandru Ioan Cuza" University of Iasi, 700554 Iasi, Romania; lavinia-maria.pop@umfiasi.ro
* Correspondence: magdalena.iorga@umfiasi.ro

Abstract: *Background and objectives*: Medical malpractice is a phenomenon that shadows current medical practice, the number of complaints following an upward trend worldwide. The background for complaints is related both to the doctor and medical practice in general, as well as to the patient. The aim of this study was to identify a profile of the Romanian doctors who are more prone to receiving complaints, by analyzing the socio-demographic, professional and institutional characteristics. *Materials and Methods*: We conducted a quantitative, prospective research, the data being collected using a newly developed questionnaire. Data analysis was performed with the IBM Statistical Package for Social Sciences (SPSS, version 24). We used counts, percentages, means and standard deviation, and comparative and correlational analyses. A logistic regression model was applied to select a statistically best-fit model to identify independent predictors for receiving complaints; a Hosmer–Lemeshow test was used to check the performance of the prediction model. *Results*: The study group consisted of 1684 doctors, of which 16.1% had been involved in a malpractice complaint. Results showed that men, senior doctors from surgical specialties who perform a greater number of on-call shifts, those who work in regional or county hospitals, those who have greater fear of receiving complaints and those whose life partner is a doctor with the same specialty are more prone to receiving complaints. *Conclusions*: The profile identified by the present research underlines the main characteristics that could be targeted with specific measures in order to prevent the ongoing increase of malpractice complaints in Romania.

Keywords: medical malpractice; complaints; doctor; Romania; socio-demographic characteristics; professional characteristics; institutional characteristics

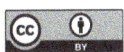

1. Introduction

The need to respect the norms of good practice in medicine has accompanied the medical profession throughout its evolution, but the perspective on failure in the medical act has undergone important changes over time. In general, complaints regarding medical professional liability are based on medical error: real, or perceived as such by the patient or his/her family.

The large number of complaints about medical professional liability all over the world is a reality that cannot be disputed, and the numerous consequences they generate sound the alarm about the need to identify prevention and reduction strategies. The data published in the literature provide an overview of the number of complaints in different countries of the world. For example, the analysis conducted in 2016 by Guardado [1] shows that 34% of members of the American Society of Medicine received at least one complaint during their career, and almost half of them (16.8%) faced at least two complaints. In Europe, Italy was the country with the highest number of complaints in 2009 [2], with an increase of 255% from 1994 to 2011 [3] and a total of about 16,000 complaints made annually by patients [4]. A study conducted in Saudi Arabia shows a tripling of the number of complaints between 1999 and 2008, with an increase from 440 to 1356 over the ten years of the study [5]. An analysis of the annual distribution of malpractice complaints filed in Romanian courts between November 2007 and April 2018 shows an increase in the number of complaints from 8 in 2008 to 65 in 2017, with 331 complaints filed during the entire study period [6]. The analysis of the complaints submitted for extra-judicial analysis in the eight counties of the Moldova region of Romania shows a total of 153 complaints in the period 2006–2019 [7].

The natural reaction of patients to the real or perceived failure of a medical procedure is the search for the culprit, and their tendency—sometimes wrong—is to put full responsibility on the shoulders of the attending physician [8]. Analyzing the human factor in medical errors, the scientific community agrees that the risk of error exists and hovers above even the most experienced physicians [9], as failure may occur despite compliance with all rules of good professional practice [10]. Failure in medical practice is often the result of complex interactions that go beyond the individual limit of the doctor involved. Thus, it is about a chain of elements that include the doctor, the institution in which he/she works, the medical system [11], the patient and the medical science itself, with its inherent limits.

Any medical act has an intrinsic risk, accepted by the medical community, about which the patient must be informed and which he/she in turn accepts once the informed consent form is signed. However, patients cannot always distinguish between the situations in which the doctor was wrong and the situations in which the failure occurred despite the fact that the doctor followed exactly the specific conduct of that medical procedure [10].

The decision of the patient or his/her family to file a complaint against the doctor is based on a combination of factors, among which the characteristics of the doctor play an important role. Thus, the data reported in the literature show that the risk of a doctor for being reported depends, on the one hand, on socio-demographic factors, such as age [1,12,13], gender [1,13] or place of birth [14], and on the other hand on educational and professional factors, such as: specialty [1,12,13], seniority in work [5,13], number of patients [15] and their level of satisfaction [15], type of medical educational institution from which they graduated (public or private), whether or not they took postgraduate training courses [5,13], the number of days off [12], the volume and location of the medical office [5], and academic activity [16]. In addition, the existence of one or more previous claims contributes to the doctor's increased risk of receiving a complaint [17].

Knowledge of the characteristics of doctors complained about by patients and the factors that influence these characteristics can be the foundation for complaints prevention strategies focused on the changeable factors, regarding both the doctor–patient relationship and the characteristics of the health care system, in terms of better cooperation between different levels of the health care system and in-depth analysis of the reasons that lead to complaints in specialties with a higher risk of complaints.

The aim of this study was to identify the socio-demographic, professional and institutional characteristics profiling the Romanian doctor prone to receiving complaints, by analyzing the characteristics of doctors involved in complaints made by patients in Romania.

2. Materials and Methods

2.1. Instruments and Data Collection

For the construction of the questionnaire, a literature data search was undertaken and supplementary information about items was suggested by the results of previous studies by the present research team: a retrospective study regarding patient complaints submitted to the Commission for monitoring and professional competence for malpractice cases within the Public Health Directorates in the Moldova region of Romania [7] and a qualitative study based on semi-structured interviews with doctors who were complained about by patients.

The questionnaire was evaluated by five experts from different specialties and was pre-tested before being distributed, with the corresponding improvements implemented based on the feedback received. The final form was approved by the research team.

A total of 88 questions were structured within three main sections: the first part included 44 questions that were addressed to all doctors, the second part included questions intended for doctors who know a colleague who was complained about, and the third part included questions for doctors who themselves were involved in a complaint from patients. The separation of the sections and the categorization of the participants regarding whether they were the subject of a complaint from a patient were made according to the answers to the question as to whether they know anyone who had received a complaint from a patient, with the following possible answers: a colleague, me, no one. In this paper we present the results of the analysis of the first part. The majority of answers were collected using a Likert-like scale and some of the items were open.

Accordingly, the data collected for this study were obtained from the questions concerning the following issues: the characteristic of being the subject of a complaint or not, socio-demographic data (such as age, gender, marital status, profession of the life partner, parenthood, working area), professional and institutional information (specialty, professional degree, seniority in the medical profession and at the current workplace, the type of medical institution in which they work, the number of work places, the number of on-call shifts, the academic degree, the type of employment contract and the performance of the full time job in a medical education institution, the type of medical education institution they graduated, holding a management position, number and type of patients they examine), characteristics related to the process of continuing medical education (participation in national/international congresses/conferences, certifications/competencies, postgraduate courses), level of personal and professional satisfaction (relationship with family, colleagues, superiors, social life, working conditions, facilities of the institution where they work, workload, financial situation, rest time), level of concern about the occurrence of adverse events (death of the patient, complications of the investigations, intraoperative and postoperative complications, adverse drug effects), characteristics connected to the relationship with patients (explaining the information from the informed consent form, explaining the results of tests, patience with difficult patients, limiting information to elderly patients, providing educational materials, offering the possibility for out-of-hours contact, consultation with colleagues in difficult cases), circumstances for disclosing the occurrence of an adverse event (never, always or depending on the severity: minor/serious) and the fear of being complained about.

2.2. Participants

The questionnaire was distributed online, using Google Docs, by the College of Physicians, to all the doctors in Romania, members of the College of Physicians, and was opened for three weeks, between 4 May and 24 May 2020. On the first page of the questionnaire the participants found a detailed presentation of the aim and objectives of the study, and a notice regarding the scientific use of the information provided and the confidentiality of data, also stating that participation was anonymous and voluntary.

2.3. Statistical Analysis

Data analysis was performed with the Statistical Package for Social Sciences (SPSS, version 24, Armonk, NY, USA). Descriptive analysis presented percentages, means and standard deviation to describe the variables. For comparative analysis a Mann–Whitney rank statistic test was performed in order to detect and describe significant differences between variables. The correlation analysis of data was done using Spearman correlation. A binomial logistic regression model was used in order to select a statistically best-fit model to identify independent predictors for being complained about. We used the Hosmer–Lemeshow test to check the performance of the prediction model. The level of statistical significance was set at $p < 0.05$.

2.4. Ethical Approval

The study was approved by the Research Ethics Commission of the Grigore T. Popa University of Medicine and Pharmacy of Iasi, Romania, registered as No. 16434/30 July 2019.

3. Results

3.1. Socio-Demographic and Professional Data

The questionnaire was filled in by 1753 doctors. Of the total number of questionnaires received, 3.9% (N = 69) were excluded from the study because they were not fully filled in. Figure 1 provides details on the response rate.

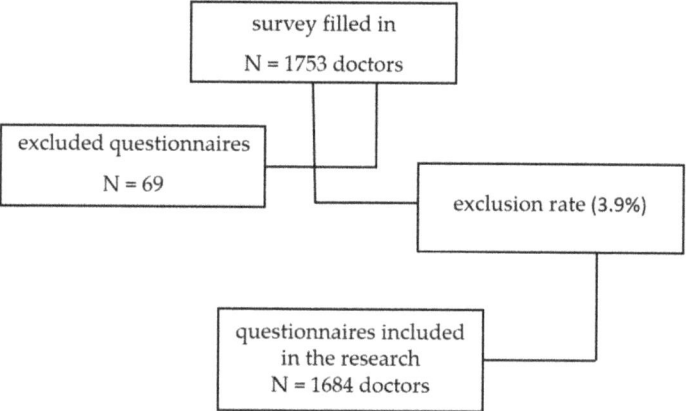

Figure 1. Study profile.

The analysis of the socio-demographic data indicated that 71.0% (N = 1196) of the participants were women; the mean age of the participants was M = 44.77 ± 10.98 years.

The research was attended by senior doctors (52.1%, N = 878), specialists (38.3%, N = 645) and residents (9.6%, N = 161). A majority of participants, 90.4% (N = 1522), practiced only in urban areas, with a length of employment in the medical system of M = 18.09 ± 11.53 years, and 16.1% of doctors (N = 271) declared that they had experienced complaints from their patients during their career.

Of the total number of doctors included in the research, just over half of them said they had more than one job (50.3%, N = 847). On average, a doctor provided medical services for a number of M = 69.20 ± 57.22 patients per week. The analysis of data showed that the number of on-call shifts/month was M = 2.26 ± 2.78.

A total of 243 doctors (14.4%) were also teaching in medical universities and 27.7% (N = 466) of the participants declared that they held a management position.

According to the nomenclature of medical specialties in the Romanian healthcare system, five categories of specialties were considered: surgical specialties, medical specialties, paraclinical-laboratory specialties, pediatric specialties (pediatrics, neonatology, pediatric surgery and orthopedics) and family medicine, and the presentation of data took these criteria into consideration. Detailed socio-demographic and professional characteristics of the participants are presented in Table 1.

Table 1. Socio-demographic characteristics and professional activity of the participants [1].

Characteristics	N (%)
Gender	
Male	488 (29.0)
Female	1196 (71.0)

Table 1. Cont.

Characteristics	N (%)
Marital status	
Single	302 (17.9)
In a relationship	1382 (82.1)
Life partner's profession	
Doctor, same specialty	96 (6.9)
Doctor, different specialty	352 (25.4)
Nurse	40 (2.8)
Other profession in the medical field	44 (3.1)
Other profession	850 (61.5)
Children	
No	543 (32.2)
Yes	1141 (67.8)
Graduating institution	
Private	50 (3.0)
Public	1634 (97.0)
Medical specialty	
Family medicine	321 (19.1)
Medical	692 (41.1)
Surgical	370 (22.0)
Pediatrics	123 (7.3)
Laboratory	178 (10.6)
Area of activity	
Urban	1522 (90.4)
Rural	88 (5.2)
Both	74 (4.4)
Type of medical institution I	
Public	749 (44.5)
Private	482 (28.6)
Both	453 (26.9)
Type of medical institution II	
Regional/county hospital	709 (42.1)
Municipality hospital	274 (16.2)
City hospital	101 (5.9)
Polyclinic/ambulatory	525 (31.1)
Private medical office	513 (30.4)
Private hospital/clinic	658 (39.0)
Type of patients	
Mostly women	260 (15.4)
Mostly men	62 (3.7)
Women and men equally	1362 (80.9)

[1] Number of answers (N) and percentage (%).

3.2. Comparative Analysis

Results of the Mann–Whitney test showed that there were significant differences depending on gender ($z = -7.960$, $p < 0.001$) and parental status ($z = -3.317$, $p = 0.001$) when we compared doctors who were/were not involved in malpractice complaints. This means that male doctors (Mean rank = 936.48) face complaints of malpractice more often than female doctors (Mean rank = 804.15). In addition, subjects who were parents declared to a higher extent (Mean rank = 859.76) that they experienced malpractice complaints than doctors without children (Mean rank = 806.24). Significant differences were also recorded in terms of partner profession ($z = -3.615, p < 0.001$) meaning that subjects whose partner was a doctor of the same specialty had received complaints of malpractice more often (Mean rank = 532.10) than subjects whose partner had another profession that was not related to the medical system (Mean rank = 466.88).

When analyzing the categories of medical specialties that had the highest risk of receiving complaints related to malpractice, the results showed that surgical specialties have the highest risk. Thus, the results of the Mann–Whitney test ($z = -6.369, p < 0.001$) showed that doctors specializing in family medicine (Mean rank = 311.06) have a lower risk of having complaints related to malpractice compared with doctors working in the field of surgery (Mean rank = 376.31). Also, there are significant differences between the specializations of surgery and pediatrics ($z = -3.031, p = 0.002$) in the sense that doctors specializing in pediatrics (Mean rank = 222.07) are less likely to be reported compared with doctors in the field of surgery (Mean rank = 255.29). Moreover, the results showed that ($z = -3.763, p < 0.001$) doctors working in the field of surgery (Mean rank = 287.29) are more likely to receive complaints related to malpractice even than doctors working in the laboratory (Mean rank = 247.90).

There are significant differences between the professional degree of doctors in terms of receiving malpractice complaints ($z = -6.560, p < 0.001$) in the sense that senior doctors are more likely to receive such complaints (Mean rank = 538.25) as opposed to resident doctors (Mean rank = 420.45). There are also significant differences between specialist and resident doctors ($z = -3.390, p = 0.001$) in the sense that specialist doctors (Mean rank = 409.86) are more likely to receive malpractice complaints as opposed to resident doctors (Mean rank = 378.01). Moreover, the results ($z = -7.466, p < 0.001$) showed that senior doctors (Mean rank = 809.64) are more likely to be sued for malpractice as opposed to specialist doctors (Mean rank = 697.16).

The Mann–Whitney test results showed that there are significant differences ($z = -4.150, p < 0.001$) in receiving malpractice complaints among doctors, depending on the type of institution in which they work, meaning that doctors working in regional or county hospitals receive more malpractice complaints (Mean rank = 879.20) than those working in smaller hospitals (Mean rank = 815.81). Data also showed that ($z = -2.325, p = 0.020$) doctors working in a hospital or private clinic (Mean rank = 864.40) are more likely to receive malpractice complaints than doctors who do not work in the private hospital environment (Mean rank = 828.46).

Significant differences ($z = -2.810, p = 0.005$) exist between the status of university teachers regarding the existence of malpractice complaints, in the sense that doctors who are at the same time teachers are more likely to receive malpractice complaints (Mean rank = 894.11) unlike doctors who do not teach at university (Mean rank = 833.80). Moreover, the results of the Mann–Whitney test ($z = -2.347, p = 0.019$) showed that doctors who are employed full time in a higher medical education unit (Mean rank = 884.79) are more likely to receive complaints related to malpractice than doctors who do not work full time in such an institution (Mean rank = 835.09).

Doctors were asked to rate their fear of being complained about from 1 (very much) to 5 (not at all). The comparative analysis ($z = -6.127, p < 0.001$) showed that the fear of complaints score is significantly higher for those who have not received any malpractice complaints (Mean rank = 872.88) compared with those who have received malpractice complaints (Mean rank = 684.10).

3.3. Correlational Results

The correlation analysis showed that there are positive correlations between the existence of a complaint among the doctors included in the research and various sociodemographic variables. It has been identified that age is positively correlated with the existence of a complaint ($p < 0.001, r = 0.194$), in the sense that as doctors age, the likelihood of dealing with malpractice complaints increases. Seniority in the medical system is positively correlated with the existence of a malpractice complaint ($p < 0.000, r = 0.202$), identifying the fact that a large number of years spent in the medical system increases the probability of r malpractice complaints among doctors. Also, the professional degree held by doctors is positively correlated with the existence of complaints ($p < 0.001$, $r = 0.230$), in the sense that the higher the professional degree, the higher the probability of malpractice complaints.

Positive correlations were identified between the existence of malpractice complaints and the number of on-call shifts performed monthly ($p = 0.001$, $r = 0.079$), in the sense that the higher the number of on-call shifts per month, the higher the likelihood of dealing with malpractice complaints. The explanation by the doctors of the results of the interventions and of the performed procedures is positively correlated with the existence of malpractice complaints ($p < 0.001$, $r = 0.101$), which means that the incomplete explanation or lack of explanation of these results can increase the probability of a malpractice complaint being filed. In addition, patience with difficult patients ($p = 0.017$, $r = 0.058$) and the distribution of educational materials among them ($p = 0.024$, $r = 0.054$) are positively correlated with the risk of being sued for malpractice, in the sense that as the patience of doctors decreases and the number of educational materials distributed is lower or even absent, the risk of doctors being sued for malpractice increases.

Spearman correlation analysis indicates that the fear of complaints is negatively correlated with the existence of a complaint related to malpractice ($p < 0.001$, $r = -0.049$) in the sense that the less worried doctors are that they might be sued, the lower the likelihood of malpractice complaints.

3.4. Assessing the Combined Effects of the Factors That Predispose to the Complaint

In order to highlight the strongest probability factors for receiving a complaint, we performed a logistic regression analysis on the characteristics of being complained about, including as predictors age, gender, parental status, professional degree, partners' profession, specialty of doctors, seniority in the medical system, the number of on-call shifts performed per month, the fear of being complained about, working in a regional/county hospital and university teacher status. The method selected for the logistic regression was the Enter method, analyzing the factorial variables simultaneously. Linearity of the continuous variables with respect to the logit of the dependent variable was assessed via the Box–Tidwell (1962) procedure. Based on this assessment, all continuous independent variables were found to be linearly related to the logit of the dependent variable.

Table 2 shows the results of the Omnibus test for the model coefficients. The results of the test χ^2 and of the likelihood rate—2LL recorded in step 1 compared with the initial step 0 allow us to reject the null hypothesis and to accept the alternative hypothesis.

Table 2. Results of the omnibus test for regression coefficients.

		Chi-Square	df	Sig.
	Step	261,043	22	0.000
Step 1	Block	261,043	22	0.000
	Model	261,043	22	0.000

Table 3 shows the results of Hosmer–Lemeshow test. This divides subjects at decile level, based on the estimated probabilities, applying in the next step the test χ^2 on the frequencies noticed. The $p = 0.473$ value indicates that the logistic model is valid from a statistical point of view, and therefore the null hypothesis can be rejected.

Table 3. Hosmer–Lemeshow Test.

Step	Chi-Square	df	Sig.
1	7.606	8	0.473

Table 4 shows the estimated values of regression coefficients of the model of logistic regression. Sig. values $p < 0.05$ showed that some factorial variables of the regression model are significant from a statistical point of view and that they influenced the status of receipt of complaints. Similarly, the Wald test values showed that the regression parameters B are different from zero. Therefore, the null hypothesis is rejected. These estimated values of the regression coefficients showed the relation between factorial variables and the dependent variable "complained": it increases (or decreases, if the coefficient sign is negative) the determined value log odds of the variable of confirmed = 1 at a change with one unit of one of the factorial variables. The influence of the other factorial is considered to be constant.

Table 4. Variables in the Equation.

		B	S.E.	Wald	df	Sig.	Exp(B)	95% C.I. for EXP(B)	
								Lower	Upper
Step 1 [a]	Gender (1)	−0.919	0.170	29.185	1	0.000	0.399	0.286	0.557
	Age	0.034	0.023	2.076	1	0.150	1.034	0.988	1.083
	Children (1)	−0.158	0.196	0.649	1	0.421	0.854	0.582	1.253
	Specialty category			20.477	4	0.000			
	Specialty category (1)	0.741	0.255	8.416	1	0.004	2.098	1.272	3.461
	Specialty category (2)	1.148	0.266	18.654	1	0,000	3.151	1.872	5.305
	Specialty category (3)	0.678	0.369	3.379	1	0.066	1.970	0.956	4.057
	Specialty category (4)	0.508	0.329	2.376	1	0.123	1.661	0.871	3.169
	Professional degree			26.542	2	0.000			
	Professional degree (1)	1.925	0.737	6.815	1	0.009	6.853	1.615	29.070
	Professional degree (2)	2.793	0.749	13.890	1	0.000	16.322	3.758	70.885
	Partner's profession			8.988	5	0.110			
	Partner's profession (1)	−0.810	0.300	7.273	1	0.007	0.445	0.247	0.802
	Partner's profession (2)	−0.531	0.516	1.058	1	0.304	0.588	0.214	1.617
	Partner's profession (3)	−0.345	0.324	1.136	1	0.286	0.708	0.375	1.336
	Partner's profession (4)	−0.930	0.543	2.933	1	0.087	0.395	0.136	1.144
	Partner's profession (5)	−0.593	0.282	4.413	1	0.036	0.553	0.318	0.961
	Fear of complaint			37.729	4	0.000			
	Fear of complaint (1)	−0.644	0.198	10.564	1	0.001	0.525	0.356	0.774
	Fear of complaint (2)	−0.880	0.264	11.108	1	0.001	0.415	0.247	0.696
	Fear of complaint (3)	−1.381	0.234	34.942	1	0.000	0.251	0.159	0.397
	Fear of complaint (4)	−1.306	0.415	9.899	1	0.002	0.271	0.120	0.611
	Seniority in medical system	0.000	0.022	0.000	1	0.995	1.000	0.958	1.043
	Number of on-call shifts monthly	0.062	0.027	5.220	1	0.022	1.064	1.009	1.122
	County/regional hospital (1)	0.338	0.166	4.145	1	0.042	1.403	1.013	1.943
	University teacher (1)	−0.045	0.201	0.049	1	0.825	0.956	0.645	1.419
	Constant	−4.635	1.039	19.882	1	0.000	0.010		

[a] Variable(s) entered on step 1: gender, age, children, specialty category, professional degree, partner's profession, fear of complaint, seniority in medical system, number of on-call shifts monthly, county/regional hospital, university teacher.

The model explained 24.6% (Nagelkerke R^2) of the variance in complaints and correctly classified 85.5% of cases. Sensitivity was 20.1% and specificity was 98.1%. Of the eleven predictor variables, seven were statistically significant: gender, specialty category, professional degree, partner's profession, fear of complaints, number of on-call shifts monthly and working in a regional hospital (as shown in Table 4). Women had 0.39 times lower odds of receiving malpractice complaints than men. An increased number of on-call shifts was associated with an increased likelihood of receiving malpractice complaints and a low level of fear about the risk of being complained about is associated with a lower likelihood of facing malpractice complaints. In addition, doctors working in regional hospitals had 1.40 times higher odds of experiencing malpractice complaints.

Professional degree is represented by two dummy variables. The first dummy variable is a comparison of specialist and resident doctor groups. The positive coefficient suggests that specialist doctors had 6.85 times higher odds of being sued for malpractice than resident doctors. Similarly, the second dummy variable compares senior doctors to residents, with results showing that senior doctors had 16.32 times higher odds of being reported for malpractice than resident doctors.

The specialty category of doctors is represented by four dummy variables. The first dummy variable is a comparison of medical specialties with those of family medicine, with the results suggesting that doctors who practice medical specialties had 2.09 times higher odds of being reported for malpractice than doctors in the family medicine specialty. Similarly, the results show that doctors in surgical specialties had 3.15 times higher odds of being reported for malpractice than doctors in family medicine.

Although the partner's profession is represented by five dummy variables, only two of them show significant differences. Thus, the negative coefficients show that doctors who have a partner who practices a different specialty of medicine had 0.44 times lower odds of being sued for malpractice than doctors who have a partner who practices the same medical specialty as them. In addition, doctors who have a partner who does not work in the medical system had 0.55 times lower odds of being sued for malpractice than doctors whose partner practices the same medical specialty as them.

4. Discussion

The present study involved a total of 1684 doctors, of whom 16.1% were complained about at least once in their careers. The binary logistic regression showed that the doctors prone to being complained about are men, with senior doctor degree, from surgical specialties, who perform a greater number of on-call shifts, who work in regional or county hospitals, who have greater fear of being complained about and whose life partner is a doctor with the same specialty.

Regarding the gender of the doctor, both the present study and other studies identified in the literature—both older [16,18,19] and more recent [1,17,20,21]—place men at higher risk for being the subject of patients' complaints compared with women. The study conducted by Guardado [1] shows that 40% of male doctors and 22.8% of female doctors who were members of the American Medical Association faced a complaint of malpractice during their career, with 20.4% of male doctors being complained about at least twice, compared with 9.7% of female doctors. In the study performed by Tibble et al. [20], focused on surgery, it was reported that male surgeons were 1.31 times more likely to be exposed to a complaint compared with their female colleagues.

There are multiple explanations for this finding. For example, Guardado [1] analyzed the gender of doctors who received complaints in terms of age and specialty and observed after separate analyses that the women were younger than the men, which means less seniority, less experience and consequently a shorter period of time in which they were exposed to the risk of complaints compared with their male colleagues. Likewise, the same author noted that except for obstetrics & gynecology, one of the specialties recognized as frequently complained about, women had specialties in which the risk of being complained about is generally low (e.g., pediatrics, psychiatry). In the same context, Taragin et al. [16] noted that male doctors, by the nature of their specialties, have a higher risk of being complained about because they deal with more severe cases.

A more in-depth analysis identifies additional explanations for men's predisposition to be complained about and implicitly for the lower risk of complaints received by women. Thus, Hall et al. [22] and Fountain [23] link the gender of doctors with their skills regarding the doctor–patient relationship and report that women have the advantage of interacting with patients more effectively, in a manner characterized by less hostility, being more meticulous, having more humanistic attributes [22], and having greater emotional involvement and a more positive approach to the patient [22,23]. Added to these are the differences in communication style [23], women more often adopting patient-centered communication, in which the patient is actively involved in the decision-making process [22,23], and often providing psycho-emotional counseling [23] and devoting more time to the discussion with the patient [22,23]. The time allotted for the discussion with the patient can be viewed from two perspectives: on the one hand, when the doctor spends more time with the patient, the latter will have the opportunity to express his/her concerns and will be more satisfied with his/her doctor. In this sense, Taragin et al. [16] argue that when patients are satisfied with the relationship they have with their doctors, they are less tempted to complain when the result of the medical procedure does not coincide with expectations. On the other hand, the time spent in discussion with the patient allows the consultation of a smaller number of patients and thus the exposure to a lower or higher risk of being complained about, respectively [22].

Although in the present study the binary logistic regression excluded older age and higher seniority from the initial profile, these two characteristics can be related to the result that identifies the degree of senior doctors as a predisposition to receiving complaints. The first stage in the doctor's training is the residency, which in Romania lasts between three and six years, depending on the specialty [24]. Next is the degree of specialist doctor, which is obtained after an examination, at the end of the residency period [25]. The degree of senior doctor is not a mandatory step in the career of doctors, but most doctors choose to sustain the examination for this promotion. In order to sustain the examination to become a senior doctor, the candidate must have sufficient experience as a specialist, practicing for at least five years in the specialty [26]. As other studies published in the literature point out, doctors' risk of facing a patient complaint increases in direct proportion to age [1,16,18] and implicitly to seniority [13,27]. Guardado [1] found that of the total number of doctors under the age of 40, 8.2% had faced a complaint during their career, whereas among doctors over the age of 54, the percentage is close to 50%. Likewise, another peculiarity of senior doctors for the increased risk of receiving complaints is the complexity of the cases they work with, as in some specialties there is a limitation in this regard depending on the degree and experience of the doctor.

At the opposite pole, the lower risk of receiving complaints among resident doctors may be related to the fact that they work under supervision, with this aspect sometimes being erroneously viewed as a lack of responsibility in the eyes of the population and sometimes in the eyes of resident doctors as well. Indeed, during their professional training, resident doctors can practice only under supervision, carrying out their activity in the field of the specialty within the limits of the competences corresponding to their training year, under the strict supervision and guidance of a specialist or senior doctor. However, this does not mean that resident doctors are immune and not responsible for the way they perform their duties, when they exceed their competencies, when they make decisions on their own or when they do not communicate properly with other members of the medical team [28].

Another relevant result of the present study was the link between the risk of complaints and the number of on-call shifts, doctors who perform more shifts being more likely to be complained about. This result can be interpreted in the context of overload and overnight work schedule. The Regulation on working time, organization and performance of on-call shifts in public medical institutions in Romania provides that "normal working time [...] is 7 h on average per day, respectively 35 h on average per week", being reduced by an hour for a series of specialties such as those in which the doctors perform postmortem examinations (pathology, forensic medicine) and those involving the risk of irradiation (e.g., radiology, radiotherapy, nuclear medicine) [29], but often this program is exceeded, doctors being forced to work over the schedule—either because of the shortage of doctors or because of the very large number of patients.

In order to ensure the permanence of medical assistance in hospitals, the doctors carry out an on-call shifts program, which in Romania starts after the usual working schedule and ends at the beginning of the working schedule of the next day, and on weekends and other official days off, the program for on-call shifts begins in the morning and ends the next day, after 24 h. Normally, after 24 h of work, doctors should rest, but often after on-call shifts doctors continue the regular schedule, so they may work up to 32 h without interruption during the week. There is no maximum number of on-call shifts allowed, the legislation in the field only specifying that it is forbidden to work two consecutive shifts [29]. Extrapolating, we can estimate that a doctor can perform a maximum of 15 on-call shifts in a month with 30 days. In the present survey, doctors reported 0 to 15 on-call shifts per month, with a mean of 2.26 ($\pm$2.78). Although the on-call schedule is not as demanding in all specialties, the shortage of doctors means that in many hospitals doctors have to perform a large number of on-call shifts, so they have little time to rest.

Similarly, a study conducted in Japan, where the normal work schedule is 40 h per week, showed that pediatricians often work over the working program, and 8% of them end up working more than 79 h a week, with a mean of 86.7 overworking hours each month and 32 consecutive hours of work when performing on-call shifts. Moreover, in Japan an overwork-related cause of death is recognized, which is known as karoshi [30].

Ensuring the continuity of health care services is an imperative of many health systems [31], even if the way it is done may differ from country to country: 24 h hospital shifts, home on-call shifts, shifts of 12 h, night shifts. However, regardless of how it is performed, the work schedule, night shift and extension of the regular work schedule can cause increased levels of stress and fatigue among physicians by interfering with their sleep schedule or sleep duration, can lead to decreased work performance, and may predispose them to chronic disease [31] or anxiety and depression [32]. Under these conditions, the risk of errors increases as well, endangering the proper care of the patient [31].

Luckhaupt et al. [33] reported that between 1985 and 1990 and later, between 2004 and 2007, there was an increase in the percentage of medical professionals who did not get enough sleep during the entire day (i.e., $\leq$6 h), from 28% to 32%.

The consequences of insufficient sleep and fatigue for medical practice can be important: the state of alertness decreases, periods of involuntary micro-sleep may occur (lasting several seconds, in which although the person has their eyes open, the brain is blocked and attention disappears), reaction time increases, the ability to concentrate, store and process new information decreases [31], and the skills are reduced [34]. Studies on resident doctors show that these negative effects of sleep deprivation can occur despite ambition, training and experience [31]. Additionally, the effects of a lack of proper rest can interfere with the ability to relate to and communicate with patients [31,35], with doctors becoming irritable and experiencing mood swings, as well as with the decision-making process, leading to a tendency to take too many risks in the activity [31]. A study on 301 anesthesiologists in New Zealand, which looked at the evaluation of fatigue errors caused by the work schedule, showed that 86% of participants confirmed the existence of errors in practice due to fatigue [36], and the study by Landrigan et al. [37] shows that during the extended work schedule of more than 24 h, the number of errors made by interns/trainees was 35.9% higher compared with the number of errors in the work schedule in shifts of maximum 16 h.

Moreover, doctors who have more shifts examine more patients, and there is again a higher risk of being exposed to complaints from patients [30].

The results of the current study show that out of the first six most risky specialties in relation to the number of doctors complained about in the total number of respondents in each specialty, five are major surgical specialties: plastic surgery, pediatric surgery, neurosurgery, general surgery and orthopedics & traumatology. In addition, when the categories of specialties (surgical, medical, pediatric, paraclinical-laboratory and family medicine) are compared, doctors working in the category of surgical specialties were the most complained about, and those working in family medicine received the fewest complaints. Malpractice complaints are incidents that surgeons frequently face in their careers [38], with numerous literature studies placing surgical specialties at the top of the list of specialties receiving the most complaints [1,13,20], along with obstetrics & gynecology [1,13]. In the study published by Jena et al. [38], in which the authors assessed the risk of complaints by specialty in the USA, the first three places are occupied by neurosurgery, cardiovascular surgery and general surgery. Taragin et al. [16] (New Jersey) identified neurosurgery as taking first place, along with orthopedics and obstetrics & gynecology, these specialists accumulating seven to nine times more complaints per year than psychiatry, the specialty least prone to complaints. Tibble et al. [20] ranks the first three places among the surgical specialties receiving complaints in Australia as neurosurgery, plastic surgery and orthopedic surgery, sustaining that they pose a higher risk compared with general surgery. In the study performed by Boyll et al. [27], of 129 plastic surgeons who were members of the American Society of Plastic and Aesthetic Surgery, nearly three-quarters stated that they had faced at least one complaint from patients. In Italy, between 1996 and 2000, the two specialties receiving the most complaints were orthopedics & traumatology and obstetrics & gynecology [2].

A possible explanation for the increased predisposition of surgeons to be complained about by patients is the intrinsic risk of the specialty [1,20], given the invasive nature of the treatment [39] and the generally high severity of the diseases they treat [20,40]. In addition, given that patients sometimes suffer from multiple comorbidities, and technological progress allows the use of increasingly advanced and complex procedures, the associated risks are directly proportional [41], but in turn, society is constantly changing and has increasing expectations, accepting these risks less and less [42]. The first place being occupied by neurosurgery in some studies can be explained by the small number of doctors working in this specialty [43]. In Romania, neurosurgeons are less than 1% of the total number of doctors (0.63%) [44], and in the group in the present study they represented 0.83%—of the 14 participating doctors, six had received complaints from patients. However, the higher risk for neurosurgeons also stems from special features, such as neurological complications resulting in functional disorders being difficult to accept by patients [42,45]. For plastic surgery, studies show that most complaints are related to patients' dissatisfaction with the results of cosmetic interventions [27,46]. In this regard, some authors suggest that complaints arise due to poor and unclear information about the expectations that patients should have after cosmetic interventions [27,47]. In addition, studies that targeted only plastic surgeons showed a 2.5 times higher risk among doctors who focus on cosmetic interventions in their practice, compared with others [27].

To these explanations can be added the relatively poor relationship skills among surgeons, which predisposes them to poor communication with patients and consequently to complaints [20].

The present study indicates that family medicine is one of the specialties in which doctors receive the fewest complaints, which is partly consistent with the results obtained in a previous study [7]. Although there are studies in the literature that place a generally high risk for family medicine [48,49], the fact that this specialty received fewer complaints in the present and the previous studies is not a situation limited to Romania, as there are other authors who have obtained similar results [38]. What is, however, particular for Romania is the general context in which patients often avoid using the services of the family doctor, instead requesting in excess the emergency services—either by calling the unique emergency number 112, which involves driving an ambulance at the patient's home, or by presenting directly to the emergency unit for conditions that could be resolved by the family doctor [50]. This preference of patients for the emergency services to the detriment of family doctors creates an imbalance in the health system, often resulting in doctors in the emergency services becoming overworked. As well as this, due to more urgent situations being prioritized, patients who abuse this service feel neglected, become irritated and thus the favorable context for a complaint is created [51].

Another characteristic of doctors prone to receiving complaints is their activity in regional or county hospitals. The explanations are multiple and related to those discussed above. Regional or county hospitals are large hospitals, which have superior competences, better equipment for diagnosis and treatment, thus having opportunities to care for patients with conditions of high complexity [52,53]. Thus, doctors are exposed to risk through the care provided to a large number of patients, who often have complex pathologies. In this way, the overloading of doctors reduces the time allotted to patients, with the subsequent dissatisfaction of the latter. Similar results were obtained by Hwang et al. [54], who found in their study that more than 70% of complaints concerned large medical centers and regional hospitals.

Fear of complaints as a factor that predisposes doctors to receiving complaints may be related to the fact that fear of complaints can cause the doctor to make decisions for their personal protection, which in turn can lead to complaints, for example by decreasing the patient's adherence to treatment [55]. At the same time, other authors claim that requesting too many investigations could raise some questions about the competence of the doctor or the quality of care [21]. This could explain the result of the present study which shows that the greater fear of complaints—which induces changes in medical practice—predisposes doctors to complaints from patients. Nevertheless, there are studies that show that supplementation of investigations gives patients the impression that they are better cared for, without considering the fact that more care does not necessarily equate to better quality of care [56].

The results of the present study indicate there is a higher risk of receiving complaints for doctors whose life partner is a doctor with the same specialty. The relevance of this characteristic requires more in-depth analysis in future studies, as no other studies found in the literature focused specifically on this issue. Consequently, a comparison to corroborate our results was not possible in the present paper.

5. Reflections and Planning

Many of the characteristics found to compose the profile of the Romanian doctor prone to receiving complaints swing around the same core, i.e., doctor–patient communication. Therefore, specific activities aiming to improve this essential component of the medical practice may help to reduce the number of complaints.

Examples of such activities would be enhancement of awareness regarding this issue starting at the university level, with periodic updates throughout the doctor's career through participation in training specifically dedicated to various issues connected to doctor–patient communication (e.g., manner in which to reveal the occurrence of a mistake or a complication, manner in which to hold discussions with different types of patients, how to address each patient when the waiting room is crowded, the limits of the new technology in medicine).

The results reflect the situation related to malpractice complaints in Romania. The fact that doctors at higher risk of receiving complaints are those in the category of surgical specialties (plastic surgery, pediatric surgery, neurosurgery, general surgery, orthopedics & traumatology) makes it necessary to study them further in depth, to identify specific risks and implicitly to implement targeted measures to prevent them.

In addition, we found that the specialty with the lowest risk is family medicine, a finding that could be explained by the under-use of the primary health care services to the detriment of emergency medical services, suggesting the need for measures aiming to improve the appropriate access of health services by patients.

The increased risk of being complained about among doctors who perform more on-call shifts raises an alarm about the risks of overload and suggests the need for collaboration between the relevant bodies to protect overworked doctors and implicitly patients requesting their services.

The results obtained are important for doctors, medical institutions and policy makers in order to implement new rules and practices to diminish the risk for malpractice complaints.

6. Strengths and Limitations of the Study

A significant strength of the present study is its pioneering character, being the first research in Romania that aims to analyze complaints regarding professional responsibility, being addressed directly to doctors, at the national level. Second, this study allowed the outlining of the profile of the Romanian doctor prone to receiving complaints from patients. In this way, the study highlighted common aspects shown by studies conducted in other countries, but also particular aspects explained by the characteristics of the medical practice in Romania and the organization of the medical system in this country.

A limitation of this study is the fact that the results concern doctors in Romania, so they cannot be generalized, or extrapolated to the situation of other countries. A second limitation could be related to the arbitrary choices of bins of the HL test.

7. Conclusions

The present study allowed us to outline the socio-demographic, professional and institutional characteristics of the Romanian doctor prone to being complained about by patients and, implicitly, highlighted aspects where interventions can be made at the national level to reduce the risk of malpractice complaints. The results outline the profile of the Romanian doctor prone to being complained about: male, senior doctor, from surgical specialties, who performs a larger number of on-call shifts, who works in regional or county hospitals, who has a higher level of fear of complaints and whose life partner is a doctor with the same specialty.

Author Contributions: Conceptualization, B.H., M.I. and B.G.I.; methodology, M.I. and L.M.P.; validation, L.M.P.; formal analysis, L.M.P.; data curation, B.H. and B.G.I.; writing—original draft preparation, B.H.; writing—review and editing, B.H. and B.G.I.; supervision, M.I. and B.G.I.; project administration, B.H. All authors equally contributed to the research. All authors have read and agreed to the published version of the manuscript.

Funding: This research received no external funding.

Institutional Review Board Statement: The study was approved by the Research Ethics Commission of the "Grigore T. Popa" University of Medicine and Pharmacy of Iasi, No. 16434/30 July 2019.

Informed Consent Statement: Informed consent was obtained from the participants before their inclusion in the study.

Data Availability Statement: Data are available, on request, from the corresponding author.

Acknowledgments: This study is part of a larger piece of doctoral research, aimed at identifying methods to prevent complaints made by patients regarding the professional responsibility of doctors and to reduce the impact of the complaints on the doctors involved.

Conflicts of Interest: The authors declare no conflict of interest.

References

1. Guardado, J.R. Medical liability claim frequency among US physicians. In *Policy Research Perspectives*; American Medical Association: Chicago, IL, USA, 2017. Available online: https://www.ama-assn.org/media/21976/download (accessed on 13 August 2021).
2. Traina, F. Medical malpractice. *Clin. Orthop. Relat. Res.* **2009**, *467*, 434–442. [CrossRef] [PubMed]
3. Miglioretti, M.; Mariani, F.; Vecchio, L. Could patient engagement promote a health system free from malpractice litigation risk? In *Promoting Patient Engagement and Participation for Effective Healthcare Reform*; An Imprint of IGI Global; Graffigna, G., Ed.; Medical Information Science Reference: Hershey, PA, USA, 2006; pp. 240–264.
4. Toraldo, D.M.; Vergari, U.; Toraldo, M. Medical malpractice, defensive medicine and role of the "media" in Italy. *Multidiscip. Respir. Med.* **2015**, *10*, 12. [CrossRef] [PubMed]
5. Oyebode, F. Clinical errors and medical negligence. *Med. Princ. Pract.* **2013**, *22*, 323–333. [CrossRef] [PubMed]
6. Dumitrescu, R.M. Litigious side of the medical malpractice in Romania. *Mod. Med.* **2019**, *26*, 197–211. [CrossRef]

7. Hanganu, B.; Iorga, M.; Muraru, I.D.; Ioan, B.G. Reasons for and Facilitating Factors of Medical Malpractice Complaints. What Can Be Done to Prevent Them? *Medicina* **2020**, *56*, 259. [CrossRef]
8. Pioger, C.; Jacquet, C.; Abitan, A.; Odri, G.A.; Ollivier, M.; Sonnery-Cottet, B.; Boisrenoult, P.; Pujol, N. Litigation in arthroscopic surgery: A 20-year analysis of legal actions in France. *Knee Surg. Sports Traumatol. Arthrosc.* **2021**, *29*, 1651–1658. [CrossRef]
9. Chukwuneke, F.N. Medical incidents in developing countries: A few case studies from Nigeria. *Niger. J. Clin. Pract.* **2015**, *18*, S20–S24. [CrossRef]
10. Hanganu, B.; Ioan, B.G. Malpraxisul medical: Cauze si consecinte asupra personalului medical. In *Psihologie Medicala Studii Clinice*; Iorga, M., Rosca, C., Eds.; Editura Universitara: Bucharest, Romania, 2019; pp. 183–188. (In Romanian)
11. Verhoef, L.M.; Weenink, J.W.; Winters, S.; Robben, P.B.M.; Westert, G.; Kool, R.B. The disciplined healthcare professional: A qualitative interview study on the impact of the disciplinary process and imposed meadures in the Netherlands. *BMJ Open* **2015**, *5*, e009275. [CrossRef]
12. Charles, S.C.; Gibbons, R.D.; Frisch, P.R.; Pyskoty, C.E.; Hedeker, D.; Singha, N.K. Predicting risk for medical malpractice claims using quality-of-care characteristics. *West. J. Med.* **1992**, *157*, 433–439.
13. Tan, E.C.; Chen, D.R. Second victim: Malpractice disputes and quality of life among primary care physicians. *J. Formos. Med. Assoc.* **2019**, *118*, 619–627. [CrossRef]
14. Adamson, T.E.; Baldwin, D.C., Jr.; Sheehan, T.J.; Oppenberg, A.A. Characteristics of surgeons with high and low malpractice claims rates. *West. J. Med.* **1997**, *166*, 37–44.
15. Wu, C.Y.; Lai, H.J.; Chen, R.C. Patient characteristics predict occurrence and outcome of complaints against physicians: A study from a medical center in central Taiwan. *J. Formos. Med. Assoc.* **2009**, *108*, 126–134. [CrossRef]
16. Taragin, M.I.; Wilczek, A.P.; Karns, M.E.; Trout, R.; Carson, J.L. Physician demographics and the risk of medical malpractice. *Am. J. Med.* **1992**, *93*, 537–542. [CrossRef]
17. Studdert, D.M.; Bismark, M.M.; Mello, M.M.; Singh, H.; Spittal, M.J. Prevalence and Characteristics of Physicians Prone to Malpractice Claims. *N. Engl. J. Med.* **2016**, *374*, 354–362. [CrossRef]
18. Gibbons, R.D.; Hedeker, D.; Charles, S.C.; Frisch, P. A random-effects probit model for predicting medical malpractice claims. *J. Am. Stat. Assoc.* **1994**, *89*, 760–767. [CrossRef]
19. Waters, T.M.; Lefevre, F.V.; Budetti, P.P. Medical school attended as a predictor of medical malpractice claims. *BMJ Qual. Saf.* **2003**, *12*, 330–336. [CrossRef]
20. Tibble, H.M.; Broughton, N.S.; Studdert, D.M.; Spittal, M.J.; Hill, N.; Morris, J.M.; Bismark, M.M. Why do surgeons receive more complaints than their physician peers? *ANZ J. Surg.* **2018**, *88*, 269–273. [CrossRef]
21. Unwin, E.; Woolf, K.; Wadlow, C.; Potts, H.W.W.; Dacre, J. Sex differences in medico-legal action against doctors: A systematic review and meta-analysis. *BMC Med.* **2015**, *13*, 172. [CrossRef]
22. Hall, J.A.; Blanch-Hartigan, D.; Roter, D.L. Patients' satisfaction with male versus female physicians: A meta-analysis. *Med. Care.* **2011**, *49*, 611–617. [CrossRef]
23. Fountain, T.R. Ophtalmic malpractice and physician gender: A claims data analysis (an American ophtalmological society thesis). *Trans. Am. Ophtalmol. Soc.* **2014**, *112*, 38–49.
24. Order No. 1109 of October 6, 2016, For the Modification of the Order of the Minister of Public Health No. 1509/2008 Regarding the Approval of the Nomenclature of Medical, Medico-Dental and Pharmaceutical Specialties for the Health Care Network, Published in the Official Gazette of Romania, Part I, No. 786 of 6 October 2016. Available online: https://legislatie.just.ro/Public/DetaliiDocument/182341 (accessed on 24 July 2021).
25. Ministry of Health. Publication on the Organization and Conduct of the Examination for Obtaining the Title of Specialist Physician, Dentist and Pharmacist, from the Session of 16 October 2019. Available online: http://www.ms.ro/wp-content/uploads/2019/08/Publicatie16.10.2019.pdf (accessed on 24 July 2021).
26. Ministry of Health. Examination Publication on the Organization and Conduct of the Examination for Obtaining the Professional Degree of Senior Physician, Dentist and Pharmacist, from the Session of 6 July 2020. Available online: http://www.ms.ro/wp-content/uploads/2020/05/Publica%C8%9Bia-de-examen-privind-organizarea-%C8%99i-desf%C4%83%C8%99urarea-examenului-pentru-ob%C8%9Binerea-gradului-profesional-de-medic-medic-dentist-respectiv-farmacist-primar-din-sesiunea-06-iulie-2020.pdf (accessed on 24 July 2021).
27. Boyll, P.; Kang, P.; Mahabir, R.; Bernard, R.W. Variables That Impact Medical Malpractice Claims Involving Plastic Surgeons in the United States. *Aesthet. Surg. J.* **2018**, *38*, 785–792. [CrossRef] [PubMed]
28. Hochberg, M.S.; Seib, C.D.; Berman, R.S.; Kalet, A.L.; Zabar, S.R.; Pachter, H.L. Perspective: Malpractice in an Academic Medical Center: A Frequently Overlooked Aspect of Professionalism Education. *Acad. Med.* **2011**, *86*, 365–368. [CrossRef] [PubMed]
29. Regulation of 1 June 2004 on Working Time, Organization and Performance of On-call Shifts in Public Units in the Sanitary Sector, Approved by Order No. 870/2004, Published in the Official Gazette of Romania No. 671 of 26 July 2004. Available online: https://legislatie.just.ro/Public/DetaliiDocument/53836 (accessed on 24 July 2021).
30. Ehara, A. Are long physician working hours harmful to patient safety? *Pediatr. Int.* **2008**, *50*, 175–178. [CrossRef] [PubMed]
31. Caruso, C.C. Negative impacts of shiftwork and long work hours. *Rehabil. Nurs.* **2014**, *39*, 16–25. [CrossRef]
32. Nicol, A.M.; Botterill, J.S. On-call work and health: A review. *Environ. Health* **2004**, *3*, 15. [CrossRef]
33. Luckhaupt, S.E.; Tak, S.; Calvert, G.M. The prevalence of short sleep duration by industry and occupation in the National Health Interview Survey. *Sleep* **2010**, *33*, 149–159. [CrossRef]

34. Dawson, D.; Chapman, J.; Thomas, M.J. Fatigue-proofing: A new approach to reducing fatigue-related risk using the principles of error management. *Sleep Med. Rev.* **2012**, *16*, 167–175. [CrossRef]
35. Holm, H.A. Postgraduate education. In *International Handbook of Research in Medical Education*; Norman, G.R., van der Vleuten, C.P.M., Newble, D.I., Eds.; Springer: Berlin/Heidelberg, Germany, 2002.
36. Gander, P.; Merry, A.; Millar, M.M.; Wellers, J. Hours of work and fatigue-related error: A survey of New Zealand Anaesthetists. *Anaesth. Intensive Care* **2000**, *28*, 178–183. [CrossRef]
37. Landrigan, C.P.; Rothschild, J.M.; Cronin, J.W.; Kaushal, R.; Burdick, E.; Katz, J.T.; Lilly, C.M.; Stone, P.H.; Lockley, S.W.; Bates, D.W.; et al. Effect of reducing interns' work hours on serious medical errors in intensive care units. *N. Engl. J. Med.* **2004**, *351*, 1838–1848. [CrossRef]
38. Jena, A.B.; Seabury, S.; Lakdawalla, D.; Chandra, A. Malpractice risk according to physician specialty. *N. Engl. J. Med.* **2011**, *365*, 629–636. [CrossRef]
39. Bourne, T.; Wynants, L.; Peters, M.; Van Audenhove, C.; Timmerman, D.; Van Calster, B.; Jalmbrant, M. The impact of complaints procedures on the welfare, health and clinical practise of 7926 doctors in the UK: A cross-sectional survey. *BMJ Open* **2015**, *5*, e006687. [CrossRef]
40. Gualniera, P.; Mondello, C.; Scurria, S.; Oliva, A.; Grassi, S.; Pizzicannella, J.; Alibrandi, A.; Sapienza, D.; Asmundo, A. Experience of an Italian Hospital Claims Management Committee: A tool for extrajudicial litigations resolution. *Leg. Med.* **2020**, *42*, 101657. [CrossRef]
41. Wienke, A. Errors and pitfalls: Briefing and accusation of medical malpractice—The second victim. *GMS Curr. Top. Otorhinolaryngol. Head Neck Surg.* **2013**, *12*. [CrossRef]
42. Debono, B.; Hamel, O.; Guillain, A.; Durand, A.; Rue, M.; Sabatier, P.; Lonjon, G.; Dran, G. Impact of Malpractice Liability Among Spine Surgeons: A National Survey of French Private Neurosurgeons. *Neurochirurgie* **2020**, *66*, 219–224. [CrossRef]
43. Agarwal, N.; Gupta, R.; Agarwal, P.; Matthew, P.; Wolferz, R., Jr.; Shah, A.; Adeeb, N.; Prabhu, A.V.; Kanter, A.S.; Okonkwo, D.O.; et al. Descriptive Analysis of State and Federal Spine Surgery Malpractice Litigation in the United States. *Spine* **2018**, *43*, 984–990. [CrossRef]
44. Ioniță, A.; Rădoi, S.; Gusicov, D.M.; Militaru, A. The Activity of the Sanitary Units in 2018. Available online: https://insse.ro/cms/en/content/activity-sanitary-units-2018 (accessed on 24 July 2021).
45. Din, R.S.; Yan, S.C.; Cote, D.J.; Acosta, M.A.; Smith, T.R. Defensive Medicine in U.S. Spine Neurosurgery. *Spine* **2017**, *42*, 177–185. [CrossRef]
46. Svider, P.F.; Keeley, B.R.; Zumba, O.; Mauro, A.C.; Setzen, M.; Eloy, J.A. From the operating room to the courtroom: A comprehensive characterization of litigation related to facial plastic surgery procedures. *Laryngoscope* **2013**, *123*, 1849–1853. [CrossRef]
47. Feola, A.; Minotti, C.; Marchetti, D.; Caricato, M.; Capolupo, G.T.; Marsella, L.T.; La Monaca, G. A Five-Year Survey for Plastic Surgery Malpractice Claims in Rome, Italy. *Medicina* **2021**, *57*, 571. [CrossRef]
48. Patanavanich, R.; Suriyawongpaisal, P.; Aekplakorn, W. Characteristics of Medical Malpractice Litigation in Thailand: Cases from Government-Run Hospitals. *World Med. Health Policy* **2018**, *10*, 259–271. [CrossRef]
49. Birkeland, S.; Bogh, S.B. Malpractice litigation, workload, and general practitioner retirement. *Prim. Health Care Res. Dev.* **2019**, *20*, e23. [CrossRef]
50. Vladescu, C.; Scintee, S.G.; Olsavszky, V.; Hernandez-Quevedo, C.; Sagan, A. Romania: Health System Review. *Health Syst Transit.* **2016**, *18*, 1–170.
51. Shen, Y.; Lee, L.H. Improving the wait time to consultation at the emergency department. *BMJ Open Qual.* **2018**, *7*, e000131. [CrossRef]
52. The Mandatory Minimum Criteria for the Classification of Hospitals according to Competence from 18 April 2011, Published in the Official Gazette of Romania, Part I, No. 274 of 19 April 2011. Available online: https://legislatie.just.ro/Public/DetaliiDocument/127826 (accessed on 24 July 2021).
53. Order No. 1408/2010 Regarding the Approval of the Criteria for Classifying Hospitals according to Competence Published in the Official Gazette of Romania, Part I, No. 769 of 17 November 2010. Available online: https://legislatie.just.ro/Public/DetaliiDocumentAfis/123677 (accessed on 24 July 2021).
54. Hwang, C.Y.; Wu, C.H.; Cheng, F.C.; Yen, Y.L.; Wu, K.H. A 12-year analysis of closed medical malpractice claims of the Taiwan civil court: A retrospective study. *Medicine* **2018**, *97*, e0237. [CrossRef]
55. Seger, T.; Harpaz, I.; Meshulam, I. Israeli physicians manage risk of litigation: Predicting empowerment role model. *Int. J. Human Resour. Manag.* **2011**, *22*, 2442–2462. [CrossRef]
56. Raposo, V.L. Defensive Medicine and the Imposition of a More Demanding Standard of Care. *J. Leg. Med.* **2019**, *39*, 401–416. [CrossRef]

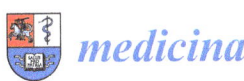

Article

The Impact of COVID-19 on Behavior and Physical and Mental Health of Romanian College Students

Sînziana Călina Silișteanu [1], Maria Totan [2,*], Oana Raluca Antonescu [3,*], Lavinia Duică [2], Elisabeta Antonescu [2] and Andrei Emanuel Silișteanu [4]

1. Faculty of Medicine and Biological Sciences, "Stefan cel Mare" University of Suceava, 13 Universitatii Str., 720229 Suceava, Romania; sinziana.silisteanu@usm.ro
2. Faculty of Medicine, "Lucian Blaga" University of Sibiu, 2A Lucian Blaga Str., 550169 Sibiu, Romania; lavinia.duica@ulbsibiu.ro (L.D.); elisabeta.antonescu@ulbsibiu.ro (E.A.)
3. County Clinical Emergency Hospital, 2-4 Corneliu Coposu Str., 550245 Sibiu, Romania
4. Faculty of Political, Administrative and Communication Sciences of Cluj-Napoca, 71 Traian Mosoiu Street, 400132 Cluj Napoca, Romania; silisteanuandrei10@yahoo.com
* Correspondence: maria.totan@ulbsibiu.ro (M.T.); oana.raluca.antonescu@gmail.com (O.R.A.)

Abstract: *Background and Objectives*: The COVID-19 pandemic caused by SARS-CoV-2 significantly marked people's lives with respect to their behavior, and their physical and mental health. *Materials and Methods*: This is a cross-sectional study that was conducted in 2021 for a period of 5 months. The study sample included 218 students from the College of Physical Education and Sports of the University of Suceava who filled in a questionnaire on mental, physical and behavioral symptoms caused by the COVID-19 pandemic, as well as the Anxiety Assessment Questionnaire (STAI). *Results*: The responses indicated increased anxiety, physical symptoms, altered behavior, and increased perception of social restrictions. Regression analyses indicated that the levels of anxiety during the COVID-19 outbreak were strongly correlated with cognitive, physical and behavioral symptoms of the students. These were influenced by the living arrangements, location (urban vs. rural), age group and study year. *Conclusions*: The results show that first-year students did not exhibit significant physical and cognitive symptoms despite reporting anxiety, probably due to their enthusiasm as beginners. The 3rd year students were prone to anxiety and reported cognitive symptoms, possibly due to the prospects of an uncertain future.

Keywords: students; psycho-emotional moods; behavioral problems; academic performance; COVID-19 pandemic

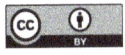

1. Introduction

The COVID-19 pandemic caused by the SARS-CoV-2 marked people's lives significantly by influencing their behavior, but also their physical and mental health. The World Health Organization issued specific guidelines and urged an analysis on the effects of the pandemic on mental health and possible psycho-social consequences [1]. Social isolation, restrictions on physical and social contact, fear of illness and the loss of loved ones are just some of the aspects caused by the pandemic [2,3]. It has been well documented that quarantine and self-isolation can affect the daily activities of the population by worsening their anxiety, depression, loneliness, insomnia and development of behavior that can lead to increased alcohol consumption, tobacco or substance use, and even suicide [4].

Previous studies have consistently shown the psychosocial impact of the COVID-19 pandemic on mental health and in particular on women and children of young age [3,5,6]. For example, one study [7] showed that approximately 1.5 billion young people, of which 90% were students enrolled in schools worldwide, did not attend classes. In China, more than 220 million children and adolescents stayed at home during long periods of times because of the pandemic [8], and 18.6% showed symptoms characteristic of anxiety disorders [9]. Thus, Chinese students were found to be at higher risks in comparison to the adult population in terms of anxiety, stress or depression [3] and were very sensitive to the negative effects of the quarantine [10–12].

The unprecedented situation created by the COVID-19 pandemic in Romania has transformed the educational system by forcing teachers as well as students to adapt within a very short time to the new social conditions and to the online learning process [13–15]. Suceava county, situated in the north-east region of Romania, saw the first and the largest COVID-19 outbreak that originated at Suceava regional county hospital. As a consequence, Suceava county was placed under complete lockdown, which had a major impact on all ages, including young individuals. Being the first region in the country under sheltering-in-place measures, students in this area were also the first ones subject to the social restrictions and sudden changes in the curriculum delivery. Therefore, we hypothesized that these measures had a negative impact on students' health due to increased stress and anxiety since there was no history on how to successfully cope with such sudden and adverse environmental factors [16]. To address this, we evaluated the impact of the first COVID-19 outbreak on physical, mental and behavioral manifestations of first-, second- and third-year college students under complete lockdown conditions in the county of Suceava, Romania.

2. Materials and Methods

The study was cross-sectional and was conducted in 2021 for a period of 5 months at "Ștefan cel Mare" University of Suceava.

The target population was represented by first-, second- and third-year students from the College of Physical Education and Sports at "Ștefan cel Mare" University in Suceava. Off the 412 students contacted, 242 responded to our online questionnaire, and 218 actually completed the questionnaires. All participants received the information package about the study and signed informed consent. The study was conducted online, and students received one questionnaire as well as the self-evaluation STAI (State-Trait Anxiety Inventory Spielberger) questionnaire, via e-mail, using Google Docs.

The study was approved by the Research Ethics Committee of the University of Suceava nr. 34/20.05.2021, in compliance with the ethical principles on human medical research according to the Declaration of Helsinki. The collected data were anonymous and confidential, and were used only for this study.

The general questionnaire was designed to evaluate the impact of the COVID-19 pandemic during the lockdown/isolation period on the emotional, cognitive and physical status of the students and also its influence on their quality of life. The questions were closed type, with multiple answer choices. The students had to choose from the options provided, with the used terms being easy to understand without creating confusion. The questions were short and precise, meant to elicit a direct answer and to be easily processed for analyses. The questions focused on mental reactions (emotional and cognitive) and physical and behavioral reactions reported by students in response to the lockdown (isolation, online courses) by assessing stress, fear, anxiety and panic. For cognitive evaluation, the questionnaire aimed to determine whether or not the student had difficulties in concentration/attention and coping with catastrophic events. For physical evaluation, the symptoms presented and recorded were headache, fatigue, myalgia, anorexia and malaise. The questionnaire also included questions that assessed changes in the general behavior of the students, such as eating, sleep, alcohol consumption, tobacco use, physical activity and social restrictions.

Students also completed the STAI questionnaire that included 40 items, assessed on a 4-point Likert scale (e.g., from "Almost Never" to "Almost Always"). The scale has 2 subscales: one for the state, with 20 items that reflects the person's condition "at this moment" and the trait subscale, also with 20 items, that reflects the person's condition "in general" [17]. This questionnaire had been used and validated in previous Romanian studies, albeit in other models [18]. It has been often used in assessing anxiety and is a sensitive predictor of distress. State anxiety items include: "I am tense; I am worried" and "I feel calm; I feel secure." The possible scores vary from a minimum of 20 points (signs are not present at all) to a maximum of 80 points (signs are very present). Trait anxiety items include: "I worry too much over something that really doesn't matter" and "I am content; I am a steady person". Likewise, the possible scores vary from a minimum of 20 points (signs are not present at all) to a maximum of 80 points (signs are very present). Data were analyzed with Student's t-test and regression analysis using Microsoft Excel and IBM SPSS Statistics for Windows version 24.0 (Armonk, NY: IBM Corp) statistical software. Data are presented as absolute numerical values, mean (±SD) as well as proportions. Values with $p < 0.05$ were considered statistically significant.

3. Results

Of the 218 students who completed the questionnaires, 155 (71.11%) were female and 63 (28.89%) were male. The proportion by study years was 75 (34.40%), 72 (33.03%) and 71 (32.57%), for the first, second and third year, respectively (Table 1).

Table 1. Socio-demographic characteristics of the study group.

	Students	1st Year		2nd Year		3rd Year	
		F	M	F	M	F	M
		59 (78.67%)	16 (21.33%)	51 (70.83%)	21 (29.17%)	45 (63.38%)	26 (36.62%)
Age	<20 years	17	4	11	8	-	-
	21–25 years	22	6	14	3	15	7
	26–30 years	9	2	12	5	16	10
	31–35 years	8	3	8	3	8	5
	>36 years	3	1	6	2	6	4
Location	University dorms	25	8	20	7	21	7
	Living with family	19	4	15	8	14	8
	Living alone	15	4	16	6	10	11
Geographical Area	Urban	40	10	21	11	22	16
	Rural	19	6	30	10	23	10

Our analyses showed that anxiety due to stress, fear, and panic attacks were observed more in females than in males (57.79% vs. 19.72%) while 72.93% of students reported difficulty in concentration/attention. A similarly high percentage of students complained of various physical symptoms, such as fatigue, myalgia, headache, malaise and anorexia. Additionally, prolonged sitting position at the computer caused pain in the lumbar and dorsal spine in a greater proportion than visual acuity disorders and low limb pain (Table 2).

Table 2. Results from the questionnaire on mental, physical and behavioral symptoms caused by COVID-19 pandemic.

Question	Answer	1st Year (n,%)		2nd Year (n,%)		3rd Year (n,%)	
		Female	Male	Female	Male	Female	Male
What was your first reaction when you found out from mass media about the COVID 19 infection?	Fear	20 (26.67)	3 (4)	8 (11.11)	5 (6.94)	12 (16.91)	5 (7.04)
	Frustration	15 (20)	5 (6.67)	6 (8.33)	3 (4.16)	12 (16.91)	8 (11.27)
	Panic attack	8 (10.6)	3 (4)	20 (27.78)	6 (8.33)	12 (16.91)	5 (7.04)
	Stress	14 (18.6)	4 (5.33)	15 (20.83)	6 (8.33)	7 (9.86)	6 (8.45)
	I don't know	2 (2.67)	1 (1.33)	2 (2.78)	1 (1.38)	2 (2.82)	2 (2.82)

Table 2. Cont.

Question	Answer	1st Year (n,%)		2nd Year (n,%)		3rd Year (n,%)	
		Female	Male	Female	Male	Female	Male
What symptoms did you experience when classes were moved online?	Fatigue	11 (14.67)	2 (2.67)	14 (19.44)	4 (5.56)	8 (11.27)	4 (5.63)
	Anorexia	12 (16)	2 (2.67)	10 (13.88)	2 (2.78)	8 (11.27)	3 (4.23)
	Myalgia	14 (18.67)	4 (5.33)	13 (18.05)	5 (6.94)	4 (5.63)	7 (9.86)
	Headache	10 (1.33)	4 (5.33)	6 (8.33)	6 (8.33)	8 (11.27)	4 (5.63)
	Malaise	12 (16)	4 (5.33)	8 (11.11)	4 (5.56)	7 (9.86)	8 (11.27)
Did lockdown cause the appearance or worsening of cognitive/attention disorders?	Difficulty in concentration	27 (36)	7 (9.33)	16 (22.22)	7 (9.72)	18 (25.35)	7 (9.86)
	Difficulty in attention	21 (28)	4 (5.33)	24 (33.33)	8 (11.11)	12 (16.91)	8 (11.27)
	Catastrophic events	10 (13.33)	4 (5.33)	10 (13.89)	6 (8.33)	15 (21.13)	10 (14.08)
	I don't know	1 (1.33)	1 (1.33)	1 (1.38)	0	0	1 (1.41)
Which food categories did you eat more often during lockdown?	Fats	16 (21.33)	4 (5.33)	23 (31.94)	6 (8.33)	12 (16.91)	8 (11.27)
	Proteins	13 (17.33)	6 (8)	12 (16.67)	8 (11.11)	20 (28.17)	7 (9.86)
	Carbohydrates	30 (40)	6 (8)	14 (19.44)	7 (9.72)	13 (18.31)	11 (15.49)
Describe the quality of your sleep during the lockdown	Sleep difficulty	16 (21.33)	4 (5.33)	20 (27.78)	6 (8.33)	12 (16.91)	6 (8.45)
	Insomnia	12 (16)	5 (6.67)	6 (8.33)	6 (8.33)	12 (16.91)	9 (12.68)
	Deep sleep	22 (29.33)	3 (4)	20 (27.78)	5 (6.94)	12 (16.91)	6 (8.45)
	No change	5 (6.67)	4 (5.33)	3 (4.17)	3 (4.17)	9 (12.68)	5 (7.04)
	I don't know	4 (5.33)	0	2 (2.78)	1 (1.38)	0	0
How did you perceive the restrictions during the lockdown?	Physical restriction	14 (18.67)	5 (6.67)	16 (22.22)	8 (11.11)	16 (22.54)	8 (11.27)
	Social restriction	25 (33.33)	8 (10.67)	20 (27.78)	6 (8.33)	18 (25.35)	8 (11.27)
	Imposed self-isolation	20 (26.67)	3 (4)	14 (19.44)	6 (8.33)	9 (12.68)	6 (8.45)
	I don't know	0	0	1 (1.38)	1 (1.38)	2 (2.82)	2 (2.82)
Was your alcohol/tobacco/coffee consumption influenced by the lockdown?	Tobacco	15 (20)	8 (10.67)	10 (13.89)	8 (11.11)	14 (19.72)	15 (21.13)
	Alcohol	2 (2.67)	6 (8)	3 (4.17)	5 (6.94)	3 (4.23)	6 (8.45)
	Tobacco and alcohol	10 (13.33)	5 (6.67)	3 (4.17)	3 (4.17)	3 (4.23)	6 (8.45)
	Coffee	12 (16)	4 (5.33)	14 (19.44)	7 (9.72)	16 (22.54)	10 (14.08)
What symptoms did you experience during online education?	Cervical spine pain	14 (18.67)	4 (5.33)	12 (16.67)	3 (4.17)	11 (15.49)	4 (5.63)
	Dorsal spine pain	18 (24)	5 (6.67)	10 (13.89)	6 (8.33)	15 (21.13)	3 (4.23)
	Lumbar spine pain	13 (17.33)	5 (6.67)	16 (22.22)	10 (13.89)	12 (16.91)	8 (11.27)
	Visual acuity disorders	6 (8)	2 (2.67)	7 (9.72)	1 (1.38)	4 (5.63)	5 (7.04)
	Low limb pain	8 (10.67)	0	6 (8.33)	1 (1.38)	3 (4.23)	6 (8.45)

A high number of students reported increased consumption of carbohydrates (37.15%) and fats (31.65%), tobacco use (32.11%) and coffee (28.89%) during lockdown. The number of students with sleeping difficulty (was quite similar with those who slept well (29.35% vs.

31.19%). Students perceived the restrictions imposed by the COVID-19 pandemic more in terms of social restrictions than physical restriction (38.99% vs. 30.73%).

When comparing students' responses by the study year, there were significant differences within each age group and between study year for most emotional, cognitive, behavioral, and physical manifestations. However, with very few exceptions, the physical activity was not significantly impacted by the lockdown (Table 3).

Table 3. Effects of age group on students' symptoms between study years (*t*-test).

Signs	Age	1st Year/2nd Year p	2nd Year/3rd Year p	1st Year/3rd Year p
Affective symptoms	<20 years	0.0171	-	-
	21–25 years	0.0026	0.0565	0.0541
	26–30 years	0.0115	0.0492	0.0601
	31–35 years	0.0487	0.0465	0.0023
	>36 years	0.1062	0.0496	0.0631
Cognitive symptoms	<20 years	0.0328	-	-
	21–25 years	0.0192	0.0049	0.0241
	26–30 years	0.0571	0.0081	0.0495
	31–35 years	0.0419	0.0238	0.0185
	>36 years	0.0172	0.0764	0.0607
Behavioral symptoms	<20 years	0.0086	-	-
	21–25 years	0.0688	0.0619	0.0076
	26–30 years	0.0527	0.0866	0.0372
	31–35 years	0.0003	0.0143	0.0141
	>36 years	0.0364	0.0039	0.0402
Physical symptoms	<20 years	0.0021	-	-
	21–25 years	0.0269	0.0052	0.0219
	26–30 years	0.0407	0.0053	0.0459
	31–35 years	0.0015	0.0858	0.0845
	>36 years	0.1061	0.0163	0.0929
Physical activity	<20 years	0.2721	-	-
	21–25 years	0.2370	0.2172	0.2217
	26–30 years	0.3102	0.0069	0.3128
	31–35 years	0.2965	0.0012	0.2965
	>36 years	0.0758	0.0824	0.1417

When examining the effect of living arrangements on students' symptoms, again there are significant differences between each study year for most categories. However, there were no significant differences in physical symptoms between first and second year for students living in the dorm, nor there were any effects on physical activity for students living alone or with their families. Similarly, there were no significant effects on physical activity between first and third year for all living arrangements (Table 4). When examining the effects of urban *versus* rural, it seems that urban environment had a greater impact on all symptom categories compared to rural area. Again, the least affected was the physical activity between study year (Table 4).

Table 4. Effects of living arrangements and geographical area on students' symptoms between study year during lockdown (*t*-test).

Signs		Living Arrangements				Geographical Area		
		1st Year/ 2nd Year	2nd Year/ 3rd Year	1st Year/ 3rd Year		1st Year/ 2nd Year	2nd Year/ 3rd Year	1st Year/ 3rd Year
		p	*p*	*p*		*p*	*p*	*p*
Affective symptoms	Living in dorms	0.0318	0.0264	0.0055	Urban	0.0184	0.0428	0.0248
	Living with family	0.0284	0.0262	0.0022	Rural	0.0114	0.0052	0.0166
	Living alone	0.0108	0.0396	0.0499				
Cognitive symptoms	Living in dorms	0.0196	0.0471	0.0281	Urban	0.0021	0.0321	0.0341
	Living with family	0.0407	0.0044	0.0365	Rural	0.0017	0.0333	0.0349
	Living alone	0.0474	0.0111	0.0367				
Behavioral symptoms	Living in dorms	0.0325	0.0346	0.0022	Urban	0.0206	0.0267	0.0062
	Living with family	0.0520	0.0304	0.0223	Rural	0.3578	0.0261	0.0098
	Living alone	0.0188	0.0351	0.0165				
Physical symptoms	Living in dorms	0.1781	0.0025	0.1796	Urban	0.0057	0.0044	0.0013
	Living with family	0.0016	0.0468	0.0483	Rural	0.0298	0.0361	0.0645
	Living alone	0.0462	0.0256	0.0212				
Physical activity	Living in dorms	0.0113	0.2096	0.2067	Urban	0.0409	0.0013	0.0422
	Living with family	0.2771	0.0072	0.2759	Rural	0.0802	0.1786	0.2074
	Living alone	0.4261	0.0027	0.4237				

Anxiety scores using STAI for state anxiety were 50.08, 49.28 and 49.66 for first, second, and third year, respectively, and for trait anxiety they were 49.97, 48.65 and 47.23 for first, second, and third year, respectively. This indicates a moderate-to-high anxiety level in the students. Linear regression analyses show a significant enhancement of the affective and physical symptoms for the 26–30 age category, of cognitive symptoms for the 21–25 age category and of physical activity for the 18–20 age category (Table 5).

Table 5. Effects of age on STAI and students' symptoms.

Age (Years)	STAI (State Anxiety)		STAI (Trait Anxiety)		Affective Symptoms		Cognitive Symptoms		Behavioral Symptoms		Physical Symptoms		Physical Activity	
	F	P	F	P	F	P	F	P	F	P	F	P	F	P
18–20	0.006	0.939	0.164	0.688	0.250	0.620	0.16	0.900	2.130	0.153	0.472	0.496	8.184	0.007
21–25	0.162	0.689	0.418	0.520	3.522	0.065	5.045	0.028	2.576	0.113	0.022	0.884	0.107	0.744
26–30	0.116	0.735	1.712	0.196	29.049	0.000	0.530	0.470	0.665	0.418	7.375	0.009	0.937	0.337
31–35	0.247	0.623	0.004	0.950	0.571	0.456	0.067	0.798	0.207	0.652	1.098	0.303	0.002	0.968
>36	0.924	0.348	0.567	0.460	0.342	0.565	0.024	0.878	2.276	0.147	2.861	0.106	3.460	0.078

Regression analyses also revealed significant differences between urban and rural environments. As such, the urban environment had a significant effect on cognitive symptoms, while the rural environment affected affective, cognitive, behavioral and physical symptoms as well as STAI trait anxiety (Table 6).

Table 6. Effects of geographical area on STAI and students' symptoms.

Geographical Area	STAI (State Anxiety)		STAI (Trait Anxiety)		Affective Symptoms		Cognitive Symptoms		Behavioral Symptoms		Physical Symptoms		Physical Activity	
	F	P	F	P	F	P	F	P	F	P	F	P	F	P
Urban	0.004	0.950	0.586	0.446	0.003	0.957	23.454	0.000	3.241	0.074	0.791	0.376	0.633	0.428
Rural	0.004	0.951	5.994	0.016	6.651	0.011	11.003	0.001	6.570	0.012	12.258	0.0001	0.963	0.328

Finally, compared to students who lived with the family or alone, more students who lived in the dorm reported affective, cognitive and behavior symptoms as well as a significant increase in trait anxiety (Table 7).

Table 7. Effects of living arrangements on STAI and students' symptoms.

Living Arrangements	STAI (State Anxiety)		STAI (Trait Anxiety)		Affective Symptoms		Cognitive Symptoms		Behavioral Symptoms		Physical Symptoms		Physical Activity	
	F	P	F	P	F	P	F	P	F	P	F	P	F	P
Living in dorms	0.095	0.759	7.061	0.009	4.967	0.028	9.545	0.003	9.573	0.003	0.461	0.499	3.877	0.052
Living with family	0.126	0.724	0.002	0.962	1.567	0.215	15.371	0.000	3.825	0.055	0.141	0.709	0.475	0.493
Living alone	0.652	0.422	1.224	0.273	0.861	0.357	9.658	0.003	2.236	0.140	0.921	0.341	2.418	0.125

4. Discussions

This study was conducted to determine the extent to which the lockdown during the first and largest COVID-19 outbreak in the county of Suceava, Romania, had on psychological, physical and behavioral manifestations of first-, second- and third-year college students. Overall, our findings show a significant increase in anxiety, as measured by STAI, as well as in reporting affective, cognitive, behavioral and physical symptoms by the students following physical restriction, quarantine and self-isolation.

The negative health-related conditions caused by the COVID-19 pandemic coupled with the public measures taken to slow the spread of the virus resulted in significant lifestyle changes in the majority of the population. Adaptability to changes was reflected by an increase in stress levels of many individuals that can trigger emotional, behavioral and physiological responses. Within the student population, anxiety has significantly increased primarily due to the fear of being infected and by the cancellation of on-site academic activities. In other words, the individual emotional reactions were caused, on one hand, by the restrictions imposed due to the COVID-19 pandemic and, on the other hand, by exposure to a demanding, competitive environment, without direct physical and social participation [19]. In our study, anxiety, under many forms was encountered in 73.39% of the total number of students. This is in line with the study of Wang et al. [20] who found that the most common emotional response of people during the pandemic was anxiety. Another study also found that the prevalence of anxiety among college students during this pandemic was 27% [6].

During the COVID-19 pandemic, the mental health of university healthcare students was affected negatively. For example, the Hospital Anxiety and Depression Scale (HADS) revealed that only 43.8% and 40.0% of participants had normal anxiety and depression scores, while 22.4% showed borderline abnormal anxiety/depression scores, with many students (33.8%) being identified with abnormal anxiety scores [21]. Among these psychological effects, other studies showed intense stress, irritability, anxiety, fear, complaints of depression and post-traumatic stress disorder as well as sleep disorders [10,22].

Besides changes in affectivity, our students reported cognitive alterations, such as difficulties in concentration (72.93%) and catastrophic thinking (25.22%). Intolerance of uncertainty includes the belief that uncertain events are unfair, unacceptable and threatening [23]. In such situations, catastrophic cognitions occur, which mediate the relationship between information seeking and health anxiety [24]. It was also found that catastrophic thinking about COVID-19 can contribute to various psychiatric symptoms associated with depression, agoraphobia and panic disorder [25].

We also assessed several psychosomatic symptoms in students during lockdown such as fatigue, anorexia, myalgia, headache, and malaise, which were reported by over 20% of the students. COVID-19 threat negatively affected the biological rhythm through intolerance of ambiguity, which then increases somatic symptoms both directly and through biological rhythm. A review of 13 articles showed that the COVID-19 pandemic had a negative impact on physical and mental health in healthcare workers, and headaches have been associated to psychological stress and work overload during the pandemic [26].

Other behaviors, such as sleep, eating, daily activities (sports) and social activities, have all been impacted or restricted due to changes in working conditions, and enforcement of quarantine or curfews. In our study, 50% of students reported at least one unhealthy habit, such as alcohol consumption and tobacco use or insomnia. In the United Kingdom, the alcohol consumption increased by 4.5% increase during April to October 2020, compared to the same period in the previous year [27]. In a study involving students, however, there was a reduction in alcohol drinking during COVID-19 pandemic. Thus, living with parents during emerging adulthood may be protective against heavy drinking [28]. A large study ($n = 3396$) on current tobacco users showed a 28% increase in cigarette use during the pandemic, while 15% reported a decrease in their tobacco use. The most common reasons for increased use were increased stress, more time at home, and boredom while quarantined, while the most common reasons for reduced use were health concerns and more time around non-smokers [29]. Students decreased smoking and vaping frequency from the week prior to their campus closing; however, decreased frequency did not correspond to reduced quantity. Higher anxiety and moving home (versus living independently) were related to the decrease [30].

Our study showed that students increase their food consumption. Some studies showed a marked increase in body mass index during the quarantine [31]; however, in a study conducted in Serbia, most students did not feel a constant need for food (63.2%), nor did they consume larger amounts of food than usual (67.5%). Students (36.0%) were careful about the nutritional and energy value of food, and they had well-balanced meals that had a beneficial effect on their immune responses [32].

Our students were more affected by the social restrictions (38.99%) than the physical restrictions (30.73%), which is in line with other studies showing student dissatisfaction with social restrictions [33]. Physical symptoms were also present in this study to a great extent, with half of students reporting dorsal and lumbar pain. The low back pain (LBP) was the most common musculoskeletal pain area that increased after the quarantine. LBP was a highly prevalent health problem in medical students in Serbia, too [34]. In other recent studies conducted in Saudi Arabia, the point prevalence of LBP found was 40.5% in medical students [35], 21.2% among health sciences students [36], in comparison with 80% in nurses [37], and 31.4% in office workers [38]. This could be related to the burden of work, type of professional or academic activity carried out by each group, and poor posture at work [39].

Regression analyses indicated that the levels of anxiety during the COVID-19 outbreak were strongly correlated with cognitive, physical and behavioral symptoms of the students. These were influenced by the living arrangements, location (urban vs. rural) and age group. Our study has several limitations that include a relatively small number of participants as well as the use of the general questionnaire that has not been internally validated. The fact that the questionnaires used to measure human feelings and emotions are self-reported is another limitation of this study. Notwithstanding this, our study reveals a significant impact on students' affective, cognitive, behavioral and physical symptoms following the first largest COVID-19 outbreak in Suceava county, Romania.

5. Conclusions

The impact of the COVID-19 pandemic on the students' physical and mental state resulted in a state of anxiety coupled with a complex of physical, emotional, cognitive and behavioral symptoms. The results also show that first-year students showed less anxiety, perhaps due to their enthusiasm, while third-year students were more prone to anxiety and experienced cognitive symptoms to a greater extent, possibly due to the prospects of an uncertain future, such as final exams and starting a career.

Author Contributions: Conceptualization, S.C.S. and A.E.S.; methodology, S.C.S. and E.A.; software, O.R.A. and A.E.S.; validation, S.C.S., M.T. and E.A.; formal analysis, L.D. and O.R.A.; investigation, S.C.S. and A.E.S.; re-sources, S.C.S.; data curation, S.C.S.; writing—original draft preparation, S.C.S. and L.D.; writing—review and editing, M.T. and O.R.A.; visualization, L.D. and E.A.; supervision, S.C.S., E.A., L.D. and M.T. All authors have read and agreed to the published version of the manuscript.

Funding: This research was funded by Lucian Blaga University of Sibiu & Hasso Plattner Foundation research grants LBUS-IRG-2021-07.

Institutional Review Board Statement: The study was carried out in accordance with the guidelines of the Helsinki Declaration. The approval was requested and received from the "Stefan cel Mare" University of Suceava, (No. 34/20.05.2021). All procedures were performed according to the regulations of the institutional ethics commission.

Informed Consent Statement: Before starting the study, the students were informed about its content, ensuring the anonymity and confidentiality of the answers.

Data Availability Statement: Data are contained within the article.

Acknowledgments: Project financed by Lucian Blaga University of Sibiu & Hasso Plattner Foundation research grants LBUS-IRG-2021-07.

Conflicts of Interest: The authors declare no conflict of interest.

References

1. World Health Organization. Mental Health and Psychosocial Considerations during the COVID-19 Outbreak, 18 March 2020. Available online: https://apps.who.int/iris/handle/10665/331490 (accessed on 30 October 2021).
2. Wang, C.; Pan, R.; Wan, X.; Tan, Y.; Xu, L.; Ho, C.S.; Ho, R.C. Immediate psychological responses and associated factors during the initial stage of the 2019 coronavirus disease (COVID-19) epidemic among the general population in China. *Int. J. Environ. Res. Public Health* **2020**, *17*, 1729. [CrossRef] [PubMed]
3. Wang, C.; Pan, R.; Wan, X.; Tan, Y.; Xu, L.; McIntyre, R.S.; Choo, F.N.; Tran, B.; Ho, R.; Sharma, V.K.; et al. A longitudinal study on the mental health of general population during the COVID-19 epidemic in China. *Brain Behav. Immun.* **2020**, *87*, 40–48. [CrossRef] [PubMed]
4. World Health Organization. Mental Health and COVID-19. Available online: http://www.euro.who.int/en/health-topics/health-emergencies/coronavirus-covid-19/novel-coronavirus-2019-ncov-technical-guidance/coronavirus-disease-covid-19-outbreak-technical-guidance-europe/mental-health-and-covid-19 (accessed on 29 October 2021).
5. Ma, Z.; Zhao, J.; Li, Y.; Chen, D.; Wang, T.; Zhang, Z.; Chen, Q.; Yu, J.; Jiang, F.; Liu, X. Mental health problems and correlates among 746,217 college students during the coronavirus disease 2019 outbreak in China. *Epidemiol. Psychiatr. Sci.* **2020**, *29*, 1–10. [CrossRef] [PubMed]
6. Chang, J.; Yuan, Y.; Wang, D. Mental health status and its influencing factors among college students during the epidemic of new coronavirus pneumonia. *J. South. Med. Univ.* **2020**, *40*, 171–176.
7. Lee, J. Mental health effects of school closures during COVID-19. *Lancet Child Adolesc. Health* **2020**, *4*, 421. [CrossRef]
8. Xiao, C.; Li, Y. Analysis on the Influence of the Epidemic on the Education in China. In Proceedings of the 2020 International Conference on Big Data and Informatization Education (ICBDIE), Zhangjiajie, China, 23–25 April 2020; pp. 143–147.
9. Xie, X.; Xue, Q.; Zhou, Y.; Zhu, K.; Liu, Q.; Zhang, J.; Song, R. Mental health status among children in home confinement during the coronavirus disease 2019 outbreak in Hubei province, China. *JAMA Pediatrics* **2020**, *174*, 898–900. [CrossRef]
10. Brooks, S.K.; Webster, R.K.; Smith, L.E.; Woodland, L.; Wessely, S.; Greenberg, N.; Rubin, G.J. The psychological impact of quarantine and how to reduce it: Rapid review of the evidence. *Lancet* **2020**, *395*, 912–920. [CrossRef]
11. Zhan, H.; Zheng, C.; Zhang, X.; Yang, M.; Zhang, L.; Jia, X. Chinese College Students' Stress and Anxiety Levels under COVID-19. *Front. Psychiatry* **2021**, *12*, 1–9. [CrossRef]

12. Wathelet, M.; Fovet, T.; Jousset, A.; Duhem, S.; Habran, E.; Horn, M.; D'Hondt, F. Prevalence of and factors associated with post-traumatic stress disorder among French university students 1 month after the COVID-19 lockdown. *Transl. Psychiatry* **2021**, *11*, 1–7. [CrossRef]
13. Butnaru, G.I.; Niță, V.; Anichiti, A.; Brînză, G. The Effectiveness of Online Education during Covid 19 Pandemic—A Comparative Analysis between the Perceptions of Academic Students and High School Students from Romania. *Sustainability* **2021**, *13*, 5311. [CrossRef]
14. Potra, S.; Pugna, A.; Pop, M.D.; Negrea, R.; Dungan, L. Facing COVID-19 Challenges: 1st-Year Students' Experience with the Romanian Hybrid Higher Educa-tional System. *Int. J. Environ. Res. Public Health* **2021**, *18*, 3058. [CrossRef]
15. Ionescu, C.A.; Paschia, L.; Gudanescu Nicolau, N.L.; Stanescu, S.G.; Neacsu Stancescu, V.M.; Coman, M.D.; Uzlau, M.C. Sustainability analysis of the e-learning education system during pandemic period—COVID-19 in Romania. *Sustainability* **2020**, *12*, 9030. [CrossRef]
16. Lucheș, D.; Saghin, D.; Lupchian, M.M. Public Perception of the First Major SARS-CoV-2 Outbreak in the Suceava County, Romania. *Int. J. Environ. Res. Public Health* **2021**, *18*, 1406. [CrossRef] [PubMed]
17. Spielberger, C.D.; Gorsuch, R.L.; Lushene, R.E. *Manual for the State-Trait Anxiety Inventory*; Consulting Psychologists Press: Polo Alto, CA, USA, 1970.
18. Pitariu, H.; Peleașă, C. *Manual for the Romanian version of State-Trait Anxiety Inventory form Y*; Sinapsis: Cluj Napoca, Romania, 2007.
19. Azuri, J.; Ackshota, N.; Vinker, S. Reassuring the medical students' disease—Health related anxiety among medical students. *Med. Teach.* **2010**, *32*, 270–275. [CrossRef] [PubMed]
20. Wang, J.; Gao, W.; Chen, M.; Ying, X.; Tan, X.; Liu, X. Survey report on social mentality under the COVID-19 based on the data analysis from January 24 to 25, 2020. *Natl. Gov. Wkly.* **2020**, *5*, 55–64.
21. Basheti, I.A.; Mhaidat, Q.N.; Mhaidat, H.N. Prevalence of anxiety and depression during COVID-19 pandemic among healthcare students in Jordan and its effect on their learning process: A national survey. *PLoS ONE* **2021**, *16*, 1–16. [CrossRef] [PubMed]
22. Huang, Y.; Zhao, N. Generalized anxiety disorder, depressive symptoms and sleep quality during COVID-19 outbreak in China: A web-based cross-sectional survey. *Psychiatry Res.* **2020**, *288*, 112954. [CrossRef] [PubMed]
23. Carleton, R.N.; Sharpe, D.; Asmundson, G.J. Anxiety sensitivity and intolerance of uncertainty: Requisites of the fundamental fears? *Behav. Res. Ther.* **2007**, *45*, 2307–2316. [CrossRef]
24. Jagtap, S.; Shamblaw, A.L.; Rumas, R.; Best, M. Information seeking and health anxiety during the COVID-19 pandemic: The mediating role of catastrophic cognitions. *Clin. Psychol. Psychother.* **2021**, *28*, 1379–1390. [CrossRef]
25. Rosebrock, L.; Cernis, E.; Lambe, S.; Waite, F.; Rek, S.; Petit, A.; Ehlers, A.; Clark, D.M.; Freeman, D. Catastrophic cognitions about coronavirus: The Oxford psychological investigation of coronavirus questionnaire [TOPIC-Q]. *Psychol. Med.* **2021**, 1–10. [CrossRef]
26. Romero, J.G.D.A.J.; de Salles-Neto, F.T.; Stuginski-Barbosa, J.; Conti, P.C.R.; Almeida-Leite, C.M. COVID-19 pandemic impact on headache in healthcare workers: A narrative review. *Headache Med.* **2021**, *12*, 75–82. [CrossRef]
27. HM Revenue and Customs. National Statistics: Alcohol Bulletin Commentary (August to October 2020). Available online: https://www.gov.uk/government/publications/alcohol-bulletin/alcohol-bulletin-commentary (accessed on 22 December 2021).
28. White, H.R.; Stevens, H.K.; Hayes, R.; Jackson, K.M. Changes in Alcohol Consumption among College Students Due to COVID-19: Effects of Campus Closure and Residential Change. *J. Stud. Alcohol Drugs* **2020**, *81*, 725–730. [CrossRef] [PubMed]
29. Yingst, J.M.; Krebs, N.M.; Bordner, C.R.; Hobkirk, A.L.; Allen, S.I.; Foulds, J. Tobacco use changes and perceived health risks among current tobacco users during the COVID-19 pandemic. *Int. J. Environ. Res. Public Health* **2021**, *18*, 1795. [CrossRef] [PubMed]
30. Sokolovsky, A.W.; Hertel, A.W.; Micalizzi, L.; White, H.R.; Hayes, K.L.; Jackson, K.M. Preliminary impact of the COVID-19 pandemic on smoking and vaping in college students. *Addict. Behav.* **2020**, *115*, 106783. [CrossRef]
31. Barrea, L.; Pugliese, G.; Framondi, L.; Di Matteo, R.; Laudisio, D.; Savastano, S.; Colao, A.; Muscogiuri, G. Does Sars-Cov-2 threaten our dreams? Effect of quarantine on sleep quality and Body Mass Index. *J. Transl. Med.* **2020**, *18*, 318. [CrossRef]
32. Stanojevic, S.; Kostic, A.; Pesic, M. Nutritional behavior of students during COVID-19 quarantine. *Hrana I Ishr.* **2020**, *61*, 36–44.
33. Thorp, H.H. Time to pull together. *Science* **2020**, *367*, 1282. [CrossRef] [PubMed]
34. Ilic, I.; Milicic, V.; Grujicic, S.; Macuzic, I.Z.; Kocic, S.; Ilic, M.D. Prevalence and correlates of low back pain among undergraduate medical systems in Serbia, a cross-sectional study. *PeerJ* **2021**, *9*, e11055. [CrossRef]
35. Algarni, A.D.; Al-Saran, Y.; Al-Moawi, A.; Bin Dous, A.; Al-Ahaideb, A.; Kachanathu, S.J. The Prevalence of and Factors Associated with Neck, Shoulder, and Low-Back Pains among Medical Students at University Hospitals in Central Saudi Arabia. *Pain Res. Treat.* **2017**, *2017*, 1235706. [CrossRef]
36. AlShayhan, F.A.; Saadeddin, M. Prevalence of low back pain among health sciences students. *Eur. J. Orthop. Surg. Traumatol.* **2018**, *28*, 165–170. [CrossRef]
37. Jradi, H.; Alanazi, H.; Mohammad, Y. Psychosocial and occupational factors associated with low back pain among nurses in Saudi Arabia. *J. Occup. Health* **2020**, *62*, e12126. [CrossRef] [PubMed]
38. Ahmad, I.; Balkhyour, M.A.; Abokhashabah, T.M.; Ismail, I.M.; Rehan, M. Occupational Musculoskeletal Disorders among Taxi Industry Workers in Jeddah, Saudi Arabia. *Biosci. Biotechnol. Res. Asia* **2017**, *14*, 593–606. [CrossRef]
39. Wami, S.D.; Abere, G.; Dessie, A.; Getachew, D. Work-related risk factors and the prevalence of low back pain among low wage workers: Results from a cross-sectional study. *BMC Public Health* **2019**, *19*, 1072. [CrossRef] [PubMed]

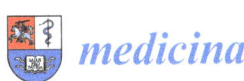 *medicina*

Case Report

Borderline Personality Disorder "Discouraged Type": A Case Report

Lavinia Duică [1,2], Elisabeta Antonescu [1,*], Maria Totan [1], Gabriela Boța [1] and Sînziana Călina Silișteanu [3]

1. Faculty of Medicine, "Lucian Blaga" University of Sibiu, 550169 Sibiu, Romania; lavinia.duica@ulbsibiu.ro (L.D.); maria.totan@ulbsibiu.ro (M.T.); gabriela.bota@ulbsibiu.ro (G.B.)
2. "Dr. Gheorghe Preda" Clinical Psychiatric Hospital, 550082 Sibiu, Romania
3. Faculty of Medicine and Biological Sciences, "Stefan cel Mare" University of Suceava, 720229 Suceava, Romania; sinziana.silisteanu@usm.ro
* Correspondence: elisabeta.antonescu@ulbsibiu.ro

Abstract: Borderline Personality Disorder (BPD) is a mental illness associated with a significant degree of distress and impairment because of the difficulties in effectively regulating emotions. BPD is frequently associated with Depressive Disorders, most commonly Major Depressive Disorder and Dysthymia. Here, we present a case report of an 18-year-old female patient hospitalized with a severe depressive episode and psychotic symptoms. A few months after discharge, the interpersonal difficulties, unstable self-image, fear of chronic abandonment, feeling of emptiness, paranoid ideation, helplessness, obsessive-compulsive elements, perfectionism, and social retreat led to the patient's impaired functionality. The spectrum of signs and symptoms presented were characteristic of BPD. The specific presentation of mixed dependent/avoidant pattern of personality, with persistent feelings of guilt and shame, social anxiety, emotional attachments, obsessions, and feelings of inadequacy have further narrowed the diagnosis to discouraged BPD, as described by Theodore Millon. In our case, this particular subtype of personality disorder can be understood as BPN associated with social perfectionism. Both BPD and perfectionism, as a trait personality, were thought to exacerbate issues with self-conception and identity formation in this patient.

Keywords: Borderline Personality Disorder; depression; perfectionism; obsessive-compulsive symptoms; fearfulness; dependency

Citation: Duică, L.; Antonescu, E.; Totan, M.; Boța, G.; Silișteanu, S.C. Borderline Personality Disorder "Discouraged Type": A Case Report. *Medicina* 2022, *58*, 162. https://doi.org/10.3390/medicina58020162

Academic Editors: Beatrice Gabriela Ioan and Magdalena Iorga

Received: 22 December 2021
Accepted: 18 January 2022
Published: 21 January 2022

Publisher's Note: MDPI stays neutral with regard to jurisdictional claims in published maps and institutional affiliations.

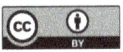

Copyright: © 2022 by the authors. Licensee MDPI, Basel, Switzerland. This article is an open access article distributed under the terms and conditions of the Creative Commons Attribution (CC BY) license (https://creativecommons.org/licenses/by/4.0/).

1. Introduction

Borderline Personality Disorder (BPD) is associated with significant emotional suffering and functional impairment [1], including low occupational and educational attainment, difficulty in forming long-term relationships, increased partner conflict, sexual risk-taking, low levels of social support, low life satisfaction, and increased service use [2]. The most frequently co-occurring psychiatric disorders with BPD are Depressive Disorders (DD), most commonly Major Depressive Disorder (MDD) and Dysthymia. Between 70 and 90% of individuals with BPD go through at least one major depressive episode or exhibit another depressive disorder throughout the course of their lives [3]. According to Linehan's biopsychosocial model, BPD has also been associated with childhood maltreatment and an invalidating family environment [4]. Indeed, childhood maltreatment, including family adversity, exposure to physical and sexual abuse, or neglect, has been found to be a robust and predictive risk factor for BPD [5].

The high prevalence of comorbid pathology amongst patients with BPD is widely recognized [6]. Therefore, a large variation in the expression of BPD pathology is apparent in clinical practice. For example, Critchfield et al. [7] describe three subtypes of BPD patients: those with co-occurring cluster A Personality Disorder (PD) traits (elevated schizotypal and paranoid features), those with cluster B traits of PD (elevated narcissistic and histrionic features), and those with cluster C traits of PD (elevated avoidant and obsessive-compulsive features). In Theodore Millon's evolutionary model of personology, subtypes describe variations of each of the prototypical personality disorders derived from research and clinical observation [8]. Each subtype, or prototypical variant, shares the core features of the main prototype with one, two, or three other different PD. Millon's four subtypes of Borderline Personality Disorder are: discouraged, self-disruptive, impulsive, and petulant.

In a recent study, the profile of the "inhibited" subtype resembled the "Discouraged" subtype characterized by avoidant, dependent features and unexpressed anger. These patients internalize more, are less impulsive, and are less likely to communicate their emotions [9]. The case brought to our attention was a patient who presented to the hospital with a recurrent, major depressive episode with psychotic symptoms, who, after the resolution of the acute symptomatology, was diagnosed with BPD, discouraged type. This is an interesting clinical case that resembles both features of cluster B Personality Disorder (dramatic, emotional, or erratic disorders) and perfectionism, a trait associated with cluster C Personality Disorder (anxious or fearful disorders) [1] as seen from the psychopathological features presented below. This combination posed significant challenges in accurately determining diagnosis and will aid clinicians in treatment recommendation.

2. Case Presentation

An 18-year-old female patient, from the rural region of Romania, was brought by her father to the emergency department for severe anxiety, suspiciousness, weight loss, food negativism, complex auditory and visual hallucinations, and fragmentary paranoid ideas. At age 16, the patient had a hospital admission to the pediatric psychiatric department with depressive and obsessive-compulsive symptoms and general low functionality in daily and school activities. She was diagnosed with a severe depressive episode and obsessive-compulsive disorder (OCD). At age 17, she was again diagnosed as an outpatient with OCD for obsessive-compulsive symptoms, low functionality, and school dropout. She was treated with Olanzapine 15 mg; however, after a few weeks, the treatment was discontinued at the request of her father because he considered that the treatment was "too strong", and that his daughter did not need a psychiatric treatment, although there were no adverse reactions to the drug.

Life and family history showed that the patient lived in the rural area with her parents and two brothers with whom she had relatively harmonious relationships. She studied for three years at the High School for Arts, painting section, and, at some point, she developed a good reputation for her artistic talent. Her father told us that he considered that a major trauma in his daughter's life was her deep disappointment at the inability of her family to afford the financial costs for studying anime in Japan, which was her exclusive life project during that period of time. When admitted to the hospital, the patient had no occupation and had dropped out of school for the past year.

Sometime after her first admission to the adult psychiatric ward, the patient communicated to us some information about her life history. She had tense interactions with her former and current classmates, who considered her "weird", and "different from others", because of her social inhibition and psychomotor slowness, and mockingly calling her "the little painter". She felt sexually abused by her classmates (indecent gestures of sexual nature, use of trivial language), culminating in a psycho-traumatic event after she witnessed an erotic act of someone close to her. She felt that she did not have the protection and warmth from her family, and she did not feel sufficiently understood.

After being exposed to multiple psycho-traumatic events, which can be referred to as "emotional bullying" based on the patient's statements, in a couple of years, the patient gradually became socially withdrawn and dropped out of school in the 11th grade. At the same time, she became addicted to watching anime, stating that "I was beginning to think I was a character". The persistence of this situation over time led to psychiatric symptoms such as depression and obsessive-compulsive symptoms that have been associated with impaired functionality and dropping out of school. The patient described herself as shy, emotionally unstable, sensitive to criticism, and perfectionist, rigid, hesitant, undecided, and being critical of herself.

At admission, clinical examination revealed very low facial expressions and gestures, distracted gaze, severe anxiety, carelessness, weekly cooperating, reduced verbal contact in simple sentences (partial verbal negativity), low tone of voice, present consciousness, and temporally-spatially oriented. In terms of perception, the patient presented with complex visual and hallucinations ("I see small, black monsters with fiery eyes telling me what to do"), auditory hallucinations ("I hear voices criticizing me"). Examination of cognitive functions indicated spontaneous and voluntary hypoprosexia, fixation hypomnesia determined by distractibility, bradyphrenia, fragmentary paranoid ideas. Volition was low/absent and activity was characterized by major difficulties in performing daily tasks. Laboratory tests, including thyroid functions, were unremarkable and within normal limits. Computerized brain tomography did not reveal any significant findings.

A few days after admission, when the patient communicated more efficiently, the psychological examination using Symptom Checklist-90 (SCL-90) showed mild levels on psychoticism scale, ambivalence, insecurity, indecision, increased vulnerability in the control and testing of reality, difficulties in differentiating the imaginary from the real, accentuated regression and dependence. The anamnesis, physical, psychiatric and psychologic examination and the lack of somatic pathology led to the diagnostic "Major recurrent depressive disorder, severe depressive episode with psychotic symptoms" according to DSM-5 criteria [1]. The patient was treated with Escitalopram 10 mg/day, Risperidone 4 mg/day, Valproic acid 600 mg/day, and Clonazepam 0.5 mg/day. A lower dose of Valproic acid was given as a mood stabilizer, and because the patient was underweight the results were positive after 2 weeks of treatment [10,11]. Similarly, 10 mg, instead of 20 mg, of Escitalopram was administered as this drug is an SSRI (selective serotonin reuptake inhibitor) with great efficacy and high doses have been associated with increased agitation and suicidal thoughts in adolescent depression [12].

During hospitalization, the psychotic symptoms decreased significantly, although the suspicion persisted, as well as the depressed mood. When communication increased and the patient became aware of the disorder, she said that before admission, she had ideas of self-depreciation and guilt and obsessive, aggressive impulses (shouting ugly words, insults, cursing people, included loved ones). At discharge, she had no psychotic symptoms, and her depression improved. The obsessive impulsive symptoms seldom appeared, and psychological examination showed a MADRS score of 20. We did not measure the obsessive-compulsive symptoms since they were manifested during the acute stage of psychotic depression at and before admission, and the patient did not report them. She reported these symptoms in the course of hospitalization when psychosis decreased significantly.

The patient was periodically evaluated in the ambulatory care service. The pharmacologic treatment was well tolerated and consisted of Escitalopram 10 mg/day, Valproic acid 500 mg/day, and Risperidone 3 mg/day for six months following discharge. Subsequently, after the patient's symptoms improved, Valproic acid was withdrawn due to its reported teratogenic effects [13]. The patient was also referred to a psychotherapist. According to existential analysis, [14] psychotherapeutic sessions focused on the fundamental "value of life" in order to accommodate the patient with the present, by structuring her everyday life, by discussing the very structure of each day, easing the burden of tasks (the stress caused by academic papers and exams), and cultivating abilities such as drawing.

During the first six months after discharge, the patient continued to show psycho-emotional lability, paranoid ideation, social anxiety, low sociability, restricted activities (only under parental guidance) that were performed only if she did not feel pressured (i.e., having contact with people that may criticize her) or if the situation involved an effort to concentrate. She behaved childishly with an increased dependence on her mother and showed excessive insecurity regarding self-image that included gestures, words, the meaning of words, and activities.

Six months from the initial hospitalization, the patient re-enrolled in high school (12th grade). Unfortunately, she encountered many difficulties in school and performed poorly due to attention and memory disorders. Moreover, she considered that there were more interesting things to do than school ("there are other more beautiful things in life, I like to know, to discover ... "). Secondly, she faced relational difficulties with colleagues and teachers, saying that "people are bad, I feel bad". Due to these challenges, the patient failed the baccalaureate exam. However, a positive sign during this period was an increased involvement in the domestic activities with her family and regaining her ability to draw. Unfortunately, the patient could not enter a psychotherapy program like cognitive behavioral therapy [15] or dialectical behavioral therapy [16] due to psychosocial causes.

Because the patient continued to display impaired functionality in her personal and professional life, after resolving the acute psychiatric disorder, the diagnostic of a Personality disorder was considered [1]. This was based on the following: marked and persistently unstable self-image, fear of abandonment, emotional instability, chronic feeling of emptiness, and paranoid ideation. Differential diagnostic with Avoidant personality disorder (APD) [1] was considered since this personality disorder includes many criteria that correspond with the patient's personality traits such as social inhibition, fear of being criticized, feelings of inadequacy in social relationships.

Currently, the patient manages to carry out house chores, has not been able to focus on her studies for the baccalaureate, no longer feels able to carry out more complex activities alone, does not watch anime anymore, and she draws infrequently, but with a lot of talent. The prognosis is mixed. On the one hand, it is reserved due to some degree of impaired functioning and persistence of obsessive-compulsive symptoms with no possibility for psychotherapy and, on the other hand, the prognosis could turn out to be good due to the relatively good cognitive potential and artistic talent, if allowed psychotherapy and is able to capitalize on her talent.

3. Discussion

This case highlights several important issues and challenges. The medical history showed that the patient had been diagnosed, at an early age, with major recurrent depressive disorder, a severe depressive episode with psychotic symptoms, and OCD accompanied by important social and school dysfunctions. One of the most important challenges of this case was establishing an accurate diagnosis and the right course of treatment. The co-occurrence of severe depressive episodes and OCD in the medical history led us to consider the common association between Bipolar Disorder (BD) and OCD as 50 to 75% of OCD cases are limited to mood episodes in BD. The majority of comorbid OCD cases appear to be secondary to mood episodes, and obsessive-compulsive symptoms occur more often, and sometimes exclusively, during depressive episodes [17] that can be as high as 75% in BD type II [18]. Notwithstanding this common association, we made the differential diagnosis between major recurrent depressive disorder with severe depressive episode psychotic elements, BP comorbidity, and OCD, based on the fact that there was no history of manic or hypomanic episode prior to the depressive episode in order to consider the diagnosis of BD. We also considered the patient's difficulties in performing school activities, the acute and chronic stress linked with her social relations, and hypersensitivity to rejection that can lead to dissociative symptoms [19]. The patient became gradually more relaxed in the family environment, and her functioning improved significantly. It is known that dissociative states have been linked to maladaptive functioning in BPD [20] and they are likely to disrupt information processing, learning, and memory on various levels [21].

In the ambulatory care service, the differential diagnosis between BPD and Avoidant Personality Disorder (APD) was made, given that life history contained multiple negative experiences, including several with sexual content, exclusive focus on the relationships and image, mood swings, infantilism, a tendency to idealism/accusations against others, and, more importantly, immaturity and an extremely fragile self-concept because adolescence was absent from the patient's life. Avoidance and inhibition are the most persisting and intense patient personality traits, as behavioral acts came from an incompletely developed self. Such a fragile ego that stems from multiple encountered trauma have led to splitting, a common defense mechanism characteristic of BPD [9].

When considering the diagnostic of BPD and its subtypes, the patient's history and symptomatology did not reflect the irritable or petulant BPD subtype [22]. Despite its heterogeneity, BPD is well-characterized by "stable instability". This means that individuals with this disorder often show instability in the areas of effect, interpersonal relationships, self-image, and behavior [23]. The current DSM-5 criteria [1] for BPD include frantic efforts to avoid abandonment, unstable interpersonal relationships alternating between idealization and devaluation, identity disturbance including unstable self-image or sense of self, impulsivity, recurrent suicidal behavior or self-harm, affective instability, chronic feelings of emptiness, inappropriate anger, and transient paranoid ideation or dissociation related to stress.

T. Millon's 2004 classification [22] of BPD includes the "discouraged" beside "irritable", "petulant", and "self-destructive" types. The discouraged type represents a mixed dependent/avoidant pattern where the attachment/submissiveness is significantly represented. It is characterized by avoiding competition, having humble behavior, constantly preoccupied with insecurity, helplessness, and doubts about one's abilities. Simple tasks seem very difficult, and life generally seems difficult and "empty". The individual looks for evidence of affection, and if not found, becomes selfish and angry, followed by rapprochement. The obsessive-compulsive symptoms were present during the severe depressive episode and throughout this patient's medical history. Studies showed that the comorbidity between BPD and OCD might be seen in patients with BPD [24]. Although clinical data show that the comorbidity rate of OCD in patients with BPD is less than 10% [25], more recent studies found a higher than expected overlap between OCD and BPD, reaching rates of up to 15–35% [26]. The obsessive-compulsive symptoms were isolated, thus ruling out the diagnosis of OCD in comorbidity with Major recurrent depressive disorder, as it did not meet the DSM 5 criteria [1].

Another important issue to consider in the diagnosis is the co-existence of BPD and the obsessive-compulsive symptoms due to the fact that each of them come from two different nosological group of disorders: cluster B personality disorder vs. cluster C personality disorders. There is, however, a connection between the "discouraged" type that involves features from cluster C personality disorders, that is avoidant, depressive, or dependent [27]. When considering the anamnesis, the origins of the obsessive-compulsive symptoms did not fit with the Obsessive-Compulsive Personality Disorder (OCPD) from cluster C personality disorder, but instead could derive from perfectionisms [28], a trait of personality that can, or cannot be part of OCPD. From early childhood and later on, this patient showed perfectionism, which was evident in all activities, but especially in her drawing. Perfectionism is a transdiagnostic process involved in the occurrence and maintenance of many mental health problems such as depression, bipolar disorder, and personality disorders [29]. While social perfectionism (i.e., thinking that others need self-perfection) is associated with borderline personality (Cluster B), as measured by the Millon Multiaxial Clinical Inventory [30], a study that used Minnesota Multiphasic Personality Inventory (MMPI) showed that perfectionism was mainly related to paranoid, schizotypal, antisocial, avoidant, compulsive, dependent, and passive-aggressive behavior [31] (Cluster A and C). From a psychopathological perspective, if Borderline Personality refers to a lack of an integrated self-concept and self-integration in relation to others [32], negative emotional experiences characteristic of perfectionists (shame and guilt) can be responsible for the observed relationships between perfectionism and identity processes [33,34]. This results in a synergy of similar defense mechanisms, with integration deficits or insufficient ego functions.

4. Conclusions

An 18-year-old female patient presents with Major recurrent depressive disorder, a severe depressive episode with psychotic symptoms. The decreased functionality before and after the depressive episode, together with the clinical symptomatology, life, and family history, led to the diagnostic of Borderline Personality Disorder-discouraged type. The diagnosis of BPD was difficult to make as it does not fall into the typical type of BPD [35], and it was derived from the association of the features of BPD, cluster B, with social perfectionism, a trait associated with cluster C of PD. Both BPD and perfectionism are associated with problems with self-conception and identity formation. This case report underlines the clinical and psychopathological particularities of BPD that, if not carefully and thoroughly evaluated, may lead to misdiagnosis. Thus far, research on BPD subtypes and their treatment have been sparse and await further validation [36].

Author Contributions: Conceptualization, L.D.; investigation, L.D. and S.C.S.; writing original draft preparation, S.C.S.; Writing, review and editing, E.A. and M.T.; supervision, G.B. All authors have read and agreed to the published version of the manuscript.

Funding: This study was supported by Lucian Blaga University of Sibiu, and Hasso Plattner Foundation research grants LBUS-IRG-2021-07.

Institutional Review Board Statement: All procedures performed in the study were in accordance with the ethical standards of the institution and with the 1964 Helsinki Declaration and its later amendments or comparable ethical standards.

Informed Consent Statement: Written informed consent was obtained from the guardian (i.e., parent) to publish this paper.

Conflicts of Interest: The authors declare no conflict of interest. The funders had no role in the design of the study; in the collection, analyses, or interpretation of data; in the writing of the manuscript, or in the decision to publish the results.

References

1. American Psychiatric Association. *Diagnostic and Statistical Manual of Mental Disorders: DSM-5*; American Psychiatric Association: Washington, DC, USA, 2013.
2. Bohus, M.; Stoffers-Winterling, J.; Sharp, C.; Krause-Utz, A.; Schmahl, C.; Lieb, K. Borderline Personality Disorder. *Lancet* **2021**, *398*, 1528–1540. [CrossRef]
3. Skodol, A.E.; Grilo, C.M.; Keyes, K.M.; Geier, T.; Grant, B.F.; Hasin, D.S. Relationship of personality disorders to the course of major depressive disorder in a nationally representative sample. *Am. J. Psychiatry* **2011**, *168*, 257–264. [CrossRef]
4. Crowell, S.E.; Beauchaine, T.P.; Linehan, M.M. A biosocial developmental model of borderline personality: Elaborating and extending Linehan's theory. *Psychol. Bull.* **2009**, *135*, 495–510. [CrossRef]
5. Stepp, S.D.; Lazarus, S.A.; Byrd, A.L. A systematic review of risk factors prospectively associated with Borderline Personality Disorder: Taking stock and moving forward. *Pers. Disord.* **2016**, *7*, 316–323. [CrossRef]
6. Lewis, K.; Caputi, P.; Grenyer, B.F.S. Borderline Personality Disorder subtypes: A factor analysis of the DSM-IV criteria. *Pers. Ment. Health* **2012**, *6*, 196–206. [CrossRef]
7. Critchfield, K.L.; Clarkin, J.F.; Levy, K.N.; Kernberg, O.F. Organization of co-occurring Axis II features in Borderline Personality Disorder. *Br. J. Clin. Psychol.* **2008**, *47*, 185–200. [CrossRef]
8. Millon, T.; Davis, R.D. *Disorders of Personality: DSM-IV and Beyond*, 2nd ed.; John Willey and Sons: New York, NY, USA, 1996.
9. Sleuwaegen, E.; Claes, L.; Luyckx, K.; Berens, A.; Vogels, C.; Sabbe, B. Subtypes in borderline patients based on reactive and regulative temperament. *Pers. Individ. Differ.* **2017**, *108*, 14–19. [CrossRef]
10. Smith, L.A.; Cornelius, V.R.; Azorin, J.M.; Perugi, G.; Vieta, E.; Young, A.H.; Bowden, C.L. Valproate for the treatment of acute bipolar depression: Systematic review and meta-analysis. *J. Affect. Disord.* **2010**, *122*, 1–9. [CrossRef]
11. Ruberto, V.L.; Jha, M.K.; Murrough, J.W. Pharmacological Treatments for Patients with Treatment-Resistant Depression. *Pharmaceuticals* **2020**, *13*, 116. [CrossRef]
12. Edinoff, A.N.; Akuly, H.A.; Hanna, T.A.; Ochoa, C.O.; Patti, S.J.; Ghaffar, Y.A.; Kaye, A.D.; Viswanath, O.; Urits, I.; Boyer, A.G.; et al. Selective Serotonin Reuptake Inhibitors and Adverse Effects: A narrative Review. *Neurol. Int.* **2021**, *13*, 387–401. [CrossRef]
13. Gotlib, D.; Ramaswamy, R.; Kurlander, J.E.; DeRiggi, A.; Riba, M. Valproic Acid in Women and Girls of Childbearing Age. *Curr. Psychiatry Rep.* **2017**, *19*, 58. [CrossRef]
14. Längle, A. Existenzanalyse der Depression: Entstehung, Verständnis und phänomenologische Behandlungszugänge. *Existenzanalyse* **2004**, *21*, 4–17.

15. Matusiewicz, A.K.; Hopwood, C.J.; Banducci, A.N.; Lejuez, C.W. The effectiveness of cognitive behavioral therapy for personality disorders. *Psychiatr. Clin. N. Am.* **2010**, *33*, 657–685. [CrossRef]
16. May, J.M.; Richardi, T.M.; Barth, K.S. Dialectical behavior therapy as treatment for Borderline Personality Disorder. *Ment. Health Clin.* **2016**, *6*, 62–67. [CrossRef]
17. Amerio, A.; Odone, A.; Liapis, C.C.; Ghaemi, S.N. Diagnostic validity of co-morbid bipolar disorder and obsessive-compulsive disorder: A systematic review. *Acta Psychiatr. Scand.* **2014**, *129*, 343–358. [CrossRef]
18. Tukel, R.; Oflaz, S.B.; Ozyildirim, I.; Aslantaş, B.; Ertekin, E.; Sözen, A.; Alyanak, F. Comparison of clinical characteristics in episodic and chronic obsessive-compulsive disorder. *Depress. Anxiety* **2007**, *24*, 251–255. [CrossRef]
19. Haaland, V.Ø.; Landrø, N.I. Pathological dissociation and neuropsychological functioning in Borderline Personality Disorder. *Acta Psychiatr. Scand* **2009**, *119*, 383–392. [CrossRef]
20. Şar, V. The many faces of dissociation: Opportunities for innovative research in psychiatry. *Clin. Psychopharmacol. Neurosci.* **2014**, *12*, 171–179. [CrossRef]
21. Frewen, P.A.; Lanius, R.A. Neurobiology of dissociation: Unity and disunity in mind-body-brain. *Psychiatr. Clin. N. Am.* **2006**, *29*, 113–128. [CrossRef]
22. Millon, T.; Grossman, S.D.; Millon, C.; Meagher, S.; Ramnath, R. *Personality Disorders in Modern Life*; John Wiley & Sons: New York, NY, USA, 2004.
23. Hooley, J.M.; Masland, S.R. Borderline Personality Disorder. In *Encyclopedia of Mental Health*, 2nd ed.; Friedman, H., Ed.; Elsevier Press: Amsterdam, The Netherlands, 2016.
24. Kernberg, O.F. Neuroses, psychosis and the borderline states. In *Comprehensive Textbook of Psychiatry, Vol III*; Kaplan, H.I., Freedman, A.M., Sadock, B.J., Eds.; Williams and Wilkins: Baltimore, MD, USA, 1980; pp. 1079–1082.
25. Zanarini, M.C.; Gunderson, J.G.; Frankenburg, F.R.; Chauncey, D.L. Discriminating Borderline Personality Disorder from other axis II disorders. *Am. J. Psychiatry* **1990**, *147*, 161–167.
26. Joshi, G.; Wozniak, J.; Petty, C.; Vivas, F.; Yorks, D.; Biederman, J.; Geller, D. Clinical characteristics of comorbid obsessive-compulsive disorder and bipolar disorder in children and adolescents. *Bipolar. Disord.* **2010**, *12*, 185–195. [CrossRef]
27. Fuste, E.A.; Ruiz, R.J. Clinical features of the 'Discouraged' Borderline personality subtype. In Proceedings of the 5th International Congress on Borderline Personality Disorder and Allied Disorders.Rethinking Borderline Personality Disorder: Improving Treatment and Training, Sitges, Barcelona, Spain, 27–29 September 2018.
28. Moretz, M.W.; Mc Kay, D. The role of perfectionism in obsessive-compulsive symptoms: "not just right" experiences and checking compulsions. *J. Anxiety Disord.* **2009**, *23*, 640–644. [CrossRef]
29. Egan, S.J.; Hattaway, M.; Kane, R.T. The relationship between perfectionism and rumination in post-traumatic stress disorder. *Behav. Cogn. Psychother.* **2014**, *42*, 211–223. [CrossRef]
30. Millon, T.; Everly, G.S.; Millon, T. *Personality and Its Disorders: A Biosocial Learning Approach*; Wiley: New York, NY, USA, 1985.
31. Morey, L.C.; Waugh, M.H.; Blashfield, R.K. MMPI scales for DSM-III personality disorders: Their derivation and correlates. *J. Personal. Assess.* **1985**, *49*, 245–251. [CrossRef]
32. PDM Task Force. *Psychodynamic Diagnostic Manual*; Alliance of Psychoanalytic Organizations: Silver Spring, MD, USA, 2006; p. 59.
33. Luyckx, K.; Schwartz, S.J.; Berzonsky, M.D.; Soenens, B.; Vansteenkiste, M.; Smits, I.; Goosens, L. Capturing ruminative exploration: Extending the four-dimensional model of identity formation in late adolescence. *J. Res. Personal.* **2008**, *42*, 58–82. [CrossRef]
34. Piotrowski, K. *Dimensions of Parental Identity and Their Relationships with Adult Attachment and Perfectionism in Mothers*; University of Social Sciences and Humanities: Poznań, Poland, 2019.
35. Stone, M.H. Personal reflections: Borderline Personality Disorder-contemporary issues in nosology, etiology, and treatment. *Psychiatr. Ann.* **1990**, *20*, 8–10. [CrossRef]
36. Smits, M.L.; Feenstra, D.J.; Bales, D.L.; de Vos, J.; Lucas, Z.; Verheul, R.; Luyten, P. Subtypes of Borderline Personality Disorder patients: A cluster-analytic approach. *Bord. Pers. Disord. Emot. Dysregul.* **2017**, *4*, 16. [CrossRef]

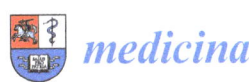

Article

Mature Adults at the GP: Length of Visit and Patient Satisfaction—Associations with Patient, Doctor, and Facility Characteristics

Marta Rzadkiewicz [1,*], Gorill Haugan [2,3] and Dorota Włodarczyk [1]

1. Department of Health Psychology, Medical University of Warsaw, Litewska 14/16, 00-575 Warsaw, Poland; dwlodarczyk@wum.edu.pl
2. Department of Public Health and Nursing, Norwegian University of Science and Technology, P.O. Box 8905, 7491 Trondheim, Norway; gorill.haugan@ntnu.no
3. Faculty of Nursing and Health Science, Nord University, 7600 Levanger, Norway
* Correspondence: mrzadkiewicz@wum.edu.pl

Abstract: *Background and objectives*: The consultation time for more mature adults is often perceived as longer, increasing with the patient's age and boosting their satisfaction with the visit. However, factors determining patient satisfaction (PS) or the consultation time (CT) in the population aged 50+ are not clearly identified. A cross-sectional design was used to identify factors specific to the facility (e.g., size, staff turnover), doctor (e.g., seniority, workload), and patient (e.g., self-rated health, impairment of activities) that are related to PS and the CT. Our secondary focus was on the relation of PS to the CT along with the role of the patient's age and gender for both. *Materials and Methods*: Doctors (n = 178) and their 1708 patients (aged 50–97) from 77 primary care facilities participated in the study. The Patient Satisfaction with Visit Scale score and the CT were the outcome measures. *Results*: We identified associations with the CT in terms of the facility-related factors (number of GPs, time scheduling); doctors' workload and health; and patients' education, time attending GP, and impairments. PS was additionally governed by doctors' perceived rate of patients aged 65+, as well as the patients' hospitalization in the prior year, frequency of visits, and impairments. For adults aged 50+ the CT was unrelated to PS and both remained independent of patients' age. *Conclusions*: Specific factors in terms of the facility, GP, and patient were identified as related to PS and the CT for participating adults in primary care. During visits of patients aged 50+ at their GP, there is scope for both time-savings and patient satisfaction improvements, when paying attention, e.g., to the time scheduled per visit, the number of doctors employed, and the patients' impairments.

Keywords: length of the visit; patient satisfaction; health status; appointments and schedules; general practice; adult; aging; primary care; physicians

1. Introduction

Patient satisfaction (PS) among adults in primary care increases with age and, on average, reflects positive experiences [1,2]. Factors determining PS are identified as representing three main domains related to the facility [3–5], doctor (including the patient-doctor relationship) [5–7], and patient [4,8]. Established correlates of satisfaction are represented, for example, by lower staff turnover [3,4] or facility size [9]; the GP's gender, workload, and work satisfaction [2,6]; or the patient's age, health status, or the continuity of the GP's care [1,8].

Many of the PS determinants are potential predictors of the consultation time (CT). Thus, exploration of this context could provide important organizational information for primary care. In turn, the CT indicates the quality of care associated with health outcomes; hence its association with PS is worth considering [6,10,11]. However, here too, characteristics of a patient (e.g., multimorbidity, deprivation status [12,13]), doctor (e.g., gender, workload, and experience [11,12]), or facility often explain the CT better than the nature of the medical problem a patient presents with [8,14].

At the same time, reports remain ambiguous regarding the relationship between the CT at the GP and patients' age [12,13,15], or between PS and their self-rated health (SRH) [13,14], yet only a handful of studies cover a wider range of CT and/or PS predictors [10,12]. Studies examining associations between the CT and PS also report discrepant findings—from none to strong [6,10,11,15–18]. Moreover, we thought that studies illustrating the above relationships are particularly important, yet they are scarce when it comes to more mature primary care users.

Primary care in Poland—with its healthcare system based on health insurance and a free choice of physician (which is similar to the British and Scandinavian systems)—is facing the same demographic trends as across Europe. The population of seniors is growing rapidly, but a gap still exists in identifying the CT and/or PS determinants among mature adults. Understanding these associations is important for the efficiency and quality of primary care.

Objective

To investigate what determines PS and the CT in relation to GP consultation, we considered factors from three domains characterizing facilities, doctors, and patients. To the best of our knowledge, analyses encompassing such a broad perspective on PS and CT determinants in primary care are scarce, and such outcomes have not been assessed among adults aged 50+ in contemporary European society. Thus, we analyzed them both contextually (separately for each domain of factors) and comprehensively (including mutual relationships between factors from different domains). The following three research questions were analyzed in parallel in this cross-sectional study:

1. With regard to the facility, the physician, and the patient, which characteristics determine PS with a visit to the GP and the CT among mature adults?
2. How does PS with a visit to the GP relate to the CT in this study group?
3. Does a patient's age or gender diversify PS and/or the CT?

The main aim of the research was to identify factors jointly affecting PS and the CT as a potential focus of efforts to improve the quality and cost-effectiveness of primary care practice for aging adults.

2. Materials and Methods

The present data came from the PRACTA—activating the elderly in medical practice—research project, conducted between 2013 and 2016 in primary healthcare facilities (PHFs) located in central Poland (Figure 1), [19,20]. Using a cross-sectional design, PS and the CT were analyzed with reference to selected characteristics of the PHFs ($n = 77$), GPs ($n = 178$), and their patients aged 50+ ($n = 1708$; with response rates of 20%, 50%, and 74.6%, respectively). The PHF-related information and agreement were obtained in advance. The patient inclusion criteria were: aged 50+, had an appointment with a participating GP on the given day, and had the ability to fill in the questionnaire. The GPs were approached earlier on in their offices; and patients were approached in the PHF waiting room before and directly after the appointment. The institutional bioethics committee approved this study; all participants signed the informed consent form to participate.

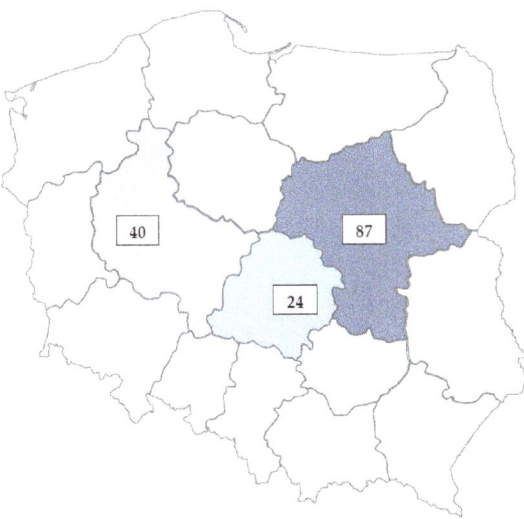

Figure 1. Map of Poland with marked districts where PHFs were involved in PRACTA study. Out of all 151 PHFs participating, 77 were randomly chosen for present analysis.

2.1. Independent Variables

PHF-specific determinants were rated by the managing staff and included: the organizational structure (state/privately owned); location; staff turnover (1 = *very high* to 5 = *very low*); time formally scheduled per visit; number of GPs employed; and average number of patients seen daily at the clinic.

All doctor-specific and patient-specific independent variables are presented in detail in Table 1. Since we aimed to capture the effect of aging on the CT and PS, the Doctors' Work Satisfaction scale (Appendix A) concerned their experience with the care of adults aged 65+. The starting phrase was: "*Regarding only your work with elderly patients (65+), please respond to the following statements . . .* ". This scale contains five items and was inspired by the Satisfaction with Life Scale [21], but modified to reflect professional experiences (e.g., *The conditions of my work are excellent*) [22]. The Cronbach's alpha reliability coefficient ($\alpha = 0.78$) was good in this study. We expected that doctors gaining more satisfaction when working with seniors would have more satisfied patients post visit, and we were keen to explore the relationship between work satisfaction and the CT.

Table 1. Descriptive variables related to physicians.

Characteristic of Physicians (n = 178)	Scale, Range, or Units	Statistics	Remarks
Age	Range 27–87	M = 50.14, SD = 1.64	
Gender		64.6% women	
Marital status	4 choices	81% married	
Geriatric training	0 = *none*, 1 = *once*, 2 = *many times*	M = 0.75, SD = 0.75	Majority had no training
Declared rate of patients aged 65+ last year	From 1 = *about 25%* to 4 = *more than 75%*	M = 2.78, SD = 0.73	The mean is close to: *more than 50%, but less than 75%* answer

Table 1. Cont.

Characteristic of Physicians (n = 178)	Scale, Range, or Units	Statistics	Remarks
Professional seniority	Range 1–60 years	M = 23.60, SD = 12.60	
Seniority in given PHF	Range 1–50	M = 12.88, SD = 12.79	
Hours of work/week	Range 8–72	M = 42.29, SD = 10.61	
Hours in PHF/week	Range 4–50	M = 33.05, SD = 10.73	
Self-rated health	Range 1–4	M = 1.83, SD = 0.70	Scale from 1 = *very good* to 5 = *very poor*
Satisfaction of work with seniors	Range 1.00 to 7.00	M = 5.11, SD = 1.06	Five items (scale from 1 = *strongly disagree* to 7 = *strongly agree*)

PHF: primary healthcare facility; M: mean; SD: standard deviation.

For patients, the Health Impact on Activities (HIA) scale was used [23], (Appendix B), describing ten everyday activities evaluated on a four-point scale, indicating the level of restraint and showing good reliability ($\alpha = 0.95$).

2.2. Outcome Variables

To assess PS, the PRACTA Patients' Satisfaction with Visit Scale was developed, consisting of seven items (e.g., "Would you recommend this doctor to your family/friends?") scored on a seven-point scale (Appendix C). A higher score indicated a higher PS (reliability coefficient $\alpha = 0.93$). The CT was noted in minutes immediately post visit.

2.3. Statistical Analysis

A generalized linear model—GENLIN, distribution Gamma, link identity [24]—was applied using IBM SPSS 24 software to test the determinants of PS and CT, separately for each outcome. First, groups of factors specific to PHFs, GPs, and patients were analyzed contextually. Next, all factors identified as significant in contextual models entered one comprehensive model, separately for the CT and PS. Effects with a significance value of 0.05 or lower were presented.

3. Results

3.1. Descriptive Statistics

Some 59.2% of the participating PHFs were public, mostly located in big towns (M = 4.41, SD = 1.64, range 1 to 6), employed more than five GPs (M = 5.74, SD = 3.37, range 1–20), and admitted M = 156.27 (SD = 84.65, range 25–400) patients per day. The staff turnover was rated between *average* and *low* (M = 3.85, SD = 0.76), and the time assigned per visit was M = 13.11 min (SD = 2.80, range 7–20). Tables 1 and 2, respectively, present the descriptive statistics for GPs and their patients.

On average, the GPs were in their fifties, had more than 20 years of professional experience, and worked more than 40 hours a week. Nevertheless, doctors' SRH was often good, as was their satisfaction with their work with patients aged 65+. Despite the fact that doctors declared that the proportion of their patients aged 65+ usually exceeded 50%, only some of the GPs had geriatric training.

Patients' mean age approached 70 years, two-thirds were married, and nearly one fifth had a higher level of education or were living alone. The majority had been hospitalized during the previous year and had presented to a GP for a medical reason.

PS showed a mean of M = 5.68 with SD = 0.82 and a range of 2.29–7.00. The average CT was 15.83 min (SD = 5.81, range 1–90), which is comparable with other countries [3]. To answer the first research question on the CT and PS, three groups of specific determinants of the CT and PS were screened independently.

Table 2. Descriptive variables related to patients.

Characteristics of Patients (n = 1708)	Answer Examples, Range	Mean, SD, or % (n)	Remarks
Age	Range 50–97	M = 69.59, SD = 8.98	
Gender		57.3% (960) women	
Education	1 = *primary* to 5 = *higher*	M = 3.31, SD = 1.29	19.4% with higher
Marital status	4 choices	63.4% (1061) married	Marriage/partnership, single, widowed, separated/divorced
Living not/alone		19.1% (326) alone	
Work status	5 choices	7% (119) working	
Financial status	1 = *poor* to 5 = *good*	M = 3.21, SD = 0.77	M indicates above *average*
Hospital use the year prior	Yes/no	71.3% (1194) used hospital	Included emergency room visits, observation, etc.
Non/medical visit	Medical/other	84.6% (1417) came for a medical reason	*Other* means formal (e.g., documents, reference) reasons
Self-rated health	1 = *very good* to 5 = *very poor*	M = 2.88, SD = 0.72	M indicates close to *average*
Number of diseases	0 = *none* to 4 = *4 or more*	M = 1.51, SD = 0.83	M falls between *one* and *2–3 diseases*
Health Impact on Activities (HIA)	Mean score range 1–4	M = 1.45, SD = 0.60	10 items (scale from 1 = *doesn't limit at all* to 4 = *limits very much*)
Waiting time	1 = *same day* to 5 = *more than 2 weeks*	M = 1.89, SD = 1.06	M indicates close to *up to 3 days*
Ease of scheduling	1 = *very easy* to 5 = *very difficult*	M = 2.29, SD = 0.85	M indicates less than *easy*
Length of attendance	Year range 0–40	M = 6.41, SD = 7.04	0 means *first visit*
Visits last 12 months	1 = *Not at all* to 4 = *8 or more times*	M = 1.48, SD = 0.75	50.6% indicated *2 or less visits*

3.2. Contextual Analysis—Determinants of CT

Facility-specific predictors yielded relationships with the CT (Wald's $\chi^2 = 78.727$, $p < 0.001$ for the model; the intercept in the model was 177.091, $p < 0.001$) in terms of the number of GPs, staff turnover, and time scheduled per visit (relevant detailed statistics for this paragraph are available in Appendix D).

Among the doctor-related variables, the self-rated health was the most notable predictor of the CT, with healthier doctors spending less time with their patients. Additionally, a set of other factors was also associated with the CT: the doctors' training in geriatrics, professional seniority, seniority within the facility, working hours in the facility, hours worked in total, and satisfaction with their work with seniors. That model yielded Wald's $\chi^2 = 69.691$, $p < 0.001$, with an intercept equal to 130.078, $p < 0.001$.

Patient-related factors that were associated with the CT include (Wald's $\chi^2 = 75.730$, $p < 0.001$ for the model; the intercept in the model was 59.189, $p < 0.001$) their education, hospital use in the last 12 m, HIA, waiting time, and attendance in years.

3.3. Contextual Analysis—Determinants of PS

Facility-specific predictors yielded relationships with the CT (Wald's $\chi^2 = 78.727$, $p < 0.001$ for the model; the intercept in the model was 177.091, $p < 0.001$) in terms of the number of GPs, staff turnover, and time scheduled per visit (relevant detailed statistics for this paragraph are available in Appendix D).

Among the doctor-related variables, the self-rated health was the most notable predictor of the CT, with healthier doctors spending less time with their patients. Additionally, a set of other factors were also associated with the CT: their training in geriatrics, professional seniority, seniority within the facility, working hours in the facility, working hours in total, and satisfaction with their work with seniors. That model yielded Wald's 69.691, $p < 0.001$; with an intercept equal to 130.078, $p < 0.001$.

Patient-related factors that were associated with the CT include (Wald's $\chi^2 = 75.730$, $p < 0.001$ for the model; the intercept in the model was 59.189, $p < 0.001$) patients' education, hospital use in the last 12 m, HIA, waiting time, and attendance in years.

3.4. Comprehensive Analysis—Determinants of CT and PS
3.4.1. Consultation Time

Three determinants from each domain—facility, doctor, and patient—predicted the CT in the comprehensive model (Table 3). The turnover of staff, number of doctors, and time scheduled per visit were the most significant PHF-specific predictors of CT. The visits were shorter when the staff turnover was lower, the number of GPs higher, and the scheduled time shorter. The strongest CT predictor among the GPs' features was their SRH—worse doctor's health increased the CT. Additionally, doctors who were working more hours weekly in a given facility spent more time with their patients, while those working more hours in general did the opposite. The comprehensive model did not confirm the effects of doctors' professional seniority, training in geriatrics, and satisfaction with their work with mature patients, which were observed in the contextual analysis. The level of impairment (a higher HIA score increasing the CT), education (a reversed relationship), and years of attendance with a specific GP represented the patient-specific predictors.

Table 3. Significant facility-, factor-, and patient-specific determinants of PS and CT. The results from GENLIN modeling for comprehensive models (patient-specific variables after inclusion of facility-specific and doctor-specific factors).

	Patient Satisfaction		Consultation Time	
	Wald's χ^2 (β)	Wald's CI †	Wald's χ^2 (β)	Wald's CI †
	Facility characteristic			
Location	21.000 *** (−0.060)	−0.086 to −0.034		
Number of GPs	8.571 *** (−0.015)	−0.024 to −0.005	5.371 * (−0.085)	−0.157 to −0.013
Staff turnover			17.585 *** (−0.892)	−1.309 to −0.475
Time reserved per visit	33.589 *** (−0.043)	−0.057 to −0.028	4.086 * (0.119)	0.004 to 0.235
	Doctor characteristic			
Marital status	9.529 *			
Self-rated health			13.219 *** (0.725)	0.334 to 1.116
% patients aged 65+	16.417 *** (−0.095)	−0.141 to −0.049		
Working hours general			5.626 * (−0.032)	−0.058 to −0.006
Working hours facility			18.932 *** (0.052)	0.029 to 0.076
	Patient characteristic			
Education			7.084 ** (−0.309)	−0.535 to −0.081
Visit aim: medical	15.168 *** (−0.043)			
Hospital use	7.179 ** (−0.112)	−0.193 to −0.030		
HIA	13.409 *** (−0.136)	−0.208 to −0.063	6.329 ** (0.583)	0.129 to 1.037
Waiting time for visit	121.564 *** (−0.216)	−0.255 to −0.178		
Easily scheduled	19.587 *** (−0.289)	−0.122 to −0.456		
Attendance years			4.625 * (−0.046)	−0.088 to −0.004
Attendance 12 m	60.884 *** (0.228)	0.171 to 0.285		

† All CIs refer to Wald's 95% evaluation, *** $p \leq 0.005$, ** $p \leq 0.01$, and * $p \leq 0.05$. The Wald's χ^2 values for the comprehensive models concerning the CT and PS are $\chi^2 = 149.793$ *** and $\chi^2 = 452.333$ ***, respectively; HIA—Health Impact on Activities score.

3.4.2. Patient Satisfaction

For PS, among facilities' characteristics, the location, number of working GPs, and the time scheduled per visit showed significant effects, with smaller populations, teams, and shorter times increasing this outcome. Among GP-specific features, the GP's marital status predicted PS, although no particular differences were found (all $p > 0.06$). The GPs reporting more patients aged 65+ received lower PS scores. Their seniority in a given facility, work satisfaction, and SRH had a meaning in the contextual models only. Patient characteristics showed the most complex influence on PS. A non-medical aim of the visit, stronger HIA, no hospitalizations, fewer visits last year, longer waiting time, and less difficulty scheduling a visit all contributed to a lower PS.

The effect of the CT on PS was feeble—with the β value explaining less than 1% of the variance—in the contextual model, but it disappeared in the comprehensive model. This indicates no or only a marginal association between the CT and PS among mature PHF users (the second research question). A patient's age or gender was not found to predict the CT or PS (all Wald's $\chi^2 < 1.09$, $p > 0.25$; the third research question).

According to the main aim of the study, we found that the time formally scheduled per visit, the number of GPs in the PHF, and the health impact on a patient's activities jointly determined both outcomes (the CT and PS) within the comprehensive analyses. To summarize, in terms of the PHF's features, the comprehensive analyses of both PS and the CT confirmed the contextual effects. The GP-specific characteristics showed different effects on the CT and PS. Among patient characteristics, more health-related variables and perceived organizational aspects of the visit predicted PS than the CT in the comprehensive model.

4. Discussion

Care-related organizational aspects (the PHF location, number of GPs, time scheduled per visit, patient-rated waiting time, and easiness of scheduling an appointment) and patients' health-related variables (their HIA, hospital use, and frequency of attending GP in the last 12 months) appeared to be the two most prominent groups of variables determining PS with visits. Thus, this study contributes to the conceptualization of PS, which is still considered incomplete [25,26]. Determinants of the CT appear to reflect the continuity of care (years attending a given GP, staff turnover), PHF status (the number of GPs, time scheduled per visit), the GP's professional profile (seniority and workload) and health, and patient's disabilities (HIA). Some similar effects were found in other studies [12,13,27]. Notably, the effect on both analyzed outcomes was observed for the consultation time a PHF schedules per visit, the number of GPs in a PHF, and patients' health-related impairments (HIA).

4.1. Knowledge from Negative Results

It is important to point out that some effects that did not appear in the present study could shed light on PS and the CT in general practice. We found PS among aging adults to be relatively independent of the CT, representing new knowledge about this group of patients, yet complementing other research where similar results were observed [10,15,27,28]. Interestingly, in one study [18] the link between the CT and PS was found mainly for a CT of 15 min or less, which may explain the lack of effect over a broader time scope. Among factors featuring PHFs and GPs, some observations can be interpreted as meaningful due to their lack of statistical significance. The source of facilities' funding, the GP's professional seniority, and their training in geriatrics had no effect in the comprehensive models on either outcome. This partially confirms existing findings [27], yet warrants further investigation exploring, for example, why a GP's greater experience and work satisfaction matter only in the contextual analysis.

No relationship was observed between patients' age, gender, or SRH in the comprehensive analysis of the CT or PS, unlike in some earlier studies [2,4], yet confirming another [13]. This might be due to the large number of competing factors and/or the fact that our group had a significantly narrower age range, making it more homogeneous. In a study of adults aged 65+ only, the CT with a GP was comparable with samples including younger and mature patients [14], which is in line with our observation. Nevertheless, the present finding that neither the CT nor PS increased with mature patients' age stands in contrast to some other research [12] and stereotypes, where physicians describe visits by mature adults as more time-consuming, running more slowly, and boring [29–31]. Another common claim, that lonely senior patients tend to seek more social than medical support, was partially contested, since neither the CT nor PS increased for those living alone or among widowers, a finding similar to one recently reported by Oser and co-workers [32]. However, we did not analyze the content of the visit [27], and the measure used here only partially indicates loneliness [33].

4.2. Strengths and Limitations

Based on one large sample of mature adults taken from a basic level of healthcare, this study bridges the gap between earlier studies in which the CT and PS were usually investigated separately, and the range of their determinants has rarely encompassed all three domains related to facility, doctor, and patient. For example, this study confirms the role of the continuity of care not only for PS [33], but also for the CT, and does so similarly (in the contextual model) for GPs' work satisfaction and retention [10,11].

A twofold—contextual and comprehensive—analysis shows the meaning of specific factors in a narrower or broader context. While some of the included variables have been studied previously—this study benefits from putting them together—others were not previously analyzed in terms of PS (physician's training, rate of elderly patients) or the CT (GP's work satisfaction or staff turnover).

Despite the fact that we applied a comprehensive approach with multiple variables, many potential complex interactions (e.g., between the CT and treatment effectiveness) still need to be understood before more definitive steps can be taken. The present data were collected from three independent sources, but were mostly self-reported. This, along with the cross-sectional design, represents a limitation of this study in terms of dynamics and objective medical records. Owing to the aforementioned shortcomings, the present results should be generalized carefully.

4.3. Implications for Research and/or Practice

The World Health Organization promotes the adaptation of primary healthcare to the needs of the growing population of mature adults [34], together with actions towards active aging [35]. Nevertheless, only a very small number of research findings in the field get used in healthcare management [36]. The present results can serve as a source of evidence-based knowledge to be implemented in PHFs, but also as an inspiration for further research. Among other things, this study shows that the number of employed GPs and staff turnover, if controlled, can help to optimize the quality of primary care in terms of CT and PS. The management of PHFs focused on doctors can consider their professional seniority, satisfaction from work with adults aged 65+, and SRH, for both the CT and PS as shown in the contextual analysis. As regards patient-specific factors, the adjustment of PHFs should acknowledge the role of educational level, HIA, and perceived accessibility (waiting time, ease in scheduling, prospect of attending the same GP) for both the CT and PS. Neither the CT nor PS increased with the patient's age, and the CT was a factor only marginally predicting PS. This finding can be important for PHFs' organizational functioning, e.g., in scheduling appointments. Respecting doctor–patient interaction as a predictor of PS [7,37], the present study complements the knowledge that can serve the medical education well. Training in geriatrics especially might benefit from enriching GPs' skills in competencies to meet more mature patients' needs [20], thus enhancing PS among seniors. To summarize the practical approach, the target at which the intervention is aimed (e.g., only for doctors; or integrating effects on the facility, doctors, and patients) should be considered carefully. Depending on this choice, units responsible for the relevant programs may use the results of the contextual or comprehensive analysis of the present study.

Additionally, our study permits the comparison of a range of various measures of patient-reported health status showing that, depending on the choice, using them can allow substantially different interpretations. Interestingly, a patient's SRH and declared number of diseases were unrelated to PS and the CT, whereas the health impact on activities was an eminent determinant of both. One possible reason for this discrepancy is that only the last scale has multiple items and relates closely to everyday life. This observation explains, to some extent, the existence of other contradictory findings in this area where the patient-reported health status shows both a positive [11] and a negative relationship with PS [4].

The suggestions for further research extend from finding effective means for improving the PHFs' participation rates, through the careful choice of tools measuring subjective health status, to studies analyzing the CT and PS with respect to treatment effectiveness, which should consider specific variables presented here. Most notably, a valuable development of the above approach would be a set of research including objective medical records and a prospective design analyzing described predictors.

5. Conclusions

Participants' health-related factors and care-related organizational aspects were found to be particularly important for PS. Patients aged 50+ with health problems resulting in limited activity experienced their visits to the GP as less satisfying, as did those who were less frequent users of medical care. Allowing the continuity of the patient–physician relationship might help to improve not only patients' satisfaction but also GPs' time management. The age of patients aged 50+ did not predict either PS or the CT and the consultation length was unrelated to satisfaction with it in this group, which opposes the common stereotype concerning the needs of mature patients. If considered, many of the mentioned factors, such as the size of a practice, a physician's workload, and the degree of a patient's impairment, permit some organizational adjustment. Therefore, they should be monitored to enhance the cost-effectiveness and quality of primary care.

Key points

* The timing of, and patient satisfaction with, appointments with a GP were linked to facility-, doctor-, and patient-related characteristics, with little comprehensive research.
* Mature patients with health problems causing impairments and those less frequently using medical care could experience lower satisfaction.
* Allowing the continuity of the patient–GP relationship could improve both a patient's satisfaction and a GP's time schedule.
* Satisfaction and the length of visits appeared unrelated and were both independent of patients' age for patients aged 50+.
* The nature of the relationship between the patient's subjective health status and PS or the CT might differ according to the health measurement used.

Author Contributions: M.R.—conceptualization, methodology, formal analysis, data curation, writing—original draft, and writing—review and editing; G.H.—conceptualization, methodology, validation, and writing—review and editing; D.W.—conceptualization, methodology, validation, investigation, resources, data curation, writing—review and editing, supervision, project administration, and funding acquisition. All authors have read and agreed to the published version of the manuscript.

Funding: This research was funded by Norway Grants within the Polish-Norwegian Research Program (Pol-Nor/200856/34/2013).

Institutional Review Board Statement: The research was approved by the Bioethics Committee of the Medical University of Warsaw (ref. no KB/10/2014; 14 January 2014).

Informed Consent Statement: Written informed consent was obtained from all subjects involved in the study.

Data Availability Statement: The data presented in this study are available on reasonable request from the corresponding author.

Conflicts of Interest: The authors declare no conflict of interest.

Appendix A

Work Satisfaction Scale—Doctor
Based on Zalewska's work [22]

Below, there are statements that you may agree or disagree with. Using the 1–7 scale below, indicate your agreement with each item by placing the appropriate number on the line preceding that item. Please be honest in your responding, according to the scale:

1. Strongly disagree
2. Disagree
3. Rather disagree
4. Hard to say if I agree or disagree
5. Rather agree
6. Agree
7. Strongly agree

Regarding only your work with the elderly patients (65+), please respond to following statements:

☐ My work is close to the ideal in many ways.
☐ The conditions of my work are excellent.
☐ I'm satisfied with my job.
☐ So far, I've succeeded in achieving my work goals.
☐ If I was to decide again, I would choose the same job.

Appendix B

PRACTA—Health Impact on Activities (HIA) scale

Please specify to what extent your health limits your ability to maintain the following (one "X" for each statement):

	Doesn't Limit at All	Limits a Little	Limits Moderately	Limits Very Much
Full body hygiene	1☐	2☐	3☐	4☐
Dressing	1☐	2☐	3☐	4☐
Preparing and eating meals	1☐	2☐	3☐	4☐
Medication taking	1☐	2☐	3☐	4☐
Moving around the house	1☐	2☐	3☐	4☐
Reading and watching TV	1☐	2☐	3☐	4☐
Shopping	1☐	2☐	3☐	4☐
Commuting	1☐	2☐	3☐	4☐
Driving	1☐	2☐	3☐	4☐
Dealing with official matters	1☐	2☐	3☐	4☐

Appendix C

The PRACTA Patient's Satisfaction with a Visit Scale (SVSP)
Would you recommend this doctor to your family/friends?
1☐ ------- 2☐ ------- 3☐ ------- 4☐ ------- 5☐ ------- 6☐ ------- 7☐
definitely no   definitely yes
Would you like to come to this doctor again?
1☐ ------- 2☐ ------- 3☐ ------- 4☐ ------- 5☐ ------- 6☐ ------- 7☐

definitely no   definitely yes
If it was easy to change a clinic—would you still come to this one?
1☐ ------- 2☐ ------- 3☐ ------- 4☐ ------- 5☐ ------- 6☐ ------- 7☐
definitel no   definitely yes
How satisfied are you with this visit at the doctor?
1☐ ------- 2☐ ------- 3☐ ------- 4☐ ------- 5☐ ------- 6☐ ------- 7☐
definitel no   definitely yes
Have your hopes for this visit been fulfilled?
1☐ ------- 2☐ ------- 3☐ ------- 4☐ ------- 5☐ ------- 6☐ ------- 7☐
definitely no   definitely yes
How satisfied are you with the time the doctor has spent on the consultation?
1☐ ------- 2☐ ------- 3☐ ------- 4☐ ------- 5☐ ------- 6☐ ------- 7☐
definitely no   definitely yes
Considering registration, travel, waiting time, help you received, etc., was the visit worth coming for?
1☐ ------- 2☐ ------- 3☐ ------- 4☐ ------- 5☐ ------- 6☐ ------- 7☐
definitely no   definitely yes

Appendix D

Contextual analysis results

The following are the statistics for the effects of independent variables on CT in three contextual analysis (provided separately for facility-, doctor, and patient-related factors) presented in paragraph 3.2 of the article:

Facility (Wald's $\chi^2 = 78.727, p < 0.001$; the intercept in the model was $177.091, p < 0.001$): the number of GPs ($\chi^2 = 8.209, p = 0.004, \beta = -0.117$), staff turnover ($\chi^2 = 19.708, p < 0.001, \beta = -0.973$), and time scheduled per visit ($\chi^2 = 8.700, p = 0.003, \beta = 0.168$).

Doctor: the self-rated health ($\chi^2 = 26.815, p < 0.001, \beta = 1.018$), training in geriatrics ($\chi^2 = 3.955, p = 0.047, \beta = -0.354$), professional seniority ($\chi^2 = 3.940, 0.047, \beta = -0.066$), seniority within the facility ($\chi^2 = 11.100, p < 0.001, \beta = -0.035$), working hours in the facility ($\chi^2 = 8.389, p = 0.004, \beta = 0.036$), working hours in total ($\chi^2 = 9.010, p = 0.003, \beta = -0.039$), and satisfaction with their work with seniors ($\chi^2 = 8.977, p = 0.003, \beta = -0.417$). That model yielded Wald's $\chi^2 = 69.691, p < 0.001$, with an intercept equal to $130.078, p < 0.001$.

Patient (Wald's $\chi^2 = 75.730, p < 0.001$ for the model; the intercept in the model was $59.189, p < 0.001$): their education ($\chi^2 = 16.119, p < 0.001, \beta = -0.467$), hospital use in the last 12 m ($\chi^2 = 5.820, p = 0.016, \beta = -0.744$), HIA ($\chi^2 = 12.355, p < 0.001, \beta = 0.963$), waiting time ($\chi^2 = 9.172, p = 0,002, \beta = -0.178$), and attendance in years ($\chi^2 = 6.620, p = 0.010, \beta = -0.053$).

The following are the statistics for the effects of independent variables on PS in three contextual analyses (provided separately for facility-, doctor, and patient-related factors) presented in paragraph 3.3. of the article:

Facility (Wald's $\chi^2 = 177.057, p < 0.001$; for the model, the intercept = $2274.429, p < 0.001$): the location ($\chi^2 = 34.867, p < 0.001, \beta = -0.084$), number of GPs employed ($\chi^2 = 6.717, p = 0.01, \beta = -0.020$), and time scheduled for visit ($\chi^2 = 62.641, p < 0.001, \beta = -0.063$).

Doctor (Wald's $\chi^2 = 61.942, p < 0.001$; for the model, the intercept = $703.732, p < 0.001$): their marital status ($\chi^2 = 8.651, p = 0.034$), self-rated health ($\chi^2 = 7.797, p = 0.005, \beta = -0.091$), estimated rate of older patients aged 65+ ($\chi^2 = 8.729, p < 0.001, \beta = -0.083$), seniority in the facility ($\chi^2 = 4.476, p = 0.034, \beta = 0.005$), and satisfaction with work with seniors ($\chi^2 = 7.681, p = 0.006, \beta = 0.064$).

Patient (Wald's $\chi^2 = 350.831, p < 0.001$, for the model, the intercept = $393.723, p < 0.001$): their education ($\chi^2 = 7.265, p = 0.007, \beta = -0.043$), aim of the visit ($\chi^2 = 19.208, p < 0.001, \beta = 0.223$), hospital use ($\chi^2 = 5.868, p = 0.015, \beta = -0.110$), HIA ($\chi^2 = 15.341, p < 0.001, \beta = -0.168$), waiting time for their visit ($\chi^2 = 196.314, p < 0.001, \beta = -0.270$), easiness of scheduling ($\chi^2 = 11.215$, $p = 0.001$, $\beta = 0.078$), frequency of attendance in the last 12 m ($\chi^2 = 50.044$, $p < 0.001$, $\beta = 0.235$), and CT ($\chi^2 = 6.544$, $p = 0.011$, $\beta = -0.008$).

References

1. Oleszczyk, M.; Krztoń-Królewiecka, A.; Schäfer, W.L.A.; Boerma, W.G.W.; Windak, A. Experiences of adult patients using primary care services in Poland—A cross-sectional study in QUALICOPC study framework. *BMC Fam. Pract.* **2017**, *18*, 93. [CrossRef]
2. Sebo, P.; Herrmann, F.R.; Bovier, P.; Haller, D.M. Is patient satisfaction with organizational aspects of their general practitioner's practice associated with patient and doctor gender? An observational study. *BMC Fam. Pract.* **2016**, *17*, 120. [CrossRef] [PubMed]
3. Seboe, P.; Herrmann, F.R.; Bovier, P.; Haller, D.M. What are patients' expectations about the organization of their primary care physicians' practices? *BMC Health Serv. Res.* **2015**, *15*, 328. [CrossRef]
4. Klemenc-Ketis, Z.; Petek, D.; Kersnik, J. Association between family doctors' practices characteristics and patient evaluation of care. *Health Policy* **2012**, *106*, 269–275. [CrossRef]
5. Thornton, R.D.; Nurse, N.; Snavely, L.; Hackett-Zahler, S.; Frank, K.; DiTomasso, R.A. Influences on patient satisfaction in healthcare centers: A semi-quantitative study over 5 years. *BMC Health Serv. Res.* **2017**, *17*, 361. [CrossRef] [PubMed]
6. Schäfer, W.L.A.; van den Berg, M.J.; Groenewegen, P.P. The association between the workload of general practitioners and patient experiences with care: Results of a cross-sectional study in 33 countries. *Hum. Resour. Health* **2020**, *18*, 76. [CrossRef]
7. Peck, B.M. Age-Related Differences in Doctor-Patient Interaction and Patient Satisfaction. *Curr. Gerontol. Geriatr. Res.* **2011**, *2011*, 137492. [CrossRef]
8. Spasojevic, N.; Hrabac, B.; Huseinagic, S. Patient's Satisfaction with Health Care: A Questionnaire Study of Different Aspects of Care. *Mater. Socio-Med.* **2015**, *27*, 220–224. [CrossRef]
9. Ferreira, P.L.; Raposo, V.; Tavares, A.I. Primary health care patient satisfaction: Explanatory factors and geographic characteristics. *Int. J. Qual. Health Care* **2020**, *32*, 93–98. [CrossRef]
10. Irving, G.; Neves, A.L.; Dambha-Miller, H.; Oishi, A.; Tagashira, H.; Verho, A.; Holden, J. International variations in primary care physician consultation time: A systematic review of 67 countries. *BMJ Open* **2017**, *7*, e017902. [CrossRef]
11. Orton, P.K.; Gray, D.P. Factors influencing consultation length in general/family practice. *Fam. Pract.* **2016**, *33*, 529–534. [CrossRef]
12. Stevens, S.; Bankhead, C.; Mukhtar, T.; on behalf of the NIHR School for Primary Care Research, Nuffield Department of Primary Care Health Sciences, University of Oxford; Perera, R.; Holt, T.A.; Salisbury, C.; Hobbs, F.D.R. Patient-level and practice-level factors associated with consultation duration: A cross-sectional analysis of over one million consultations in English primary care. *BMJ Open* **2017**, *7*, e018261. [CrossRef] [PubMed]
13. Gopfert, A.; Deeny, S.R.; Fisher, R.; Stafford, M. Primary care consultation length by deprivation and multimorbidity in England: An observational study using electronic patient records. *Br. J. Gen. Pract.* **2021**, *71*, e185–e192. [CrossRef]
14. Tai-Seale, M.; McGuire, T.G.; Zhang, W. Time Allocation in Primary Care Office Visits. *Health Serv. Res.* **2007**, *42*, 1871–1894. [CrossRef]
15. Teunis, T.; Thornton, E.R.; Jayakumar, P.; Ring, D. Time Seeing a Hand Surgeon Is Not Associated With Patient Satisfaction. *Clin. Orthop. Relat. Res.* **2015**, *473*, 2362–2368. [CrossRef]
16. Kong, M.C.; Camacho, F.T.; Feldman, S.R.; Anderson, R.T.; Balkrishnan, R. Correlates of patient satisfaction with physician visit: Differences between elderly and non-elderly survey respondents. *Health Qual Life Outcomes* **2007**, *24*, 62. [CrossRef]
17. Lindfors, O.; Holmberg, S.; Rööst, M. Informing patients on planned consultation time—A randomised controlled intervention study of consultation time in primary care. *Scand. J. Prim. Health Care* **2019**, *37*, 402–408. [CrossRef]
18. Alarcon-Ruiz, C.A.; Heredia, P.; Taype-Rondan, A. Association of waiting and consultation time with patient satisfaction: Secondary-data analysis of a national survey in Peruvian ambulatory care facilities. *BMC Health Serv. Res.* **2019**, *19*, 439. [CrossRef]
19. Wlodarczyk, D.; Chylinska, J.; Lazarewicz, M.; Rzadkiewicz, M.; Jaworski, M.; Adamus, M.; Haugan, G.; Lillefjell, M.; Espnes, G.A.; Taveira-Gomes, T.; et al. Enhancing Doctors' Competencies in Communication with and Activation of Older Patients: The Promoting Active Aging (PRACTA) Computer-Based Intervention Study. *J. Med. Internet Res.* **2017**, *19*, e45. [CrossRef]
20. Jaworski, M.; Rzadkiewicz, M.; Adamus, M.; Chylinska, J.; Lazarewicz, M.; Haugan, G.; Lillefjell, M.; Espnes, G.A.; Wlodarczyk, D. Primary care patients' expectations regarding medical appointments and their experiences during a visit: Does age matter? *Patient Prefer. Adher.* **2017**, *11*, 1221–1233. [CrossRef]
21. Diener, E.; Emmons, R.A.; Larsen, R.J.; Griffin, S. The Satisfaction with Life Scale. *J. Pers. Assess.* **1985**, *49*, 71–75. [CrossRef]
22. Zalewska, A. Job Satisfaction Scale—Measuring the cognitive aspect of overall job satisfaction. *Acta Univ. Lodz. Folia. Psychol.* **2003**, *7*, 49–61. (In Polish)
23. Rzadkiewicz, M.; Chylinska, J.; Jaworski, M.; Lazarewicz, M.; Adamus, M.; Haugan, G.; Lillefjell, M.; Espnes, G.A.; Wlodarczyk, D. Activation of older patients through PRACTA intervention for primary healthcare doctors: Does the method matter? *Eur. J. Public Health* **2017**, *27*, 998–1003. [CrossRef]
24. Dobson, A.J. *An Introduction to Generalized Linear Models*, 2nd ed.; Chapman and Hall/CRC: Boca Raton, FL, USA, 2002.
25. Batbaatar, E.; Dorjdagva, J.; Luvsannyam, A.; Amenta, P. Conceptualisation of patient satisfaction: A systematic narrative literature review. *Perspect. Public Health* **2015**, *135*, 243–250. [CrossRef] [PubMed]
26. Boquiren, V.M.; Hack, T.F.; Beaver, K.; Williamson, S. What do measures of patient satisfaction with the doctor tell us? *Patient Educ. Couns.* **2015**, *98*, 1465–1473. [CrossRef]

27. Lemon, T.I.; Smith, R.H. Consultation content not consultation length improves patient satisfaction. *J. Fam. Med. Prim. Care* **2014**, *3*, 333–339. [CrossRef]
28. Elmore, N.; Burt, J.; Abel, G.; Maratos, F.A.; Montague, J.; Campbell, J.; Roland, M. Investigating the relationship between consultation length and patient experience: A cross-sectional study in primary care. *Br. J. Gen. Pract.* **2016**, *66*, e896–e903. [CrossRef]
29. Adler, R.; Vasiliadis, A.; Bickell, N. The relationship between continuity and patient satisfaction: A systematic review. *Fam. Pract.* **2010**, *27*, 171–178. [CrossRef] [PubMed]
30. Samra, R.; Griffiths, A.; Cox, T.; Conroy, S.; Gordon, A.; Gladman, J.R. Medical students' and doctors' attitudes towards older patients and their care in hospital settings: A conceptualisation. *Age Ageing* **2015**, *44*, 776–783. [CrossRef]
31. Higashi, R.T.; Tillack, A.A.; Steinman, M.; Harper, M.; Johnston, C.B. Elder care as "frustrating" and "boring": Understanding the persistence of negative attitudes toward older patients among physicians-in-training. *J. Aging Stud.* **2012**, *26*, 476–483. [CrossRef]
32. Oser, T.K.; Roy, S.; Parascando, J.; Mullen, R.; Radico, J.; Reedy-Cooper, A.; Moss, J. Loneliness in Primary Care Patients: Relationships with Body Mass Index and Health Care Utilization. *J. Patient-Cent. Res. Rev.* **2021**, *8*, 239–247. [CrossRef] [PubMed]
33. Dahlberg, L.; McKee, K.J. Correlates of social and emotional loneliness in older people: Evidence from an English community study. *Aging Ment. Health* **2014**, *18*, 504–514. [CrossRef]
34. World Health Organization. Towards age friendly primary health care. In *Active Aging Series*; WHO: Geneva, Switzerland, 2004; pp. 1–40.
35. World Health Organization. Good health adds life to years. In *Global Brief for World Health Day*; WHO Document Production Services: Geneva, Switzerland, 2012. Available online: http://apps.who.int/iris/bitstream/10665/70853/1/WHO_DCO_WHD_2012.2_eng.pdf (accessed on 6 March 2021).
36. Stolee, P.; MacNeil, M.; Elliott, J.; Tong, C.; Kernoghan, A. Seven lessons from the field: Research on transformation of health systems for older adults. *Healthc. Manag. Forum* **2020**, *33*, 220–227. [CrossRef] [PubMed]
37. Baumgardner, D.J. A Watched Pot Never Boils: Attentive Care Needs No Timer. *J. Patient-Cent. Res. Rev.* **2021**, *19*, 5–7. [CrossRef] [PubMed]

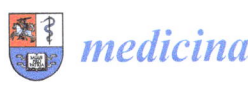

Article

Patient and Physician Perspectives on Asthma and Its Therapy in Romania: Results of a Multicenter Survey

Dragos Bumbacea [1,2,*,†], Carmen Panaitescu [3,4,†] and Roxana Silvia Bumbacea [5,6]

1. Department of Cardio-Thoracic Medicine, "Carol Davila" University of Medicine and Pharmacy, 020021 Bucharest, Romania
2. Department of Pneumology and Acute Respiratory Care, Elias Emergency University Hospital, 011461 Bucharest, Romania
3. Department of Functional Sciences, Physiology, Center of Immuno-Physiology and Biotechnologies (CIFBIOTEH), Victor Babeș University of Medicine and Pharmacy, 300041 Timisoara, Romania; cbunu@umft.ro
4. Center for Gene and Cellular Therapies in Treatment of Cancer—OncoGen Center, Pius Brinzeu County Clinical Emergency Hospital, 300723 Timisoara, Romania
5. Department of Allergology, "Carol Davila" University of Medicine and Pharmacy, 020021 Bucharest, Romania; roxana.bumbacea@umfcd.ro
6. Department of Allergology, "Dr. Carol Davila" Nephrology Clinical Hospital, 010731 Bucharest, Romania
* Correspondence: dragos.bumbacea@umfcd.ro; Tel.: +40-21-3161600; Fax: +40-21-2243895
† These authors have equal contribution as co-first authors.

Abstract: *Background and Objectives*: Patient's behaviours, attitudes and beliefs related to asthma and its treatment were shown to influence the adherence to therapy and the level of asthma control. This survey aimed to assess the level of asthma control and patient-reported behaviours, attitudes and expectations related to their disease in Romanian patients. *Materials and Methods*: This cross-sectional quantitative survey was performed in February-March 2019 and enrolled 70 specialist physicians experienced in asthma management and 433 asthma patients under their care. *Results*: Of the 433 patients enrolled, 19.4% had mild asthma, 60.5% moderate asthma and 20.1% severe asthma. For the previous 12 months, asthma symptoms, exacerbations and emergency room visits were common in the sample analysed, with significantly higher figures in severe asthma patients ($p < 0.001$). The most important treatment goal for asthma patients was participation in all activities of daily living, while for physicians this was preventing asthma exacerbations. The valuation of the treatment goals was different between patients with severe asthma and those with mild and moderate forms. Based on the patients' responses, 3 attitude clusters were identified: empowered savvy (36.5% of the patients), pessimistic non-compliers (43.2%), and anxious strugglers (20.3%). "Empowered savvy" had the lowest frequency of severe asthma, the highest adherence to maintenance therapy and the highest level of confidence in the effectiveness of asthma medication. The opposite of this attitude cluster is the "anxious strugglers", containing more patients with severe asthma, a higher score for worries about asthma therapy and better self-reported knowledge of their treatment, contrasting with a proportion of 25% taking maintenance therapy only when having breathing difficulties. *Conclusion*: Asthma control in Romania remains poor, with frequent exacerbations and hospitalizations. The differences in treatment goals found between patients and physicians and between different asthma severity groups suggest the need for more patient-centred approaches.

Keywords: asthma; asthma therapy; severe asthma; patient behaviour; patient attitudes

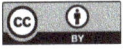

1. Introduction

Asthma is one of the most common non-communicable chronic diseases, with an estimated number of 272 million persons affected worldwide in 2017 [1]. In Europe, approximately 30 million persons are living with asthma, and the total annual costs to society due to indirect costs and direct healthcare expenditures predominantly related to outpatient treatment are estimated to be around 34 billion Eur [2]. As opposed to mild and moderate forms that can be controlled with appropriate treatment, severe asthma is refractory to maximal optimized therapy and to strategies addressing contributory factors, such as inhaler technique and adherence [3]. It affects only 3–10% of patients diagnosed with asthma but has a large impact on patients' life and is responsible for a large proportion of asthma-associated economic burden [4–6].

Despite the availability of effective asthma therapy, the adherence remains unsatisfactory, with rates ranging between 30% and 70% [7]. Non-adherence to therapy has been associated with poor asthma control and outcomes (including asthma death), increased healthcare resource utilization, and increased indirect costs [8,9]. Causes of non-adherence to asthma therapy are complex and a key factor seems to be related to patient behaviour, itself influenced by patient's attitudes and beliefs related to the disease and its management [10]. Patient surveys showed that patients overestimate the level of their asthma control [11,12]. Additionally, it has been shown that even patients with persistent asthma do not believe their disease is chronic and tend to only use as-needed medication; hence the adherence increases only when the need for symptom prevention is perceived as high [13–15]. The over-reliance on short-acting beta-agonists (SABA) and underuse of inhaled corticosteroids (ICS) due to patients' poor understanding of the chronic inflammatory nature of the disease were previously shown as some of the root causes of non-adherence [16]. To reverse this behaviour, the Global Initiative for Asthma (GINA) in its updated guidelines no longer recommends as-needed SABA as the only therapy for mild asthma in adults and adolescents [17].

In Romania, limited data is available on asthma prevalence and control [18,19] and no published data on patients' attitudes related to asthma and its therapy currently exists. Given the potential to improve asthma control by understanding and addressing patient-related factors, the aim of this survey was to assess the patient-reported behaviours, attitudes and expectations related to asthma and its treatment in Romanian patients. These data would result in a better understanding of patients' needs, providing useful insights for physicians to optimally tailor their patients' management.

2. Materials and Methods

2.1. Survey Design and Population

The SABA Trends IN Over-reliance (SABATINO) was a cross-sectional quantitative questionnaire-based survey conducted from 1st of February 2019 to 13th of March 2019. The participants were specialist physicians involved in asthma patients' management and patients under their care. The sample of physicians consisted of pulmonologists and allergists randomly selected from the national database. Physicians were recruited using computer-assisted telephone interviews (CATI) methodology. The eligible physicians which were interested in participating received an online invitation to the survey with a questionnaire to complete from patients' medical charts. The following inclusion criteria applied for physicians: between 3 and 35 years since obtaining the specialist physician degree, treating at least an average number of 20 asthma patients per month and currently monitoring at least 5 asthma patients with any type of treatment except maintenance and reliever therapy (MART) in 1 inhaler regimen. Physicians unable to fill out the survey based on patients' medical charts were excluded. To ensure national representativity, we aimed to enroll 30% of physicians from the capital of the country and the remaining from other geographical regions of Romania. The physicians which participated were asked to enroll at least 5 adult asthma patients under their current care, randomly selected over 2 weeks period, but no more than 1 patient per day. At the time of their visit to the doctor's office, the patients selected by their treating physician to participate in SABATINO were invited to complete a paper questionnaire specifically designed for this survey. Inclusion criteria for patients were: aged 18 years or older, men or women, with physician-diagnosed asthma irrespective of their disease duration and receiving any type of maintenance treatment except the MART regimen. Eligible patients should have been prescribed SABA therapy at least once or have been previously informed about reliever therapy, irrespective if at the time of the survey they were using SABA.

As this was a market research survey, no ethics committee approval was required as per local regulations. Data collection was compliant with General Data Protection Regulation (GDPR). No information allowing patient identification was collected. The information allowing physicians' identification was not transferred from the company performing the data collection to the sponsor of this survey. All of the patients and physicians were informed about data collection and their rights related to GDPR and provided written informed consent before data collection.

2.2. Data Collection

The SABATINO survey was developed by the market research organization ISRA Center (Bucharest, Romania). Questionnaires for physicians were used to collect data on medical specialty, experience (years of practice, average number of patients with asthma seen in a month) and asthma treatment goals. Patients' data collected by physicians from medical charts were anonymized and included the following variables: disease severity at the time of diagnosis and of the present survey, presence and type of allergies, number of exacerbations and hospitalizations during the past 12 months and current treatment for asthma.

Patients' questionnaire included 29 items grouped in the following main sections: socio-demographics, asthma diagnosis and manifestations, current asthma treatment, habits connected to and expectations from their asthma treatment, current status of the disease, including asthma-related healthcare use in the past 12 months and impact of the disease on their activities in the last month and year before survey enrollment, patients' attitude towards asthma and sources of information about asthma. An English version of questionnaires for physicians and patients are included in the Supplementary Table S1.

2.3. Statistical Analysis

Responses were analysed separately for patients and physicians in the overall populations and stratified by the severity of asthma of the patients and the specialty of the physicians. Patients with severe and very severe asthma were analysed together as one group (severe asthma). Descriptive analysis of the responses was provided using mean ± standard deviation (SD) and frequency. The differences in patients' responses between asthma severity groups were evaluated using analysis of variance (ANOVA) and chi-square methods and a p-value of less than 0.05 was considered significant.

To define patient typologies (clusters of attitudes) a combination of k-means and hierarchical clustering in Convergent Cluster & Ensemble Analysis System (Sawtooth Software, Provo, UT, USA) was used. The first step was to identify the efficient options from a statistical/mathematical point of view using homogeneity (respondents from each attitude cluster to be relatively similar between them on the investigated dimensions), heterogeneity (significant differences between attitude clusters, even if common pillars can exist) and segment dimension relatively balanced (for example not having 80% of the sample in one attitude cluster). Following this, the options/solutions were logically analysed to check their plausibility in the market context. Solutions with attitude clusters that had large overlaps, no coherent profile (no statements matching them) and too large groups to be compared with the others were removed.

3. Results

3.1. Socio-Demographic Characteristics

Of the 430 physicians contacted, 394 gave a positive response via phone and received further information via email. Of these, 70 fulfilled the inclusion criteria, had no exclusion criteria, and accepted to participate (15 allergists and 55 pulmonologists) and were enrolled in this survey. They had a balanced distribution of number of years of experience, geographic location and average number of asthma patients seen per month. Study physicians enrolled 433 asthma patients. Patients were mostly women, with a mean age of 49.8 years (range 18–89 years), mostly employed or retired, and with a balanced distribution of education history (Table 1).

Table 1. Respondents' demographic and clinical characteristics.

Patients Characteristics	N = 433
Women, n (%)	247 (57.0%)
Age, n (%)	
>55 years	160 (37.0%)
40–55 years	164 (37.9%)
<40 years	109 (25.2%)
Smokers, n (%)	102 (23.6%)
Education, n (%)	
University education	154 (35.6%)
High school	214 (49.4%)
Primary or secondary school	63 (14.5%)
Occupational status, n (%)	
Employed	261 (60.3%)
Retired	129 (29.8%)
Unemployed	21 (4.8%)
Pupil/student	13 (3.0%)
Housewife	8 (1.8%)
Paid leave/maternity leave	1 (0.2%)
Physicians characteristics	**N = 70**
Specialty, n (%)	
Pulmonology	55 (78.6%)
Allergology	15 (21.4%)
Years of experience, n (%)	
<15 years	29 (41.4%)
15–20 years	22 (31.4%)
>20 years	19 (27.1%)
Region of Romania, n (%)	
Bucharest	25 (35.7%)
East	14 (20.0%)
West	9 (12.8%)
South	12 (17.1%)
Center	10 (14.3%)
Average number of asthma patients/month, n (%)	
>50 patients	24 (34.3%)
30–50 patients	28 (40.0%)
<30 patients	18 (25.7%)

n/N (%), number (percentage) of patients.

3.2. Clinical Characteristics and Indicators of Asthma Symptoms Control

Of the 433 enrolled patients, 19.4% were classified as mild asthma, 60.5% as moderate asthma and 20.1% as severe asthma. The mean duration of asthma was 8.5 years, with a steady increase from mild to moderate and severe forms ($p = 0.002$). Physicians reported on average 1.8 asthma exacerbations and 1.0 hospitalizations for asthma per patient in the previous year. The average yearly number of exacerbations and hospitalizations due to asthma was higher in the more severe asthma patients ($p < 0.001$). The same trend was noticed in patient-reported outcomes. A higher percentage of severe asthma patients reported emergency room visits for asthma and overnight hospital stays during the last year ($p < 0.001$). Moreover, the number of days off-work or inability to perform usual activities during the past year was higher in severe asthma patients compared with mild-to-moderate ones ($p < 0.001$; Table 2).

Table 2. Clinical characteristics of patients and indicators of asthma symptoms and exacerbations according to asthma severity.

	Mild N = 84	Moderate N = 262	Severe N = 87	Total N = 433	p-Value for Difference between Groups
Physician Reported Characteristics					
Years since asthma diagnosis, mean ± SD	6.9 ± 6.0	8.1 ± 7.8	10.9 ± 9.2	8.5 ± 7.9	0.002
Number of exacerbations during the past 12 months, mean ± SD	1.0 ± 1.0	1.5 ± 1.3	3.2 ± 1.9	1.8 ± 1.5	<0.001
Distribution of number of exacerbations during the past 12 months, n (%)					
No exacerbation	28 (33.3%)	50 (19.1%)	2 (2.3%)	80 (18.5%)	<0.001
1 exacerbation	34 (40.5%)	85 (32.4%)	12 (14.0%)	131 (30.3%)	
2 exacerbations	11 (13.1%)	79 (30.2%)	16 (18.0%)	106 (24.5%)	
≥3 exacerbations	6 (7.1%)	42 (16.0%)	56 (64.0%)	104 (24.0%)	
Number of hospitalizations during the past 12 months, mean ± SD	0.6 ± 1.5	0.8 ± 1.2	2.0 ± 1.8	1.0 ± 1.5	<0.001
Distribution of number of hospitalizations in the past 12 months, n (%)					
No hospitalization	51 (60.7%)	127 (48.5%)	14 (16.1%)	192 (44.3%)	<0.001
1 hospitalization	17 (20.2%)	70 (26.7%)	23 (26.4%)	110 (25.4%)	
2 hospitalizations	4 (4.8%)	42 (16.0%)	26 (29.9%)	72 (16.6%)	
≥3 hospitalizations	5 (6.0%)	13 (5.0%)	23 (26.4%)	41 (9.5%)	
Patients reported characteristics					
Patients with ER visits during the past 12 months, n (%)	17 (20.2%)	66 (25.2%)	57 (65.5%)	140 (32.3%)	<0.001
Patients with overnight hospital stay during the past 12 months, n (%)	26 (31.0%)	104 (39.7%)	62 (71.3%)	192 (44.3%)	<0.001
No of days with inability to work or carry out usual activities during the past 12 months, n (%)					
0–2 days	42 (50.0%)	114 (43.5%)	9 (10.3%)	165 (38.1%)	<0.001
3–5 days	17 (20.2%)	53 (20.2%)	15 (17.2%)	85 (19.6%)	
6–9 days	8 (9.5%)	17 (6.5%)	6 (6.9%)	31 (7.2%)	
≥10 days	3 (3.6%)	14 (5.3%)	27 (31.0%)	44 (10.2%)	
Do not remember	14 (16.7%)	64 (24.4%)	30 (34.5%)	108 (24.9%)	
Asthma impact on patient's activities during last month, n (%)					
High & Very high	3 (3.6%)	17 (6.5%)	15 (17.2%)	35 (8.1%)	<0.001
Moderate	10 (11.9%)	68 (26.0%)	29 (33.3%)	107 (24.7%)	
Limited	24 (28.6%)	83 (31.7%)	32 (36.8%)	139 (32.1%)	
Very limited	21 (25.0%)	60 (22.9%)	10 (11.5%)	91 (21.0%)	
None	26 (31.0%)	34 (13.0%)	1 (1.1%)	61 (14.1%)	

ER, emergency room; n/N (%), number (percentage) of patients; SD, standard deviation.

3.3. Asthma Therapy

Overall, based on medical charts, 94.0% of patients participating in SABATINO survey had maintenance therapy with a separate reliever therapy prescribed at the time of the survey, and 6.0% had reliever therapy only. Severe asthma patients were prescribed more reliever and maintenance medication than mild-to-moderate ones, mostly biological therapy, oral steroids, anticholinergic and antileukotrienes (Table 3).

Table 3. Asthma therapy usage as reported by patients and physicians.

	Mild N = 84	Moderate N = 262	Severe N = 87	Total N = 433	p-Value for Difference between Groups
Physician Reported Characteristics					
Maintenance therapy type, n (%)					
ICS/LABA #	48 (57.1%)	200 (76.3%)	72 (82.8%)	320 (73.9%)	
ICS	23 (27.4%)	28 (10.7%)	20 (23.0%)	71 (16.4%)	
Antileukotrienes	14 (16.7%)	66 (25.2%)	39 (44.8%)	119 (27.5%)	
Anticholinergic	3 (3.6%)	10 (3.8%)	20 (23.0%)	33 (7.6%)	
Xanthines	2 (2.4%)	10 (3.8%)	4 (4.6%)	16 (3.7%)	
OCS	1 (1.2%)	15 (5.7%)	24 (27.6%)	40 (9.2%)	
Biological therapy	0 (0.0%)	2 (0.8%)	8 (9.2%)	10 (2.3%)	
Reliever therapy (SABA), n (%)	60 (71.4%)	215 (82.1%)	80 (92.0%)	355 (82.0%)	
Patients reported characteristics					
Mean number of reliever inhalers purchased in the previous 12 months, mean ± SD	3.1 ± 2.6	3.1 ± 2.2	5.1 ± 3.4	3.6 ± 2.8	<0.001
Mean number of maintenance inhalers purchased in the previous 12 months, mean ± SD	8.0 ± 4.2	8.4 ± 4.0	7.7 ± 4.3	8.2 ± 4.1	0.51
Usage of reliever inhalers during last month, n (%)					
Never	46 (54.8%)	86 (32.8%)	17 (19.5%)	149 (34.4%)	<0.001
Some weeks	26 (31.0%)	148 (56.5%)	31 (35.6%)	205 (47.3%)	
Every week	12 (14.3%)	28 (10.7%)	39 (44.8%)	79 (18.2%)	
Over-the-counter reliever therapy, n (%)	28 (33.3%)	79 (30.2%)	42 (48.3%)	149 (34.4%)	0.008

Only as combination therapy. GP, general practitioner; ICS, inhaled corticosteroids; LABA, long-acting beta agonists; n/N (%), number (percentage) of patients; OCS, oral corticosteroids; SABA, short-acting beta agonists; SD, standard deviation

Based on the patients' completed questionnaires, 86.1% of patients reported regular administration of their asthma medication. Reliever medication was used by 79.7% of patients for symptom relief only and 19.2% also used it to prevent asthma symptoms. Maintenance medication was used daily to prevent asthma symptoms by 81.3% of those using this type of medication, with 17.9% of the patients reporting the use of their maintenance medication only when experiencing asthma symptoms. Per severity groups, the use of maintenance therapy only when having asthma symptoms was reported by 10 patients (12.2%) with mild asthma, 45 patients (18.1%) with moderate asthma and 18 patients (23.4%) with severe asthma ($p = 0.390$).

3.4. Valuation of Treatment Goals

The most important treatment goals frequently identified by patients were: participation in all activities of daily living, prevention of asthma exacerbations and prevention of chronic symptoms that interfere with daily living. The most important treatment goals most frequently identified by physicians were preventing asthma exacerbations, allowing the person to participate in all activities of daily living and preventing asthma mortality. Valuation was different between pulmonologists and allergists and between patients with severe asthma and those with mild and moderate forms (Figure 1).

3.5. Patients Attitudes toward Asthma

The patients in the survey had similar attitudes on the effectiveness of the therapy and the ease of use of any medication irrespective of their asthma severity. However, patients with severe asthma had greater concerns about their therapy and the burden of asthma medication; thus, they scored higher in questions related to worries on having breathing difficulties, the use of medication when feeling well and self-adjustment of medication (Supplementary Table S2).

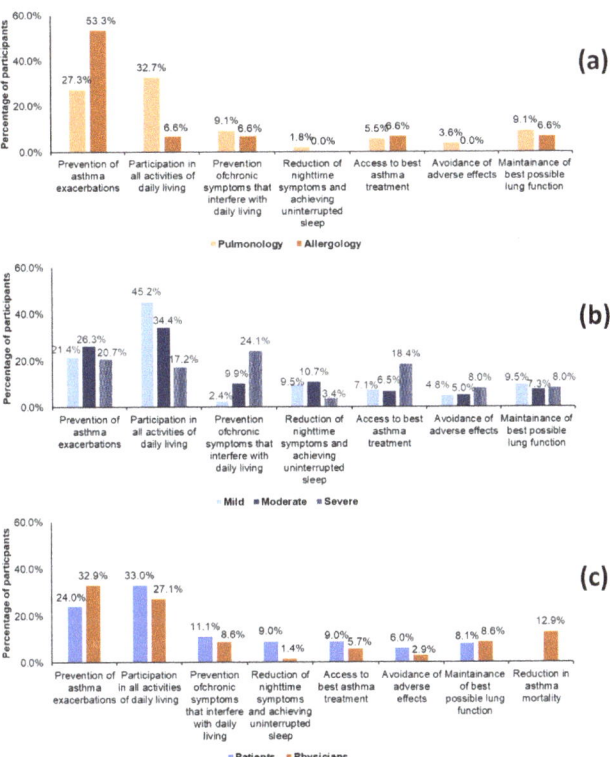

Figure 1. Valuation of treatment goals in physicians according to their specialty (**a**), in patients according to asthma severity (**b**) and in physicians as compared to patients (**c**). "Reduction in asthma mortality" was not a treatment goal in patient questionnaire due to cultural reasons.

Three attitude clusters were identified based on patients' responses to questions on attitudes towards asthma and its therapy (Supplementary Table S3): empowered savvy (36.5% of the patients), pessimistic non-compliers (43.2% of patients), and anxious strugglers (20.3% of the patients).

"Empowered savvy" patients were aware and knowledgeable of their condition and felt in control even when the worsening of their symptoms occur. Compared to the other clusters, the patients in this cluster generally had a higher level of education, were less likely to be smokers and had the lowest mean number of exacerbations and hospitalizations during the previous 12 months. Furthermore, they more frequently reported administering their asthma medication, the use of reliever therapy when coughing or having breathing difficulties and daily use of maintenance therapy to prevent asthma symptoms (Table 4).

The patients in the "pessimistic non-compliers" cluster had a limited understanding of asthma therapies and as a result, they considered the therapy a burden, leading to complaints about price and multiple inhaler usage, and embarrassment related to inhaler usage in public. Lacking the knowledge or understanding about the ways to prevent a worsening of symptoms, these patients felt scared and worried, unable to manage by themselves such situations. Compared to the other clusters, patients in this attitude cluster were older, had a lower level of higher education and reported the lowest frequency of administering their asthma medication (Table 4).

Table 4. Patient characteristics for each attitude cluster identified.

	Empowered Savvy N = 158	Pessimistic Non-Compliers N = 187	Anxious Strugglers N = 88	p-Value for Difference between Groups
Age, years	49.0 ± 13.4	52.0 ± 13.9	46.0 ± 15.7	0.002
Smokers, n (%)	28 (17.7%)	39 (20.9%)	35 (39.8%)	<0.001
Education, n (%)				0.003
University education	75 (47.5%)	49 (26.2%)	30 (34.1%)	
Highschool	62 (39.2%)	110 (58.8%)	42 (47.7%)	
Primary or secondary school	21 (13.3%)	27 (14.4%)	15 (17.0%)	
Asthma severity, n (%)				0.003
Mild	42 (26.6%)	28 (15.0%)	14 (15.9%)	
Moderate	94 (59.5%)	121 (64.7%)	47 (53.4%)	
Severe	22 (13.9%)	38 (20.3%)	27 (30.7%)	
Number of exacerbations during the past 12 months, mean ± SD	1.5 ± 1.7	1.7 ± 1.4	2.4 ± 1.4	<0.001
Number of hospitalizations during the past 12 months, mean ± SD	0.6 ± 1.7	1.1 ± 1.1	1.7 ± 1.4	<0.001
Maintenance therapy type, n (%)				
ICS/LABA *	132 (83.5%)	127 (67.9%)	61 (69.3%)	
Antihistamines	24 (15.2%)	61 (32.6%)	42 (47.7%)	
Antileukotrienes	44 (27.8%)	51 (27.3%)	24 (27.3%)	
ICS	14 (8.9%)	23 (12.3%)	34 (38.6%)	
OCS	12 (7.6%)	11 (5.9%)	17 (19.3%)	
Reliever therapy (SABA), n (%)	123 (77.8%)	165 (88.2%)	67 (76.1%)	<0.05
Usage of asthma therapy, n (%)				<0.001
Always	146 (92.4%)	147 (78.6%)	80 (90.9%)	
Sometimes	12 (7.6%)	40 (21.4%)	8 (9.1%)	
Reliever therapy use, n (%)				0.002
When coughing or having breathing difficulties	139 (88.0%)	145 (77.5%)	61 (69.3%)	
Sometimes to prevent asthma exacerbations	18 (11.4%)	38 (20.3%)	27 (30.7%)	
Usage of reliever inhalers during last month, n (%)	91 (57.6%)	125 (66.8%)	68 (77.3%)	0.007
Mean number of reliever inhalers purchased in the previous 12 months, mean ± SD	3.4 ± 2.5	3.6 ± 2.9	3.9 ± 2.8	0.448
Maintenance therapy use, n (%)				0.001
Every day	140 (88.6%)	140 (74.9%)	51 (58.0%)	
When coughing or having breathing difficulties	15 (9.5%)	36 (19.3%)	22 (25.0%)	
Mean number of maintenance inhalers purchased in the previous 12 months, mean ± SD	10.1 ± 3.3	7.3 ± 4.0	5.5 ± 4.0	<0.001

* Only as combination therapy. ICS, inhaled corticosteroids; LABA, long-acting beta agonists; n/N (%), number (percentage) of patients; OCS, oral corticosteroids; SABA, short-acting beta agonists; SD, standard deviation.

The patients in the "anxious strugglers" cluster reported a good knowledge of asthma therapies and management of symptoms but exhibited worries regarding the efficiency and potential side effects of their medication. They were worried about taking too much medication when feeling well, and therefore they preferred to adjust the doses. The patients in this attitude cluster were more likely to be smokers, with severe asthma and had more exacerbations and hospitalizations during the previous 12 months. They also more frequently reported the use of reliever medication to prevent asthma symptoms and of maintenance therapy only when coughing and having breathing difficulties and less frequently daily (Table 4).

4. Discussion

SABATINO is the first survey conducted in Romania specifically investigating the adult patients' expectations and attitudes towards asthma and its treatment. It shows that despite advances in asthma therapy, significant unmet needs persist in terms of asthma care, particularly in those with severe disease and points towards a lack of improvement in asthma control.

Asthma symptoms and exacerbations were common in the sample analysed; for almost half of the patients, physicians reported ≥ 2 exacerbations and for a quarter of them ≥ 2 hospitalizations within 12 months prior to the survey. Moreover, one-third of the patients reported ER visits. The situation was more dramatic when data were analysed according to the asthma severity, with severe asthma patients having more exacerbations and hospitalizations than mild-to-moderate ones. Unsurprisingly, severe asthma patients used significantly more reliever medication (including over-the-counter use) than mild-to-moderate patients. These results align with previously published results of surveys performed in patients with asthma, which also showed a persistence of significant exacerbations and low levels of symptom control in other European populations [11,12]. It is known that patients with severe asthma are a category characterized by a high burden of illness due to poor symptom control, experiencing frequent and often life-threatening exacerbations, associated comorbidities, and low quality of life [20–22]. A recent study evaluated the experiences and impact of severe asthma on patient's life and showed significant emotional distress in these patients because of the disease and its therapy [21]. This study identified the neglected needs of patients with severe asthma, such as "empathy and understanding" and "encouragement" (21). It also pointed towards the need for a support service that would improve adherence problems resulting in concerns about medication side effects [21].

The behaviour of SABATINO participants who reported the use of reliever therapy only to prevent exacerbation or of maintenance therapy when experiencing symptoms is not uncommon [13–15]. Previous reports suggested that low adherence to the prescribed therapy probably reflects patients' beliefs about medication and their personality traits [13,23,24]. In our survey, we identified 3 attitude clusters corresponding to different personality traits with distinct clinical characteristics. "Empowered savvy" had the lowest frequency of severe asthma, the highest adherence to maintenance therapy and the highest level of confidence in the effectiveness of asthma medication. The opposite of this attitude cluster is the "anxious strugglers" with more patients with severe asthma, a higher score for worries about asthma therapy (side effects, dose, and appropriateness especially when symptoms were absent) and better knowledge of their treatment as self-reported which was in contradiction with their behaviour, with 25% of them reporting taking maintenance therapy only when having breathing difficulties. The clusters identified in SABATINO show similarities to clusters previously identified in other populations, which reported well-controlled asthma among patients with few concerns about their medications [25,26]. The non-confidence in the effectiveness of asthma medication and negative concerns about therapy were associated with reduced adherence to therapy [16] and uncontrolled disease [26]. These findings suggest that asthma management should not only be tailored for the severity of the disease but should also consider patients' beliefs and behaviours, specifically targeting medication concerns with the aim to improve treatment adherence [24,27].

The lack of adherence to prescribed therapy and empowerment in asthma self-management may also reflect the discrepancy between treatment goals as seen by patients and physicians and between different asthma severity groups, suggesting different patients' needs. For example, the most important treatment goal reported by the highest percentage of physicians was preventing asthma exacerbations, while for patients it was the participation in activities of daily living. The difference in asthma expectations between patients and physicians when it comes to asthma control is not new, and points toward unmet patient needs [28–30]. Previous studies showed that physicians tend to focus on asthma control while patients are more concerned about long-term health and costs [28–30]. When analysed by the severity of the disease, in our survey, the most important goals identified by the highest percentage of patients was participation in daily-life activities for those with mild and moderate asthma and preventing chronic symptoms that interfere with daily lives in those with severe asthma. These results indicate a different valuation of treatment goals that vary according to the severity of the disease and the need for targeted approaches. The one-size-fit-all approach may not be suitable, and physicians should work with their respiratory patients to define individualized treatment goals through a shared-decision making process.

This survey has several limitations that may limit the generalization of our findings. This was a cross-sectional survey, and the selection bias cannot be precluded. Moreover, the sample size, especially of those with severe asthma was limited. It was not designed to compare patients with different asthma severity, but it would be of interest to observe these differences in future surveys designed for this purpose.

5. Conclusions

The results of this survey point to suboptimal asthma control in Romania and underlines the significant burden of asthma, and especially of severe asthma, in Romania, with implications for clinical practice and policymakers. The different valuations of the treatment goals observed in patients and physicians, and in different asthma severity groups suggest the need for individualized approaches, more patient-centred. Guidelines recommendations should be adapted, with practical tools more adequate for the Romanian healthcare setting to be provided for the routine use of clinicians, including patient educational programs. The ultimate common goal should be to improve patients' knowledge and self-awareness through a solid therapeutic alliance with the treating physicians, thus enabling optimal symptom control.

Supplementary Materials: The following are available online at https://www.mdpi.com/article/10.3390/medicina57101089/s1, Supplementary Table S1. Questionnaires used for physicians and patients in the SABATINO survey, Supplementary Table S2. Patients' attitudes toward asthma by severity of asthma, Supplementary Table S3. Patients' attitude toward asthma according to attitude clusters identified

Author Contributions: Conceptualization, D.B., C.P. and R.S.B.; methodology, D.B., C.P. and R.S.B.; formal analysis, D.B., C.P. and R.S.B.; writing—original draft preparation, D.B.; writing—review and editing, D.B., C.P. and R.S.B. All authors have read and agreed to the published version of the manuscript.

Funding: This research was funded by AstraZeneca Romania. The sponsor participated in the survey design and facilitated the overall operational process, including data collection and statistical analyses. The sponsor was also involved in the decision to publish this manuscript.

Institutional Review Board Statement: Ethical review and approval were waived for this study, due to the fact it was a market research survey. Data collection was compliant with GDPR. No information allowing patient identification was collected. The information allowing physicians' identification was not transferred from the company performing the data collection to the sponsor of this survey.

Informed Consent Statement: Informed consent was obtained from all subjects involved in the study.

Data Availability Statement: Research data are not shared.

Acknowledgments: Operational support and statistical analysis were provided by ISRA Center (Bucharest, Romania) and medical writing support by MedInteractiv (Bucharest, Romania) on behalf of AstraZeneca Romania.

Conflicts of Interest: D Bumbacea reports personal fees from AstraZeneca, personal fees from Chiesi, personal fees from Novartis, grants and personal fees from Sanofi, outside the submitted work; RS Bumbacea reports personal fees from AstraZeneca, personal fees from Chiesi, personal fees from Ewopharma, personal fees from Novartis, outside the submitted work; C Panaitescu has nothing to disclose.

References

1. GBD 2017 Disease and Injury Incidence and Prevalence Collaborators. Chronic Respiratory Disease Collaborators. Global, regional, and national deaths, prevalence, disability-adjusted life years, and years lived with disability for 354 diseases and injuries for 195 countries and territories, 1990–2017: A systematic analysis for the Global Burden of Disease Study 2017. *Lancet* **2018**, *392*, 1789–1858.
2. European Respiratory Society. European Lung White Book. 2013. Available online: https://www.erswhitebook.org (accessed on 27 February 2020).
3. Global Initiative for Asthma. Difficult to Treat & Severe Asthma in Adolescents and Adult Patients. Diagnosis and Management. 2019. Available online: https://ginasthmaorg/wp-content/uploads/2019/04/GINA-Severe-asthma-Pocket-Guide-v20-wms-1pdf (accessed on 19 February 2020).
4. McDonald, V.M.; Maltby, S.; Reddel, H.K.; King, G.G.; Wark, P.A.; Smith, L.; Upham, J.W.; James, A.L.; Marks, G.B.; Gibson, P.G. Severe asthma: Current management, targeted therapies and future directions-A roundtable report. *Respirology* **2017**, *22*, 53–60. [CrossRef] [PubMed]
5. Dean, B.B.; Calimlim, B.C.; Sacco, P.; Aguilar, D.; Maykut, R.; Tinkelman, D. Uncontrolled asthma: Assessing quality of life and productivity of children and their caregivers using a cross-sectional Internet-based survey. *Health Qual. Life Outcomes* **2010**, *8*, 96. [CrossRef] [PubMed]
6. Hekking, P.P.; Wener, R.R.; Amelink, M.; Zwinderman, A.H.; Bouvy, M.L.; Bel, E.H. The prevalence of severe refractory asthma. *J. Allergy Clin. Immunol.* **2015**, *135*, 896–902. [CrossRef] [PubMed]
7. Bender, B.; Milgrom, H.; Rand, C. Nonadherence in asthmatic patients: Is there asolution to the problem? *Ann. Allergy Asthma Immunol.* **1997**, *79*, 177–185. [CrossRef]
8. Bender, B.G.; Rand, C. Medication non-adherence and asthma treatment cost. *Curr. Opin. Allergy Clin. Immunol.* **2004**, *4*, 191–195. [CrossRef]
9. Royal College of Physicians. Why Asthma Still Kills: The National Review of Asthma Deaths (NRAD); Confidential Enquiry Report 2014. London: Royal College of Physicians. 2014. Available online: https://www.rcplondon.ac.uk/file/868/download (accessed on 11 June 2020).
10. George, M.; Bender, B. New insights to improve treatment adherence in asthma and COPD. *Patient Prefer. Adherence* **2019**, *13*, 1325–1334. [CrossRef]
11. Sastre, J.; Fabbri, L.M.; Price, D.; Wahn, H.U.; Bousquet, J.; Fish, J.E.; Murphy, K.; Sears, M.R. Insights, attitudes, and perceptions about asthma and its treatment: A multinational survey of patients from Europe and Canada. *World Allergy Organ. J.* **2016**, *9*, 13. [CrossRef]
12. Price, D.; Fletcher, M.; van der Molen, T. Asthma control and management in 8000 European patients: The REcognise Asthma and LInk to Symptoms and Experience (REALISE) survey. *NPJ Prim. Care Respir. Med.* **2014**, *24*, 14009. [CrossRef]
13. Kaptein, A.A.; Hughes, B.M.; Scharloo, M.; Fischer, M.J.; Snoei, L.; Weinman, J.; Rabe, K.F. Illness perceptions about asthma are determinants of outcome. *J Asthma* **2008**, *45*, 459–464. [CrossRef]
14. Halm, E.A.; Mora, P.; Leventhal, H. No symptoms, no asthma: The acute episodic disease belief is associated with poor self-management among inner-city adults with persistent asthma. *Chest* **2006**, *129*, 573–580. [CrossRef] [PubMed]
15. Bidad, N.; Barnes, N.; Griffiths, C.; Horne, R. Understanding patients' perceptions of asthma control: A qualitative study. *Eur. Respir. J.* **2018**, *51*, 1701346. [CrossRef] [PubMed]
16. O'Byrne, P.M.; Jenkins, C.; Bateman, E.D. The paradoxes of asthma management: Time for a new approach? *Eur. Respir. J.* **2017**, *50*, 1701103. [CrossRef]
17. Global Initiative for Asthma. Global Strategy for Asthma Management and Prevention. 2019. Available online: www.ginasthma.org (accessed on 29 February 2020).
18. Bumbacea, D.; Ionita, D.; Ciobanu, M.; Tudose, C.; Bogdan, M. Prevalence of asthma symptoms, diagnosis and treatment use in Romania. *Eur. Respir. J.* **2013**, *42*, 964.
19. Chereches-Panta, P.; Sorin, C.; Dumitrescu, D.; Marshall, M.; Mirestean, I.; Muresan, M.; Iacob, D.; Farcau, M.; Ichim, G.E.; Nanulescu, M.V. Epidemiological survey 6 years apart: Increased prevalence of asthma and other allergic diseases in schoolchildren aged 13-14 years in Cluj-Napoca, Romania (based on isaac questionnaire). *Maedica* **2011**, *6*, 10–16. [PubMed]

20. Chung, K.F.; Wenzel, S.E.; Brozek, J.L.; Bush, A.; Castro, M.; Sterk, P.J.; Adcock, I.M.; Bateman, E.D.; Bel, E.H.; Bleecker, E.R.; et al. International ERS/ATS guidelines on definition, evaluation and treatment of severe asthma. *Eur. Respir. J.* **2014**, *43*, 343–373. [CrossRef] [PubMed]
21. Foster, J.M.; McDonald, V.M.; Guo, M.; Reddel, H.K. "I have lost in every facet of my life": The hidden burden of severe asthma. *Eur. Respir. J.* **2017**, *50*, 1700765. [CrossRef]
22. McDonald, V.M.; Hiles, S.A.; Jones, K.A.; Clark, V.L.; Yorke, J. Health-related quality of life burden in severe asthma. *Med. J. Aust.* **2018**, *209* (Suppl. 2), S28–S33. [CrossRef]
23. Menckeberg, T.T.; Bouvy, M.L.; Bracke, M.; Kaptein, A.A.; Leufkens, H.G.; Raaijmakers, J.A.; Horne, R. Beliefs about medicines predict refill adherence to inhaled corticosteroids. *J. Psychosom. Res.* **2008**, *64*, 47–54. [CrossRef]
24. van der Molen, T.; Fletcher, M.; Price, D. Identifying Patient Attitudinal Clusters Associated with Asthma Control: The European REALISE Survey. *J. Allergy Clin. Immunol. Pract.* **2018**, *6*, 962–971. [CrossRef]
25. Unni, E.; Shiyanbola, O.O. Clustering medication adherence behavior based on beliefs in medicines and illness perceptions in patients taking asthma maintenance medications. *Curr. Med. Res. Opin.* **2016**, *32*, 113–121. [CrossRef] [PubMed]
26. Axelsson, M.; Cliffordson, C.; Lundback, B.; Lotvall, J. The function of medication beliefs as mediators between personality traits and adherence behavior in people with asthma. *Patient Prefer. Adherence* **2013**, *7*, 1101–1109. [CrossRef] [PubMed]
27. Braido, F.; Chrystyn, H.; Baiardini, I.; Bosnic-Anticevich, S.; van der Molen, T.; Dandurand, R.J.; Chisholm, A.; Carter, V.; Price, D.; Group, R.E. "Trying, But Failing"—The role of inhaler technique and mode of delivery in respiratory medication adherence. *J. Allergy Clin. Immunol. Pract.* **2016**, *4*, 823–832. [CrossRef] [PubMed]
28. Hyland, M.E.; Stahl, E. Asthma treatment needs: A comparison of patients' and health care professionals' perceptions. *Clin. Ther.* **2004**, *26*, 2141–2152. [CrossRef]
29. Gelhorn, H.L.; Balantac, Z.; Ambrose, C.S.; Chung, Y.N.; Stone, B. Patient and physician preferences for attributes of biologic medications for severe asthma. *Patient Prefer. Adherence* **2019**, *13*, 1253–1268. [CrossRef] [PubMed]
30. Williams, B.; Steven, K.; Sullivan, F.M. Tacit and transitionary: An exploration of patients' and primary care health professionals' goals in relation to asthma. *Soc. Sci. Med.* **2011**, *72*, 1359–1366. [CrossRef] [PubMed]

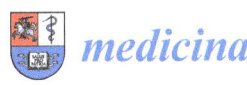

Review

The Psychosocial Role of Body Image in the Quality of Life of Head and Neck Cancer Patients. What Does the Future Hold?—A Review of the Literature

Vlad Ioan Covrig [1], Diana Elena Lazăr [2,*], Victor Vlad Costan [3], Roxana Postolică [4] and Beatrice Gabriela Ioan [5]

1. Doctoral School, Grigore T. Popa University of Medicine and Pharmacy, 700115 Iasi, Romania; vlad-ioan.d.covrig@d.umfiasi.ro
2. Department of Oncology, Regional Institute of Oncology, 700483 Iasi, Romania
3. Surgery Department, Oral and Maxillo-Facial Surgery, Faculty of Dentistry, Grigore T. Popa University of Medicine and Pharmacy, 700115 Iasi, Romania; victor.costan@umfiasi.ro
4. Department of Psychology, Regional Institute of Oncology, 700483 Iasi, Romania; roxana.postolica@yahoo.com
5. IIIrd Medical Department, Legal Medicine, Faculty of Medicine, Grigore T. Popa University of Medicine and Pharmacy, 700115 Iasi, Romania; beatrice.ioan@umfiasi.ro
* Correspondence: lazardianaelena@yahoo.com; Tel.: +40-747-693883

Abstract: *Background and Objectives:* It is well known that among all cancers, cancers of the head and neck (HNC) have a major impact on patients' quality of life. Disfigurement, anxiety and disabling physical and psychological symptoms affect people with HNC to such an extent that the suicide rate in this category of patients is exceeded only by that of patients with pancreatic cancer. The aim of this review was to summarize the published literature describing the severity of body image and quality of life impairment in patients with HNC over time, and to examine the psychosocial and functional associations and interventions implemented to improve body image and quality of life. *Materials and Methods:* We conducted a literature search from 1 January 2018 to June 2021 that included electronic searches of six major databases (PubMed, ScienceDirect, ProQuest, PsycINFO, PsychArticles and Scopus) and review of references of articles screened. Of 620 records, only 9 articles met the eligibility criteria. *Results:* Numerous studies have been conducted to analyze various psychological variables, but there is still a lack of standardization in the assessment of body image perception (BI) and quality of life, resulting in small-scale testing of interventions with poor results. *Conclusions:* Expected longitudinal studies describing the flow of body image problems and the mediation and balance factors associated with body image will allow researchers to design methods aimed at limiting body image disorders and thus improving quality of life of patients with head and neck cancer.

Keywords: head and neck cancer; quality of life; body image; psychosocial; interventions

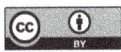

1. Introduction

Most of the major challenges posed by the need for medical care around the world are related to the long-term care of chronic diseases. Diseases that were once fatal are now treatable, but they still have a profound impact on the quality of life of patients and survivors and require ongoing medical care even after recovery. A central problem with chronic illness is emotional distress. The American Psychiatric Association has recognized the diagnosis of cancer as a traumatic stressor because it can lead to impairments in several areas of functioning (ability to work and social relationships) due to negative cognitions and moods [1].

Cancers of the head and neck are a heterogeneous group of cancers, representing the seventh most common cancer in both sexes worldwide in 2018, accounting for 3% of all cancers [2–5]. This type of cancer occurs in cosmetically and functionally critical areas and results in life-altering disfigurement, difficulty swallowing and speech problems.

Traditionally, tobacco and alcohol use have been the main risk factors for head and neck (HNC) in developing countries, and the increasing transmission of human papillomavirus (HPV) in developed countries has led to significantly more HNC cases worldwide [2–5]. Men have a higher risk of developing HNC than women [3]. Patients with HNC are four times more likely to commit suicide than other cancer patients [4]. In addition, suicide rates were highest in patients with laryngeal cancer and hypopharyngeal cancer [4].

The devastating impact of HNC on quality of life (QoL) is determined by the fact that *"the face"* is an important component of personality, self-image and interpersonal relationships [6]. Physically, the face is the most exposed, conspicuous and visible part of the body, uncovered by clothing in most people, and conveys individual identity. Functionally, it inspires intellect, communication and emotion, or the representation of the self. Cognitively, the environment is taken in through the senses of sight, hearing, taste and smell. Emotionally, an attractive face is often associated with well-being. It is also a matter of culture, where beauty, especially in women, is associated with art, social status, personal and collective well-being [6].

As a newly defined but "old as times" concept, body image has a complex meaning in contemporary society and can be defined as a multidimensional dynamic perception of the body itself (somato-perception controlled by body position in space, interoceptive and exteroceptive inputs), which is distinct from cognitive, culturally influenced representation (somato-representation or semantic knowledge about the body) [7–10]. Moreover, body image is closely related to identity, attractiveness, self-esteem, social relationships, sexual functioning and a number of social aspects that are constantly updated [11]. It largely plays out at an unconscious level and is usually regulated by the state of the body [12]. The primary changes in body image that occur during HNC surgery are caused by facial disfigurement and dysfunction.

Dissatisfaction with one's body can also affect sexuality [9]. HNC survivors are threatened in all its dimensions: in sexual identity (the highly visible changes in facial shape alter the patient's ability to show facial expressions, which are important for normal nonverbal communication) and in sexual relationships (e.g., difficulties in relating to a partner due to shame about one's body) [7].

Disfigurement due to HNC is stigmatized in society because beauty is a social goal, desire and standard. Disfigurement is significantly associated with deterioration of structures related to personal identity, communication skills, social relationships, impaired sexuality and clinical levels of depression and anxiety [13–15]. Despite the high risk of body image disturbances in HNC patients, there are no effective treatment options for these particular patients.

HNC and its treatment is often associated with significant morbidity, deformity, loss of function and high treatment costs. In daily life, the negative changes in these patients (e.g., difficulties with appearance, disturbances in swallowing, dental hygiene, digestion, speech, pain, role function, movement and psychological well-being) reported in Patient Concerns Inventory often go beyond the realm of physical health, as the disease can also cause psychological problems and increase social demands [16]. The literature reports that 75% of surgically treated HNC patients experience psychosocial problems [15].

As mentioned earlier, body image (BI) is an important psychosocial issue in head and neck oncology. Head and neck surgeons should play an important role in screening their patients for depression and anxiety. As part of the multidisciplinary team, professionally trained psychologists can assist with formal assessment and refer patients to specialist psychiatrists as needed.

The concept of psychosocial impact is defined as the effects of environmental and/or biological factors on the social and/or psychological aspects of individuals to improve understanding of the impact of disasters on people and communities [17].

Body image is an important aspect of quality of life that has been studied to a very limited extent in patients with HNC. However, a systemic review published in 2018 [18], which examined body image and perceived quality of life in HNC survivors, concluded that body image dissatisfaction is a public health concern due to its high prevalence, as it is often associated with poorer behaviors such as physical inactivity and poor dietary habits, and may be associated with poorer quality of life. In the era of personalized postoperative care for HNC, this study highlights the need to ask patients, caregivers and families what they think are the most important priorities for future research, and it also highlights the need for public health action to address these issues.

The aims of this review were to: (1) assess the impact of HNC treatments on patients' body image and quality of life; (2) evaluate the relationship between body image and quality of life; and (3) examine interventions implemented to improve body image and quality of life in this population and also identify directions for future research in this important survivorship area.

2. Materials and Methods

Publications addressing body image and quality of life in patients with HNC from all geographic regions were identified through systematic searches of PubMed, ScienceDirect, ProQuest, PsycINFO, PsychArticles and Scopus databases from 1 January 2018, to 1 June 2021. The search terms "head and neck cancer", "body image" and "quality of life" were used in all six databases (Table 1).

Table 1. Data sources and search strategies.

Database	Search Strategies
PubMed	**Search terms:** "head and neck cancer" AND "body image" AND "quality of life" **Filters:** English, publication date: from January 2018 to June 2021, species: human, article type: clinical trial, randomized controlled trial **Results:** 28 records **Relevant:** 12
Science Direct	**Search terms:** "head and neck cancer" AND "body image" AND "quality of life" **Filters:** English, publication date: from January 2018 to 2021, research articles, subject areas: medicine and dentistry, access type: open access, HNC relevant publications **Results:** 66 records **Relevant:** 1
ProQuest	**Filters:** English, publication date: January 2018 to 2021, sort by: newest first, source type: include—Scholarly Journals, Working Papers, Trade Journals; exclude: Books, Reports, Dissertations and Theses, Wire Feeds, Magazines, Newspapers **Results:** 166 records **Relevant:** 1
PsycINFO	**Filters:** English, publication date: from January 2018 to June 2021, sorted by journal article **Results:** 62 records **Relevant:** 0
PsychArticles	**Search terms:** "head and neck cancer" AND "body image" AND "quality of life" **Filters:** English, publication date: from January 2018 to June 2021, sorted by journal article **Results:** 6 records **Relevant:** 0
Scopus	**Search terms:** "head and neck cancer" AND "body image" AND "quality of life" **Filters:** English, publication date: from January 2018 to June 2021, species: humans, publication type: article, subject area: medicine **Results:** 292 records **Relevant:** 5

2.1. Data Collection Process

After introducing the above keywords and filters regarding publication date and language in all databases, a total of 620 articles were found. Finally, only 9 studies met the eligibility criteria and were included in the systematic review. Figure 1 shows the overview of the selection process using the PRISMA 2020 flowchart, where the data were extracted systematically.

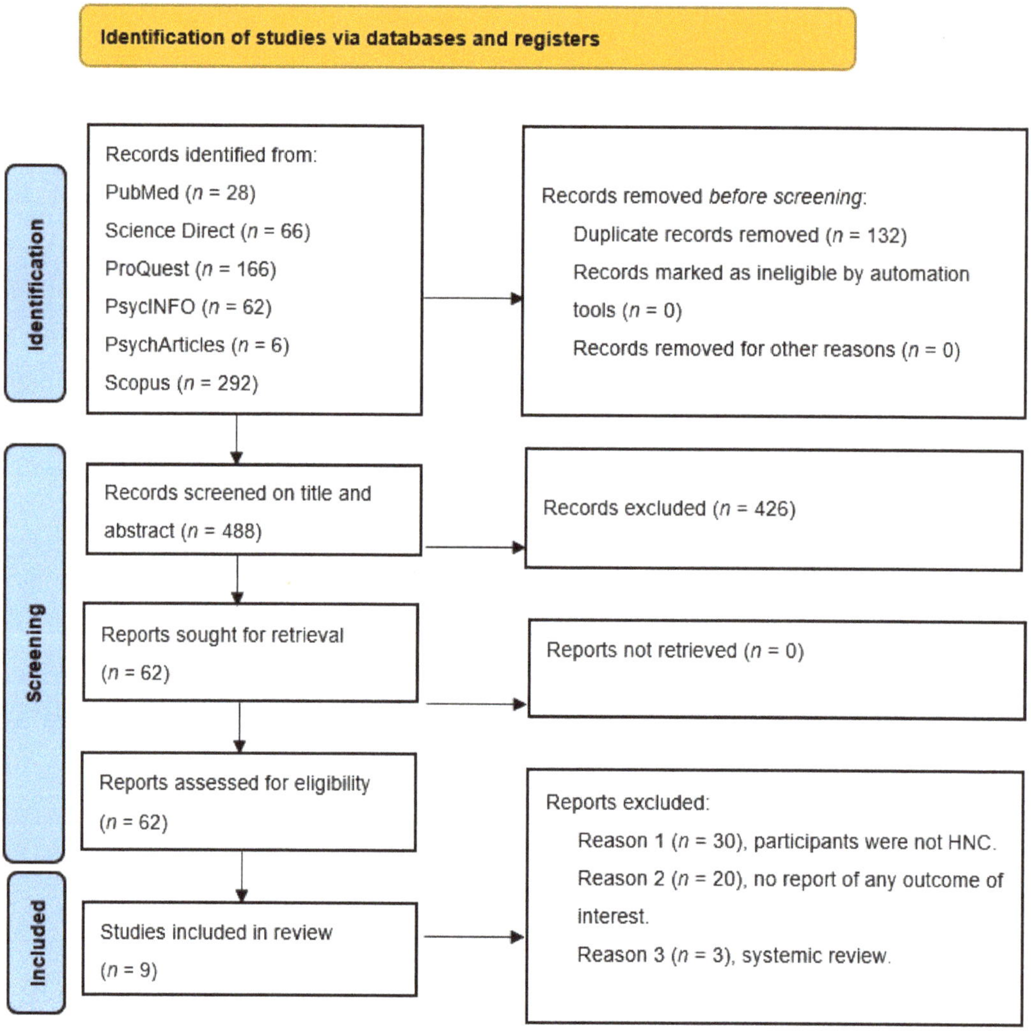

Identification of studies via databases and registers

Identification

Records identified from:
PubMed (*n* = 28)
Science Direct (*n* = 66)
ProQuest (*n* = 166)
PsycINFO (*n* = 62)
PsychArticles (*n* = 6)
Scopus (*n* = 292)

→ Records removed *before screening*:
Duplicate records removed (*n* = 132)
Records marked as ineligible by automation tools (*n* = 0)
Records removed for other reasons (*n* = 0)

Screening

Records screened on title and abstract (*n* = 488)

→ Records excluded (*n* = 426)

Reports sought for retrieval (*n* = 62)

→ Reports not retrieved (*n* = 0)

Reports assessed for eligibility (*n* = 62)

→ Reports excluded:
Reason 1 (*n* = 30), participants were not HNC.
Reason 2 (*n* = 20), no report of any outcome of interest.
Reason 3 (*n* = 3), systemic review.

Included

Studies included in review (*n* = 9)

Figure 1. Flow diagram of the selection process of the studies.

2.2. Eligibility Criteria

The inclusion criteria for this review were: (1) original research; (2) published in English as of 2018 with accessible full text; (3) measurement of body image as an outcome variable; and (4) results included reports of age-related outcomes. The definition of "younger" and "older" is not addressed by the reviewers prior to review, as no consensus was reached in the literature on the definition of "young" and "old" in cancer.

Exclusion criteria were: (1) examination of body image with respect to medical imaging; (2) disfigurement due to trauma, burns or congenital health problems, (3) review articles, systemic reviews, unpublished articles, dissertations, commentaries, meeting and conference abstracts, and case reports, book reviews, opinions and editorials.

3. Results

According to the search strategy, a total of 620 articles were identified. However, 132 records were duplicated. Of the remaining 488 articles, 426 were excluded after reading titles and abstracts, and of these, 62 were selected based on the eligibility criteria; 53 articles were further excluded (if they did not include HNC survivors, studies that did not evaluate body image and quality of life outcomes, and were systemic reviews), and finally, a total of 9 studies were selected for qualitative synthesis, indicating the scarcity of research in this area. The year 2018 was chosen as the baseline year, as this was when the last paper describing BI and the quality of life of HNC patients was published. The screening process consisted of four steps: (I) title screening; (II) abstract screening; (III) full-text screening; and (IV) critical appraisal. After the initial search, eligible titles and abstracts were analyzed by two authors (V.I.C., D.E.L.), and full-text articles were independently reviewed for eligibility by first and senior authors (V.I.C., V.V.C., B.G.I., R.P.). Three authors searched the reference lists of included publications to identify additional articles (V.V.C., B.G.I., R.P.). Disagreements between authors were resolved by referring back to the original article and discussing with the authors to reach consensus.

3.1. Characteristics of the Studies

The general characteristics of the studies included in the review ($n = 9$) can be found in Table 2. The articles were published from 2018 to 2021 in a variety of scientific journals with different aims and scopes: Indian journal of palliative care [19], Supportive care in cancer: official journal of the Multinational Association of Supportive Care in Cancer [20], Sexual Medicine [21], Psycho-oncology [22], Otolaryngology-head and neck surgery: official journal of American Academy of Otolaryngology-Head and Neck Surgery [23], Indian journal of palliative care [24], Psycho-oncology [25], Surgery [26], Medicina oral, patología oral y cirugía bucal [27]. All the records were written in English.

3.1.1. Design of the Studies

Six of the nine studies were descriptive, cross-sectional studies with pre/post design. Only one of the studies was a controlled trial. Thus, it was a quasi-experimental pretest-posttest and follow-up design.

3.1.2. Participants and Regrouping

A total of 1445 HNC patients were enrolled in the studies. The number of participants in the different studies ranged from 10 to 768 HNC patients. Study 1 [19] included 60 HNC patients (46 males/14 females), the average mean age of the patients was 43 years, who were divided into a total of 8 HNC localization groups: carcinoma of buccal mucosa ($n = 24$), carcinoma of tongue ($n = 14$), carcinoma of maxilla ($n = 3$), hard palate ($n = 3$), carcinoma postcricoid/supraglottic ($n = 5$), carcinoma of central arch /mandible ($n = 6$), carcinoma esophagus ($n = 4$) and carcinoma of lip ($n = 1$) in the Department of Pain and Palliative Medicine, Gujarat Cancer and Research Institute, India. Study 2 [20] included 87 patients, with a mean age of 66 years, divided into a total of 5 groups: oral cavity ($n = 17$), oropharynx ($n = 20$), hypopharynx ($n = 5$), larynx ($n = 29$) and others ($n = 16$), from the Department of Otolaryngology—Head and Neck Surgery at Amsterdam UMC, location VUmc. Study 3 [21] consisted of 134 HNC survivors (males = 44/females = 23), with a mean age of 66 years, who were divided into a total of 3 HNC localizations: lip/oral/cavity/oropharynx ($n = 29$), hypopharynx/larynx ($n = 21$), other head and neck cancers ($n = 17$), randomized to investigate differences in the course of sexual interest and sexual pleasure between a care program targeting psychological distress compared to usual care and a control, at the clinic of Amsterdam University Medical Centers (Amsterdam UMC), location VU University medical center. Study 4 [22] is registered at ClinicalTrials.gov (NCT03518671) and was conducted with 10 HNC survivors. Participants were predominantly female ($n = 7$)/male ($n = 3$), had oral cancer ($n = 4$), underwent microvascular reconstruction ($n = 8$) and received adjuvant therapy ($n = 7$) with BID, they were enrolled in a single-arm pilot trial designed to evaluate the feasibility, acceptability and preliminary clinical effect of BRIGHT (Building a Renewed ImaGe after Head and Neck Cancer Treatment). Study 5 [23] enrolled 68 patients (males $n = 43$/females $n = 25$), with a tumor location and histology divided into: oral squamous cell carcinoma ($n = 37$), oropharynx SCC/SCC of unknown primary ($n = 8$), larynx/hypopharynx SCC ($n = 9$) and facial cutaneous malignancy ($n = 21$), with pretreatment and 1, 3-, 6-, 9- and 12-months posttreatment and underwent microvascular reconstruction ($n = 45$); the median age was 63 years. Study 6 [24] included a total of 105 patients (male = 78/ female = 27) who were divided into a total of 6 HNC localizations: oral cavity ($n = 13$), nasopharynx ($n = 6$), oropharynx, ($n = 60$), larynx ($n = 9$), other ($n = 7$), unknown ($n = 10$) from the Henry Joyce Cancer Clinic in the Vanderbilt-Ingram Cancer Center. Study 7 [25] included a total of 168 patients aged over 30 years diagnosed with breast, cervical, head and neck, gastrointestinal tract, lung or colorectal cancer at stage III or IV and who had undergone radiotherapy, chemotherapy or surgery or a combination of both, from a total of 12 hospitals in the southern part of Karnataka (Manipal, Mangalore and Bengaluru). Study 8 [26] was performed with 1710 thyroid cancer survivors (male = 199/female = 1511), who were surveyed online, with the mean age at survey 51 years, mean age at diagnosis 44 years and mean time since surgery 6,8 years. Study 8 [26] was conducted with 1710 thyroid cancer survivors (male = 199/female = 1511) who were interviewed online. The mean age at interview was 51 years, the mean age at diagnosis was 44 years and the mean time since surgery was 68 years. Study 9 [27] included a total of 103 individuals (male = 81/female = 22) with HNC and ages ranging from 20.0 to 81.6 years, with tumor location and histology subdivided as follows: oral cavity ($n=35$), larynx ($n=26$), skin ($n=16$), pharynx ($n = 12$), others/unknown ($n = 14$).

3.2. Changes in Body Image after Head and Neck Cancer

Numerous instruments are already in use to assess various body image and quality of life variables. Among the most common are: Body Image Scale (BIS); Body Image Quality of Life (BIQL); Inventory Vanderbilt Head and Neck Symptom survey; European Organization for Research and Treatment of Cancer, Quality of Life Questionnaire, Head and Neck Cancer -specific module, etc.; others are currently being tested, but there is still no validated, comprehensive and efficient tool to correctly assess the impact of HNC on body image and quality of life and predict its future evolution.

As Chang and colleagues [25] found in their study, overall negative body image was associated with higher levels of depression, greater anxiety about social interactions, poorer social-emotional functioning, receipt of surgery, female gender and greater avoidance of social interactions. Body image is an important issue when it comes to patient acceptance of therapies and procedures. For example, in the study by Umrania et al. [19], 88.33% of those who refused a naso-gastric tube (NG) for feeding justified that "it will disrupt my body image", and also 80% said that they would be "unable to go outside/mix with people" (80%).

Melissant et al. [20] found in their intervention study that expressive writing, an exercise that performed well in people with breast cancer, had no effect on body image disturbance in people with HNC.

An interesting ongoing study, called BRIGHT (Building a Renewed ImaGe after Head and Neck Cancer Treatment) is testing a novel telemedicine-based cognitive-behavioral intervention to manage body image disturbance (BID) in head and neck cancer survivors [22]. In a pilot trial of this study, the 10 patients included presented improved image-related coping behavior [22]. In a pilot trial of this study, the 10 participating patients demonstrated improved image-related coping behaviors [22].

Table 2. Characteristics of the included studies.

Authors	Year	Design	Number of Participants	Measure of Body Image and QoL	Results	Link
1. Umrania et al. [19]	March 2021	Descriptive, cross sectional, after treatment	60 HNC patients	A questionnaire referring to most common cause for enteral feeding refusal. Variables: QoL Disrupted body image Inability of eating and feeling the tastes.	The reasons for refusal of NG tube were "it will disrupt my body image" (88.33%), "unable to go outside/mix with people" (80%) and "dependency on others for activities" (66.66%).	Survey of Psychosocial Issues of Nasogastric Tube Feeding in Head-and-Neck Cancer Patients (nih.gov)
2. Melissant et al. [20]	March 2021	Descriptive, cross sectional, after treatment	87 HNC patients	Baseline survey on body image-related distress My Changed Body—expressive writing activity Variables: Body image related distress. Self-compassion.	Expressive writing activity does not significantly improve body image-related distress, but likely increases self-compassion	A structured expressive writing activity targeting body image-related distress among head and neck cancer survivors: who do we reach and what are the effects?
3. Schutte et al. [21]	January 2021	Randomized control trial, after treatment	134 HNC survivors	"Sexuality" symptom subscale, part of the European Organization for Research and Treatment of Cancer, Quality of Life Questionnaire, Head and Neck Cancer-specific module. Variables: Psychological distress	76.1% had an unmet sexual need at baseline, and 24.6% had a psychiatric disorder (anxiety or depression). Stepwise care did not reduce problems with sexual interest and pleasure in any of the follow-up measurements	Effect of Stepped Care on Sexual Interest and Enjoyment in Distressed Patients with Head and Neck Cancer: A Randomized Controlled Trial—ScienceDirect
4. Graboyes et al. [22]	December 2020	Clinical trial	10 HNC survivors	BRIGHT (Building a Renewed ImaGe after Head and Neck Cancer Treatment), telemedicine-based cognitive-behavioral intervention to manage BID. Variables: Body image disturbance	BRIGHT was associated with a 34.5% reduction in mean Body Image Scale scores at 1 month, an effect that persisted at 3 months—post BRIGHT.	Evaluation of a novel telemedicine-based intervention to manage body image disturbance in head and neck cancer survivors—PubMed (nih.gov)
5. Graboyes et al. [23]	January 2020	Prospective cohort study	68 patients with treated HNC	Body Image Scale Variables: Body image disturbance	BID worsening after treatment before returning to pre-treatment (baseline) levels 9 months after treatment.	Temporal Trajectory of Body Image Disturbance in Patients with Surgically Treated Head and Neck Cancer (nih.gov)

Table 2. Cont.

Authors	Year	Design	Number of Participants	Measure of Body Image and QoL	Results	Link
6. Burchfield et al. [24]	December 2019	Descriptive, cross-sectional, after treatment	105 patients with treated HNC	Body Image Quality of Life Inventory Vanderbilt Head and Neck Symptom survey General Symptom Survey Neurotoxicity Rating Scale Profile of Mood States -Short Form Quality of life Variables: QoL	In addition to lower mean quality of life, it was found that a higher proportion of patients in the high systemic symptoms patient group rated quality of life as poor compared to the low systemic symptoms patient group, emotional and intellectual overall negative	Late systemic symptoms in head and neck cancer survivors
7. Chang et al. [25]	May 2019	Descriptive, cross sectional, after treatment	168 people with oral cavity cancer	HADS (Hospital Anxiety and Depression Scale), LSAS (Liebowitz Social Anxiety Scale), UW-QoL (University of Washington Quality of Life Scale) BIS (Body Image Scale) Variables: Body image Socio-emotional function. Depression. Poor perceived attractiveness Dissatisfaction with body appearance	Negative overall body image was associated with greater degree of depression, greater fear of social interactions, poorer social-emotional function, receipt of surgery, female gender and greater avoidance of social interaction.	Factors influencing body image in posttreatment oral cavity cancer patients—PubMed (nih.gov)
8. Kurumety et al. [26]	June 2018	Descriptive, cross sectional, after treatment	1710 thyroid cancer survivors	Online survey with 5-point Likert scale. QoL evaluated through Patient-Reported Outcomes Measurement Information System Variables: Self-reported appearance	Age >45, >2 years since surgery and higher quality of life were independently associated with better self-reported neck appearance.	Post-thyroidectomy neck appearance and impact on quality of life in thyroid cancer survivors—Surgery (surgjournal.com)
9. Nogueira et al. [27]	February 2018	Descriptive, cross sectional, after treatment	103 people with HNC	Functional Assessment of Cancer Therapy (FACT-H&N) questionnaire Variables: QoL, Orofacial functioning, Facial disfigurement	The ssymptoms-related domain had the major impact, while emotional domain was the least affected (79.1% of the maximum possible score)	Factors associated with the quality of life of subjects with facial disfigurement due to surgical treatment of head and neck cancer

Severity of Body Image Disturbance over Time

There were variable findings with regards to the association between the severity of body image disturbance (BID) and time since treatment. Unfortunately, none of the analyzed studies compared pre-to posttreatment BID severity. In general, surgically treated HNC survivors declared to have a disturbed body image after the diagnosis of the disease and early in the survivorship period, but the degree of disturbance varies with the type of surgical procedure. Women were more emotionally affected than men [24,25].

Disfigurement of the head and neck due to surgical cancer treatment was significantly related to the functional dimension of patients' quality of life, especially in cases of major neck and lower facial sequelae. Patients with HNC who undergo surgery usually undergo further reconstruction 6 to 12 months after the original reconstruction to improve shape, contour, appearance and function.

On the other hand, the BID may remain stable and/or improve over time, especially with continuous adjustment and surgical/flap revisions. There were significant limitations in the methods in many studies examining BID and quality of life in different areas as most of the studies were randomized (with patients in different areas for continuous treatment). These methodological limitations preclude knowledge of the longitudinal course of BID and QoL in patients with HNC. The knowledge gap about the longitudinal course of BID and QoL in patients with HNC, particularly in long-term survivors, precludes delivery of optimally timed, patient-centered preventative and therapeutic interventions for BID.

Graboyes et al. [23] have shown in one of their studies that patients treated surgically for HNC recover to pretreatment levels of body image dissatisfaction by 9 months posttreatment.

3.3. Quality of Life

"*Sexuality and sexual*" needs are often overlooked, even though they are an essential component of quality of life. Only a limited number of studies have examined sexuality in patients with HNC. These studies suggest that HNC and its treatment negatively affect these aspects of sexuality, especially immediately after oncologic treatment and particularly in patients with high levels of distress, impaired social functioning, severe disfigurement and advanced tumor stages [24–26]. Moreover, sexuality was mentioned by patients with HNC among the top 3 most distressing areas of their lives.

Using the European Organization for Research and Treatment of Cancer, Quality of Life Questionnaire, Head and Neck Cancer–specific module, Schutte et al. [21], found in their study that 76.1% of participants had an unmet sexual need at baseline, and 24.6% had a psychiatric disorder (anxiety or depression).

In a study of 103 participants, Noguiera and colleagues [27] used the Functional Assessment questionnaire from Cancer Therapy (FACT-H&N) and concluded that lower quality of life was associated with sequels in the neck and/or lower third of the face, higher degree of disfigurement and female gender. The association between facial disfigurement and quality of life was significantly greater in women, concerning the social and familiar, functional and head and neck cancer specific domains. One of the conclusions of this study is that there is no clear evidence of a linear relationship between the level of facial disfigurement and dysfunction and the impact on QoL, which suggests that other emotional and psychosocial factors may play an important role in individual patient's response.

3.4. Body Image and Quality of Life

The quality of life of patients with HNC has also been studied in relationship to body image. It has been suggested that QoL difficulties rank higher in terms of importance than the body image issues [24].

The UW-QOLv4 and the EORTC are the commonest reported QoL questionnaires in HNC and both include sections asking about appearance/disfigurement. In general, there are only a few studies where the relationship between QoL and body image is investigated. One of the possible causes is that in many instances the change in body image is considered an aspect of the QoL and it is evaluated with a subscale within the QoL instrument.

Surprisingly, a study by Burchfield et al. [24] on 105 participants with HNC found no change in body image but altered quality of life (40%) or poor quality of life (15%) and also a high frequency of neuropsychiatric symptoms: restlessness (47.6%), tension (47.5%), decreased motivation (46.7%), distractibility (38.5%), slowed movements (38.5%) and irritability (38.5%), lack of interest in other people (21.9%). The study used Vanderbilt Head and Neck Symptom survey plus the General Symptom Subscale, the Body Image Quality of Life Inventory, Neurotoxicity Rating Scale, the Profile of Mood States and a five-item quality of life measure.

3.5. Specific Interventions

An important determinant of the ability of HNC patients to cope with their disease and treatments is the perceived social support (PSS), which can be defined as the extent to which a person believes that his/her needs for support, information and feedback are fulfilled during times of need [28]. From the nine studies used in this review, some specific interventions may be of interest in the near future (Table 3).

Table 3. Specific interventions to improve body image and quality of life in people with head and neck cancer.

Authors	Date of Publication	Type of Study	Number of Patients	Intervention	Results	Link
Melissant et al. [20]	March 2021	Descriptive, Cross sectional, after treatment	87 HNC patients	Baseline survey on body image-related distress My Changed Body—expressive writing activity	Expressive writing activity does not significantly improve body image-related distress, but likely increases self-compassion.	A structured expressive writing activity targeting body image-related distress among head and neck cancer survivors: who do we reach and what are the effects?
Umrania et al. [19]	March 2021	Descriptive, cross sectional, after treatment	60 HNC patients	A questionnaire referring to most common cause for enteral feeding refusal. Variables: QoL Disrupted BI Inability of eating and feeling the tastes.	The reasons for refusing NG tube were "it will disrupt my body image"(88.33%), "unable to go outside/mix with people"(80%) and "dependency on others for activities"(66.66%).	Survey of Psychosocial Issues of Nasogastric Tube Feeding in Head-and-Neck Cancer Patients (nih.gov)
Graboyes et al. [22]	December 2020	Ongoing Clinical trial (started on 13th of June 2020, estimated completion date July 2022)	10 HNC survivors	BRIGHT (Building a Renewed ImaGe after Head and Neck Cancer Treatment), telemedicine-based cognitive-behavioral intervention to manage BID.	BRIGHT was associated with a 34.5% reduction in mean Body Image Scale scores at 1-month post-, an effect that was durable at 3-months post-BRIGHT	Evaluation of a novel telemedicine-based intervention to manage body image disturbance in head and neck cancer survivors—PubMed (nih.gov) Building a Renewed ImaGe After Head and Neck Cancer Treatment (BRIGHT) 2.0—Full Text View—ClinicalTrials.gov

Psychological counseling proved useful for 47 of 60 patients who initially refused the nasogastric tube feeding but then understood its benefits and eventually accepted it [19].

Telemedicine-based cognitive-behavioral intervention to manage body image disturbance (BID) in head and neck cancer (HNC) survivors from BRIGHT (Building a Renewed ImaGe after Head and Neck Cancer Treatment) trial presented promising results on coping behavior in the pilot study [22].

My Changed Body (MyCB) is an exercise of expressive writing pre- and post- treatment which showed an improvement in self-esteem, but no effect on body image distress, measured on Body Image Scale [20].

These results suggest that positive perception of a supportive social network may help patients with HNC better cope with the psychological impact of treatment on their body image.

3.6. Limitations, Strengths and Future Directions

Limitations of this study should be mentioned. We excluded studies published in languages other than English, which bias our results. We also excluded unpublished articles, dissertations, commentaries, conference proceedings or meeting and conference abstracts, which put our results at risk of publication bias.

The studies described and analyzed here are heterogeneous in nature with respect to country, study design and population, but there was no discussion in relation to the individual healthcare systems. Many studies were cross-sectional in design and included a heterogeneous mix of patients before and after treatment. Therefore, the relationship between key psychological outcomes and body image disturbance/QoL remains unknown. Few studies have examined the relationship between quality of life and body image, possibly because body image is considered an aspect of quality of life and is assessed with a subscale within the quality-of-life instrument.

The main gaps in the study related to BID research related to quality of life in HNC identified in this review include the following: (1) nutritional status is a factor that appears to be related to body image and thus quality of life, but it has not been analyzed, (2) the lack of an HNC-specific BID patient-reported outcome measures (PROM) and thus the reliance on PROMs developed by patient populations and validated differently, (3) the variability of PROMs used to assess BID and the lack of clear points to distinguish BID from "normal" body image concerns, (4) the nature of the relationship between body image disturbance and other psychosocial variables such as depression, anxiety and social isolation in patients with HNC over the course of treatment and during recovery, (5) the lack of evidence-based interventions in the treatment of BID in patients with HNC, (6) the body satisfaction scale was not assessed in our studies.

From the pilot studies presented in the specific intervention section, we learned that targeted psychological interventions are effective in reducing BI issues related to HNC patients. However, results are mixed as to the magnitude of these effects. It seems worthwhile to replicate the findings in larger studies of psychological support for HNC patients.

Finally, even in the face of the above-mentioned limitations, considering the severity of the disease and the significant impact of treatment side effects on HNC patients, the variety of symptoms, the need for objective evaluation scales and the paucity of possible interventions, we believe that future research and trails are expected in order to minimize symptoms and make treatment less exhausting and traumatic.

4. Conclusions

Living after receiving a diagnosis of cancer is a difficult task, but moreover living with the scars of the treatment for head and neck cancer may be extremely physically and psychologically exhausting. HNC and its treatment subside in disfigurement, neurological disorder, impaired senses, a wide variety of psychological disorders, ranging from distress to suicidal thoughts. From the results of the analyses, it can be concluded that body image is related to the quality of life of HNC patients.

While mortality after cancer may be decreasing, new morbidities and impacts on QoL and body image are increasingly recognized in HNC patients. These new morbidities have the potential to disproportionately impact the entire life span of patients, and may indirectly affect caregivers and future dependents. In addition to new disability, HNC survivors are at risk for late mortality and readmission, and often require increased health care resources. First studies in the field indicate that over a third of HNC survivors may have new disability between one to three months after HNC diagnosis and treatment, with physical effects and behavioral impacts lasting years in some cases. There is an unmet need to identify HNC patients at risk of long-term sequelae early, to better characterize the new post-HNC morbidities and their impact, define optimal approaches for post-discharge follow-up, and design effective interventions to enhance recovery and maximize quality of life in HNC survivors.

Recent evidence shows that combining psychological therapies with cosmetic and beauty treatments is important in preventing the development of illness concerns and highlights an important growth area for the future of HNC care, where complex decisions are discussed with patients and commitments are made.

Recommendations for Future Research

Regarding future research directions, more interventions are needed that focus on developing positive BI and self-esteem in this population, as these factors are important for disease progression and may predict psychological functioning and QoL in HNC patients. For example: (1) Since psychosocial problems vary by personality, behavioral patterns, culture and regional background of the patient and family, assessment of these problems requires a large multicenter longitudinal study to allow generalization; (2) Advances in therapeutic interventions targeting sexuality may increase psychological well-being, but it is not yet known whether interventions specifically targeting psychological problems also reduce sexual problems in patients with HNC; (3) Few studies have published data on patient and caregiver experiences of tracheostomy, particularly in the community. There is a need to better understand these experiences in order to formulate strategies and provide resources to improve the quality of care and overall quality of life for patients with tracheostomy and their caregivers in the hospital and community. (4) Understanding the structure and dynamics of personality should be a priority to assist these types of patients and potentially improve outcomes. Even though some authors have investigated the relationship between body image and quality of life, the role of personality traits in the deterioration of quality of life associated with HNC treatments has no received scientific attention. Qualitative studies could be evaluated to assess patients' individual perceptions with the aim of exploring deviations from body image and implementing personalized psychological interventions focused on the disease experienced. (5) Many questions related to specific interventions for HNC remain unanswered, e.g., (a) How might interventions to improve body image using technology impact body image in HNC patients? (b) Does social media have an impact on HNC patients' body image and how they perceive our own appearance? (c) How does cross-cultural perspective impact HNC survivors' body image?

Author Contributions: Conceptualization, B.G.I., V.V.C. and R.P.; methodology, V.I.C., D.E.L. and B.G.I.; validation, B.G.I., V.V.C. and R.P.; formal analysis, V.I.C. and D.E.L.; investigation, V.I.C. and D.E.L.; resources, B.G.I.; data curation, V.I.C., D.E.L. and B.G.I.; writing, V.I.C. and D.E.L.; original draft preparation, V.I.C., D.E.L. and R.P.; writing—review and editing, B.G.I. and V.V.C.; visualization, V.I.C., D.E.L. and B.G.I.; supervision, B.G.I.; project administration, B.G.I. All authors have read and agreed to the published version of the manuscript.

Funding: This research received no external funding.

Institutional Review Board Statement: Not applicable.

Informed Consent Statement: Not applicable.

Data Availability Statement: The data presented in this study are available in the main text.

Conflicts of Interest: The authors declare no conflict of interest.

References

1. Yi, J.C.; Syrjala, K.L. Anxiety and depression in cancer survivors. *Med. Clin. N. Am.* **2017**, *101*, 1099–1113. [CrossRef]
2. Bray, F.; Ferlay, J.; Soerjomataram, I.; Siegel, R.L.; Torre, L.A.; Jemal, A. Global cancer statistics 2018: GLOBOCAN estimates of incidence and mortality worldwide for 36 cancers in 185 countries. *CA Cancer J. Clin.* **2018**, *68*, 394–424. [CrossRef]
3. Siegel, R.L.; Miller, K.D.; Jemal, A. Cancer statistics, 2018. *CA Cancer J. Clin.* **2018**, *68*, 7–30. [CrossRef] [PubMed]
4. Zeller, J.L. High suicide risk found for patients with head and neck cancer. *JAMA* **2006**, *11*, 21716–21717. [CrossRef] [PubMed]
5. Mourad, M.; Jetmore, T.; Jategaonkar, A.A.; Moubayed, S.; Moshier, E.; Urken, M.L. Epidemiological Trends of Head and Neck Cancer in the United States: A SEER Population Study. *J. Oral Maxillofac. Surg.* **2017**, *75*, 2562–2572. [CrossRef] [PubMed]
6. Global Burden of Disease Cancer Collaboration. Global, regional, and national cancer incidence, mortality, years of life lost, years lived with disability, and disability-adjusted life-years for 32 *Cancer* groups, 1990 to 2015: A systematic analysis for the global burden of disease study. *JAMA Oncol.* **2017**, *3*, 524–548. [CrossRef]
7. O'Brien, K.; Roe, B.; Low, C.; Deyn, L.; Rogers, S.N. An exploration of the perceived changes in intimacy of patients' relationships following head and neck cancer. *J. Clin. Nurs.* **2012**, *21*, 2499–2508. [CrossRef] [PubMed]
8. Fawzy, N.W.; Secher, L.; Evans, S.; Giuliano, A.E. The Positive Appearance Center: An innovative concept in comprehensive psychosocial cancer care. *Cancer Pract.* **1995**, *3*, 233–238.
9. Anderson, M.S.; Johnson, J. Restoration of body image and self-esteem for women after cancer treatment: A rehabilitative strategy. *Cancer Pract.* **1994**, *2*, 345–349.
10. Manne, S.L.; Girasek, D.; Ambrosino, J. An evaluation of the im-pact of a cosmetics class on breast cancer patients. *J. Psycho Soc. Oncol.* **1994**, *12*, 83–99. [CrossRef]
11. Longo, M.R.; Azanon, E.; Haggard, P. More than skin deep: Body representation beyond primary somatosensory cortex. *Neuropsychologia* **2010**, *48*, 655–668. [CrossRef]
12. Dahl, C.A.F.; Reinertsen, K.V.; Nesvold, I.-L.; Fosså, S.D.; Dahl, A.A. A study of body image in long-term breast cancer survivors. *Cancer* **2010**, *116*, 3549–3557. [CrossRef] [PubMed]
13. Dropkin, M.J. Body image and quality of life after head and neck cancer surgery. *Cancer Pr.* **1999**, *7*, 309–313. [CrossRef]
14. Rhoten, B.A. Head and Neck Cancer and Sexuality: A Review of the Literature. *Cancer Nurs.* **2016**, *39*, 313–320. [CrossRef] [PubMed]
15. Meningaud, J.-P.; Benadiba, L.; Servant, J.-M.; Herve, C.; Bertrand, J.-C.; Pelicier, Y. Depression, anxiety and quality of life: Outcome 9 months after facial cosmetic surgery. *J. Craniomaxillofacial Surg.* **2003**, *31*, 46–50. [CrossRef]
16. Fingeret, M.C.; Vidrine, D.J.; Reece, G.P.; Gillenwater, A.; Gritz, E.R. Multidimensional analysis of body image concerns among newly diagnosed patients with oral cavity cancer. *Head Neck.* **2010**, *32*, 301–309. [CrossRef]
17. Smith, T.W.; Ruiz, J.M. Psychosocial influences on the development and course of coronary heart disease: Current status and implications for research and practice. *J. Consult. Clin. Psychol.* **2002**, *70*, 548–568. [CrossRef] [PubMed]
18. Qualizza, M.; Bressan, V.; Rizzuto, A.; Stevanin, S.; Bulfone, G.; Cadorin, L.; Ghirotto, L. Listening to the voice of patients with head and neck cancer: A systematic review and meta-synthesis. *Eur. J. Cancer Care* **2019**, *28*, e12939. [CrossRef] [PubMed]
19. Patel, B.C.; Umrania, R.; Patel, D.; Singh, M.; Sanghavi, P.; Patel, H. Survey of psychosocial issues of nasogastric tube feeding in head-and-neck cancer patients. *Indian J. Palliat. Care* **2021**, *27*, 113–117. [CrossRef]
20. Melissant, H.C.; Jansen, F.; Eerenstein, S.E.J.; Cuijpers, P.; Lissenberg-Witte, B.I.; Sherman, K.A.; Laan, E.T.M.; Leemans, C.R.; Leeuw, I.M.V.-D. A structured expressive writing activity targeting body image-related distress among head and neck cancer survivors: Who do we reach and what are the effects? *Support. Care Cancer* **2021**, *29*, 5763–5776. [CrossRef]
21. Schutte, L.E.; Melissant, H.C.; Jansen, F.; Lissenberg-Witte, B.I.; Leemans, C.R.; Sprangers, M.A.; Vergeer, M.R.; Leeuw, I.M.V.-D.; Laan, E.T. Effect of Stepped Care on Sexual Interest and Enjoyment in Distressed Patients with Head and Neck Cancer: A Randomized Controlled Trial. *Sex. Med.* **2021**, *9*, 100304. [CrossRef]
22. Graboyes, E.M.; Maurer, S.; Park, Y.; Bs, C.H.M.; McElligott, J.T.; Day, T.A.; Hornig, J.D.; Sterba, K.R. Evaluation of a novel telemedicine-based intervention to manage body image disturbance in head and neck cancer survivors. *Psychooncology* **2020**, *29*, 1988–1994. [CrossRef] [PubMed]
23. Graboyes, E.M.; Hill, E.G.; Marsh, C.H.; Maurer, S.; Day, T.A.; Hornig, J.D.; Lentsch, E.J.; Neskey, D.M.; Skoner, J.; Sterba, K.R. Temporal Trajectory of Body Image Disturbance in Patients with Surgically Treated Head and Neck Cancer. *Otolaryngol. Head Neck Surg.* **2020**, *162*, 304–312. [CrossRef] [PubMed]
24. Wulff-Burchfield, E.; Dietrich, M.S.; Ridner, S.; Murphy, B.A. Late systemic symptoms in head and neck cancer survivors. *Support. Care Cancer* **2019**, *27*, 2893–2902. [CrossRef]
25. Chang, Y.-L.; Huang, B.-S.; Hung, T.-M.; Lin, C.-Y.; Chen, S.-C. Factors influencing body image in posttreatment oral cavity cancer patients. *Psychooncology* **2019**, *28*, 1127–1133. [CrossRef] [PubMed]
26. Kurumety, S.K.; Helenowski, I.B.; Goswami, S.; Peipert, B.J.; Yount, S.E.; Sturgeon, C. Post-thyroidectomy neck appearance and impact on quality of life in thyroid cancer survivors. *Surgery* **2019**, *165*, 1217–1221. [CrossRef] [PubMed]
27. Nogueira, T.E.; Adorno, M.; Mendonça, E.; Leles, C. Factors associated with the quality of life of subjects with facial disfigurement due to surgical treatment of head and neck cancer. *Med. Oral Patol. Oral Cir. Bucal.* **2018**, *23*, e132–e137. [CrossRef] [PubMed]
28. Chang, O.; Choi, E.K.; Kim, I.R.; Nam, S.J.; Lee, J.E.; Lee, S.K.; Im, Y.H.; Park, Y.H.; Cho, J. Association between socioeconomic status and altered appearance distress, body image, and quality of life among breast cancer patients. *Asian. Pac. J. Cancer. Prev.* **2014**, *15*, 8607–8612. [CrossRef]

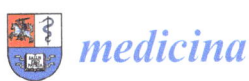

Article

Assessing the Opinion of Mothers about School-Based Sexual Education in Romania, the Country with the Highest Rate of Teenage Pregnancy in Europe

Magdalena Iorga [1,2], Lavinia-Maria Pop [2], Nicoleta Gimiga [3,4,*], Luminița Păduraru [3,5] and Smaranda Diaconescu [3,4]

1. Department of Behavioral Sciences, "Grigore T. Popa" University of Medicine and Pharmacy, 700115 Iasi, Romania; magdalena.iorga@umfiasi.ro
2. Faculty of Psychology and Education Sciences, "Alexandru Ioan Cuza" University, 700111 Iasi, Romania; lavinia.pop@student.uaic.ro
3. Department of Mother and Child, "Grigore T. Popa" University of Medicine and Pharmacy, 700115 Iasi, Romania; luminita.paduraru@umfiasi.ro (L.P.); smaranda.diaconescu@umfiasi.ro (S.D.)
4. "Saint Mary" Children Emergency Hospital of Iasi, 700309 Iasi, Romania
5. "Cuza Vodă" University Maternity Hospital, 700038 Iasi, Romania
* Correspondence: nicoleta.chiticariu@umfiasi.ro

Citation: Iorga, M.; Pop, L.-M.; Gimiga, N.; Păduraru, L.; Diaconescu, S. Assessing the Opinion of Mothers about School-Based Sexual Education in Romania, the Country with the Highest Rate of Teenage Pregnancy in Europe. *Medicina* 2021, 57, 841. https://doi.org/10.3390/medicina57080841

Academic Editor: Jimmy T. Efird

Received: 2 July 2021
Accepted: 16 August 2021
Published: 19 August 2021

Publisher's Note: MDPI stays neutral with regard to jurisdictional claims in published maps and institutional affiliations.

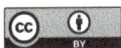

Copyright: © 2021 by the authors. Licensee MDPI, Basel, Switzerland. This article is an open access article distributed under the terms and conditions of the Creative Commons Attribution (CC BY) license (https://creativecommons.org/licenses/by/4.0/).

Abstract: *Background and Objectives:* Without mandatory school-based education, Romania is a leading European country in teen pregnancy. This survey aimed at assessing the level of knowledge and the opinions about sexual education and sexual-related issues among mothers of female teenagers aged 13–18 years old. *Material and Methods*: The survey was conducted between 2015 and 2017 and had four parts, collecting data about sociodemographic variables, the level of knowledge about sexuality, sexually transmitted diseases, and contraception. The respondents were mothers of female teenagers hospitalized in a tertiary pediatric clinic. Data were analyzed using IBM Statistical Package for Social Sciences (SPSS) Statistics for Windows, version 25 (Inc., Chicago, IL, USA). *Results*: One hundred and thirty-five mothers (42.46 ± 6.81 years old) were included in the research. Most of them were from rural areas, had graduated secondary school, were Christian-orthodox, married, and with a stable job. More than half of the mothers (61.42%) declared that they personally knew adolescents that were already mothers. In great proportion, mothers proved good knowledge about sexual education, contraception, and STDs. They considered that the minimum age for becoming married, in general, is about M = 18.62 ± 2.09 years old but in the case of their daughters, mothers appreciated that the best age would be 23.56 ± 9.37. Mothers considered that they had good communication with their daughters (M = 4.28 ± 0.99) and two-thirds sustained that they had discussed with them about sexual activity, pregnancy, sexually transmitted diseases, and contraception. In case of unwanted pregnancy of their daughters, one-third of the mothers (38.50%) would advise their girls to continue the pregnancy and 7.40% mentioned the termination of pregnancy. Two-thirds of them (74.10%) agreed to school-based sexual education. In the order of preferred sources for sexual education, mothers mentioned parents (85.90%), teachers (33.30%), and family doctors (24.40%). Comparative results regarding their own sex life and that of their daughters are presented. *Conclusions*: School-based programs should meet parental beliefs about sexuality and sexual education. School, as a creator of values and models, should find the golden ratio to better shape the personal, familial, and social needs for the healthy sexual behavior of the new generation.

Keywords: teenager; sex education; sexual health; pregnancy; teenage pregnancy; sexually transmitted diseases; contraception; communication

1. Introduction

Despite the widely recognized importance of sexual health for the normal development of a person, the education programs to promote it have remained a sensitive and sometimes controversial issue. The World Health Organization (WHO) emphasized the importance of healthy sexual development to overall mental and physical well-being [1].

One of the main controversial ideas studied in many cultures and countries was about who is more entitled to educate children and adolescents about sexuality and healthy sexual activity. Many studies point out that parents are generally not prepared to provide complete education about sexuality. Therefore, as Shtarkshall et al. (2007) identified, health and educational systems have the obligation to provide sex education for adolescents and young adults, taking into consideration the social and familial values with respect and professionalism [2].

School-based sex education is a sensitive topic that divides opinion in all nations. A study conducted by Saarreharju et al. (2020) after the 2015 curriculum reform on sex education in Canada, for example, emphasized that the most significant topics that parents and community were interested in were children's rights and adults' values, political dimensions of the curriculum reform, and appropriate timing for sex education [3]. The unsuccessful attempt of the United Kingdom (UK) Government to insert sex education as a statutory part of the National Curriculum also determined many debates. Those who were willing to introduce sex education in schools were focusing on promoting the virtue of respect for every adult's right to sexual self-determination [4]. In Japan, where sexuality education programs were implemented in junior high schools, parents appreciated that school was a more appropriate setting than home for teaching the physiological aspects of sexuality and for providing accurate information about sexual life and intimate relationship [5].

Many debates were developed in the United States of America (USA). For example, Gresle-Favier (2013) pointed that there was adult discrimination against children because the sex education presented abstinence-only programs [6]. In Argentina, Ambrosius (2019) showed that there was a position of domination that remained intact over the years, as children were still seen as passive subjects, unable to understand or reconstruct the social world around them [7]. Similarly, in Sweden, researchers found that parents sustained sex education in school and the delivery of diverse information, such as sexual-related risks and porn-related issues, but programs did not present information related to harm or how to avoid it [8].

Delivering information about sex determines a huge debate in many countries that want to implement such programs, especially because the information that is delivered to students must meet the family, community, and society's opinions. The scientific literature about this topic is not rich. Cultural aspects, community rules, sex debates propagated by media, religious issues, parents' reluctance, ethnicity, and ethical concerns usually limit the chances to conduct studies on children, teenagers, or caregivers. The topic was related to moral norms and parents' consent about the proper age when sexual education must be taught but, on the other hand, the need for delivering the truth about a consensual sexual relationship, sexual criminality, sexual abuse, human sexual traffic, child marriage, teenage pregnancy, and how to recognize abuse and look for help also generated a lot of discussions among parents' associations, non-governmental associations, and education policymakers [9]. In Sweden, parents' attitudes regarding sex education were found to be related to the sex of the parent and the sex and age of the child. Additionally, the link between parents' attitudes and young people's sexual activities, especially online ones, appeared to be mediated by parental rules [10].

Given that mothers play an important role in the sexual education of their daughters, it is important to understand their views about sexual practice and health-related problems, as well as their opinions about the implementation of educational programs in schools. In general, formal sexuality education programming falls into one of the following two categories: abstinence-only (focusing on delaying partnered sex until marriage), and comprehensive sexuality education (discussing delayed sex until marriage, information about birth control, safe sex practices, contraception, and sexually transmitted infections). The new program models must facilitate collaboration between parents, educators, and health professionals to effectively provide sex education to young people [11].

The importance of sexual education must not be neglected since teenagers must be informed that sexual-related characteristics and sexually active life are influenced by a lot of factors. Studies [12–14] have proved that early menarche is related to a high body mass index, diets, poor nutrition, and low physical activity; thus, explaining these risks could increase the quality of life among teenagers. Additionally, early sexual contact is related to a high risk of pregnancy and birth, dropping out of school, and poor socio-economic outcomes and health. Married girls are ten times more likely to drop out than their unmarried peers, and pregnant teenagers are more prone to experience pregnancy and postnatal complications. Female teenagers with an early age at their first sexual act were found to be more prone to experience non-consensual sexual relationships, unwanted pregnancy, and a high frequency of sexually transmitted diseases. Because family models and parental beliefs are important factors in shaping female teenagers' paths for education, marriage, and life, teaching sexual education in school is intrinsically related to family, community, and social norms.

Romania reported in 2011 around 34,700 teen pregnancies among females 15–19 years of age. With a pregnancy rate of 61% and a birth rate of 35%, Romania has the highest rates in Europe [15,16]. Because Romania has an increasing rate of teenage pregnancy, we wanted to identify the level of mothers' knowledge about sexuality, and to assess their opinions about sexual programs in school. About 16 million girls 15 to 19 years old, and another one million girls under 15 give birth every year, most in low- and middle-income countries [17].

Few studies are focusing on sexual education in Romania, especially among teenagers. Some of the research conducted in Romania by the same extended team pointed to the socio-economic and educational factors that increased the risks for teenage pregnancy and the medical-related problems for both adolescent mothers and babies. Additionally, we proved that usually, the partner of a pregnant teenager is traditionally an older man that used age as a reason to not utilize contraceptive methods as condoms. Similarly, our previous studies showed that the younger the pregnant adolescent was, the more prone she was to become a mother again in the very next year [16,18,19].

The goal of the present research was to identify to what extent mothers could provide a proper sexual education for their daughters, and to find their opinions about it. We collected data about sexual-related information and practices such as the age of sexual contact, contraception, the level of knowledge about sexually transmitted diseases, the role of parents and teachers in teaching sexual education, etc. The research also evaluated mothers' sexual behaviors, the knowledge about the daughter's sexual life, and sexual-related information, as well as personal experiences.

2. Materials and Methods

This survey was developed as part of larger research with the purpose to identify the level of knowledge of hospitalized female patients' mothers registered in Saint Mary University Hospital for Children about sexually transmitted diseases, the risk of pregnancy, methods of contraceptives, and to assess attitudes and behaviors related to sexual activity among daughters.

2.1. Participants and Data Collection

The survey was distributed between September 2016 and November 2017 among mothers who visited their daughters while they were hospitalized in a pediatric tertiary center. The caregivers were informed about the purpose of the research, and they were assured about the confidentiality of data. No incentives were offered to the voluntary respondents. Informed consent was previously obtained from the mothers. The inclusion criteria were parents that had at least one female teenager (aged 13–18 years) hospitalized during the considered period, agreeing to sign the informed consent. Exclusion criteria: mothers aged under 18, mothers of pregnant teenagers, mothers of normal children (with no psychological or psychiatric diagnostic, no medical disease that impacted physical growth and sexuality, such as genetic disorders).

The survey was delivered to all one hundred and fifty-two mothers who visited their daughters during hospitalization. The response rate was 95%. We excluded ten questionnaires because the respondents filled them in, but the informed consent was not signed. Finally, one hundred and thirty-five forms were included in our databases and considered for the present research.

2.2. Instruments

A questionnaire was constructed in purpose for this research and contained four parts:
- The first part collected sociodemographic data such as age, gender, religion, number of children, marital status, level of education, environment, monthly income, alcohol abuse or physical abuse, and information about the relationships between the family members.
- The second part gathered information about sexual-related data and sexual life such as the age at which they had their first menstruation, the age at which they had their first sexual contact, from whom they received the first information about menstruation, if they knew the term sex education, if they knew the term contraception, and if they used contraception, as well as if they had information about diseases with sexual transmission.
- The third part contained items to identify the extent to which mothers considered themselves informed about their daughters' lives and sexual activity and whether they had begun sexual activity. The questions focused on whether mothers knew that girls had/did not have a partner, whether girls already had menstruation, whether they had told them about menstruation, who would like to deliver sex education to their daughters, whether they had talked to their daughters about sexual activity, pregnancy, sexually transmitted diseases, or methods of contraception.
- The fourth part of the questionnaire had items that wanted to identify the mothers' opinions about specific situations, such as what advice they would give to their daughters in case they became pregnant, what contraceptive methods would be appropriate for their daughters to use, if they would agree that their daughters should have sex before marriage, at what age they would like their daughters to marry and at what age they considered as appropriate for their daughters to have their first child.

2.3. Statistical Analysis

All analyses were performed using the IBM Statistical Package for Social Sciences (SPSS) Statistics for Windows, version 25 (Inc., Chicago, IL, USA). The descriptive statistics of socio-demographic data were expressed as means and standard deviations (SD), frequencies and percentages. The Mann–Whitney test was performed for the comparative analysis among categories. The correlation analysis was performed using the Spearman correlations. The level of statistical significance was set at $p < 0.05$.

2.4. Ethical Approval

The present study was conducted in accordance with the Declaration of Helsinki and the protocol was approved by the Ethical Committee of Saint Mary Emergency Hospital for Children, number 23403/30.10.2015, as part of a larger study supported by the European Society of Contraception and Reproductive Health. The project was entitled "Identifying and tackling economic, cultural, and social factors that lead to inappropriate sexual education in Romanian teens" (P-2015-A-05). Informed consent was obtained from all mothers included in the research.

3. Results

Sociodemographic data and medical characteristics were collected. Additionally, the answers for items regarding mothers' opinions were analyzed.

3.1. Sociodemographic and Family-Related Data

Sociodemographic data were gathered, together with the financial status, environment characteristics, and family-related information. All questioned participants were mothers aged 42.46 ± 6.81 (minimum of 29, maximum of 55 years old), most of them being married or in a relationship, Christian-orthodox, and coming from rural areas.

Detailed results about marital status, level of education, number of children, employment, and the presence of adverse experiences such as alcohol consumption or physical abuse between partners are presented in Table 1.

Table 1. Sociodemographic characteristics [1].

Sociodemographic Characteristics	%/M ± SD
Age	42.46 ± 6.81
Environment	
Urban	36.60
Rural	63.40
Religion	
Christian-orthodox	92.50
Catholic	4.50
Pentecostal	3.00
Level of education	
Primary school	4.50
Secondary school	42.20
High school	39.80
University	12.50
Nationality/Ethnicity	
Romanian	97.00
Roma	2.30
Others	0.70
Number of children	
One child	20.70
Two children	37.00
Three children	18.50
Four children	3.70
Five children	5.20
Six children	5.20
More than six	9.70
Marital status	
Married/in relationship	80.92
Single/divorced/widow	19.08
Employment	
Employed (stable job)	50.81
Unemployed (temporary without job)	18.55
Housewife	30.65
Partner working abroad	20.10
Partner is an alcoholic	10.69
Partner is a physical aggressor	1.55

[1] Number of answers (N) and percentage (%); means and standard deviations (M ± SD).

3.2. Level of Knowledge about Sexually Transmitted Diseases, Sexual Education, and Contraception

A series of items were formulated to identify the level of knowledge about sexually transmitted diseases, healthy sexual behaviors, preventive measures, and sexual activity.

Most mothers had knowledge about sexually transmitted diseases (83.08%). They were also asked to declare which STD they knew and how they can be transmitted. The analysis of data revealed that mothers had knowledge about the following STDs: syphilis (61.54%), HIV (80.77%), trichomoniasis (8.46%), candidosis (25.38%), gonorrhea (20.77%), B Hepatitis (43.08%), and chlamydia (7.69%).

The analysis of data showed that more than two-thirds of the respondents (86.7%) knew what the term sex education meant and what it referred to, what contraception was (84.40%), and that they knew contraceptive methods (86.70%).

One item investigated how many contraceptive methods they knew, and 74.10% mentioned oral contraceptives, 66.70% condoms, and 43% mentioned as a contraceptive method "the use of calendar".

More than half of the mothers (61.42%) declared that they personally knew adolescents that were already mothers. Additionally, we identified that the minimum age that mothers considered proper for marriage was M = 18.62 ± 2.09 years old.

3.3. Medical and Sexual Related Characteristics of Mothers

Mothers were asked about the first age at which the menstruation occurred and at what age they had their first sexual intercourse. Data about the age of marriage, when they became mothers for the first time, or who were the sources of information (mothers, siblings, teachers, friends) were also collected. Detailed results are presented in Table 2.

Table 2. Sexual-related information data.

Items	M ± SD [1]
Age at which menstruation occurred	13.50 ± 1.64
Age of first sexual contact	19.50 ± 2.76
Age at which they married	21.27 ± 3.51
Age at which they had their first child	22.23 ± 4.71
From whom they received the first information about menstruation	
Parents	75.63
Siblings	6.72
Friends	7.54
Teachers/school staff	6.72
Others	3.39

[1] Means and standard deviations (M ± SD).

3.4. The Mother–Daughter Relationship and the Impact on Sexual Education

The mothers were asked to rate, on a five point Likert-like scale (from 1—*extremely poor*—to 5—*extremely good*), their satisfaction concerning the communication with their daughters. The statistical analysis proved a score of M = 4.28 ± 0.99, meaning that mothers appreciated that they had good communication with their offspring. Detailed results are presented in Table 3.

A series of items were formulated to investigate what kind of contraception methods they counselled their daughters to use. The most frequent mentioned contraceptives methods were condoms (36.30%) and oral pills (34.80%). A smaller percentage mentioned "the use of calendar" (8.10%) and a smaller percentage, about 7.40%, considered that the partner must take precautions to not impregnate the teenage girl.

In case of unwanted pregnancy, one-third of the mothers (38.50%) would advise their girls to continue the pregnancy, or let the adolescents choose for themselves (28.10%), 11.90% considered that in case of pregnancy their daughters must marry, 7.40% would prefer that their offspring choose termination of the pregnancy, and 1.50% mentioned that probably the girl would be sent to live with her partner. A total of 12.60% of questioned mothers mentioned that they had no idea what to tell their daughters.

The analysis of answers proved that mothers appreciated that the most frequent risks related to teen pregnancy were school dropout (68.30%) and psychological trauma (59.20%).

Table 3. Items focusing on mothers' level of knowledge about their daughters' sexuality and sexual activity.

Items	M ± SD [1]
At what age did your daughter have her first period?	12.47 ± 1.29
At what age did you tell your daughter about menstruation?	10.77 ± 2.61
Did you talk to your daughter about sexual activity, pregnancy, STD or contraception?	
Yes	72.40
Is your daughter sexually active?	
Yes	14.10
No	74.10
I do not know	11.80
Does your daughter have a partner?	
Yes	37.80
No	55.60
I do not know	6.60
Has your daughter ever become pregnant?	
Yes	3.70
No	93.30
I do not know	3.00
If your daughter became pregnant, would you share it with your spouse?	
Yes	84.40
No	0.70
I do not know	14.70
Among your daughter's friends, are there teenagers who became pregnant?	
Yes	20.00
No	54.80
I do not know	25.20
Do you agree that your daughter should have sex before marriage?	
Yes	31.10
No	37.10
I do not know	31.80
At what age would you like your daughter to marry?	23.56 ± 9.37
At what age would you like your daughter to have her first child?	24.83 ± 3.06

[1] Percentages (%); means and standard deviations (M ± SD).

3.5. The Opinion about School-Based Sexual Education

Mothers were asked if they would like their daughters to have sex education classes at school: 74.10% agreed that their daughters had sexual education in school, 10.40% disagreed with it, 12.6% sustained that they did not know, and 3% mentioned that it was too early for their daughters to have classes about sexual education.

One item investigated mothers' opinion about who would be more appropriate to teach sexual education. The frequency of answers showed that the more preferred sources were parents, teachers, and family doctors. Detailed results are presented in Table 4.

Table 4. The frequency of answers to the item who do you think should teach your daughter about sex education [1].

Who Do You Think Should Teach Your Daughter about Sex Education?	Yes (%)
Parents	85.90
Teachers/school staff	33.30
Friends	1.50
Siblings	5.09
Priest	3.70
Family doctor	24.40

[1] Percentages (%).

There were significant differences in the level of education of mothers regarding certain items. Mothers who had low levels of education, namely, lower secondary school, had on average a higher number of children (Mdn = 3) than mothers who had a university level of education (Mdn = 2), $p = 0.005$. In addition, mothers with a lower level of education married earlier and had their first child at a younger age as opposed to participants who reported a higher level of education. Family income was considerably higher for mothers with a higher level of education, and the number of methods of contraception was better known among mothers with a higher level of education. The detailed results for these items are presented in Table 5.

Table 5. Comparative results considering the level of education [1].

Items	Mann–Whitney U	Z	p	Secondary School	University Studies
The number of children you had	226.500	−2.836	0.005	3	2
At what age did you marry?	64.500	−5.069	0.000	19	24
At what age did you have your first child?	56.000	−5.238	0.000	20	24.5
The family's monthly income	71.000	−4.960	0.000	1	5
What methods of contraception did you know?	145.000	−4.112	0.000	2	3

[1] Median, Mann–Whitney results.

The correlational analysis showed that there were significant associations between the age at which mothers gave birth to their first child and certain variables. We identified that the more mothers gave birth to younger children, the higher the number of children in the family ($r = -0.395$ **, $p < 0.001$). The age at which mothers gave birth to their first child was positively correlated with the onset of menarche, in the sense that the higher the age of onset of the first menstruation, the higher the age at which mothers give birth to the first child ($r = 0.217$ *, $p = 0.029$). At the same time, the correlational analysis showed that the older the age at which mothers wanted their daughters to marry, the higher the age at which mothers wanted their daughters to become pregnant with their first child ($r = 0.824$ **, $p < 0.001$).

The results showed that the younger the mothers, the lower the level of education, the age of the first sexual contact, the age at which mothers married and gave birth to their first child were. Negative correlations existed between mothers' ages and the level of education ($r = -0.270$ *, $p = 0.049$), the age of first sexual intercourse ($r = -0.518$ **, $p < 0.001$), the age at which they married ($r = -0.479$ **, $p < 0.001$) and the age at which they had their first child ($r = -0.562$ **, $p < 0.001$). The level of education correlated positively with the mothers' age of marriage ($r = 0.629$ **, $p < 0.001$) and the age at which they gave birth to the first child ($r = 0.640$ **, $p < 0.001$). The analysis of data also revealed that the more educated the mothers were, the more they would marry and give birth to the first child later.

The family income correlated positively with the mother's level of education ($r = 0.625$ **, $p < 0.001$), the age at which the mothers married ($r = 0.419$ **, $p < 0.001$), and the age at which they gave birth to the first child ($r = 0.494$ **, $p < 0.001$), in the sense that the higher the family income, the higher the level of education and the age at which the mothers married at, respectively, gave birth to the first child. At the same time, family income correlated negatively with the number of children in the household because the higher the family income, the lower the number of children in the household ($r = -0.357$ **, $p < 0.001$).

4. Discussion

Numerous studies have pointed to the need for sexual education among children and teenagers and identified that schools and parents were the most important sources of knowledge. Many countries have implemented sexual education programs. Education for sex and sexuality was proved to positively impact adolescents' knowledge about sexual activity, safe sex behavior, contraception, and how to avoid sexual abuse, teenage pregnancy, sexually transmitted diseases, and risk for pornography and bullying. Healthy sexual activity has a great impact on physical, psychological, and social status [2,8,9].

There are many educators regarding sexuality and sexual activity: family, school, church, media, society, peers, etc. The results of the present study are important to shape the context of future school-based programs in Romania. Different results were also pointed out by the scientific literature, and they are diverse and contradictory. For example, a study conducted in Israel identified that most of both male and female students from secondary schools mentioned school as their preferred source of sex education and evaluated home as their last choice. The same study identified that only one-quarter of teenagers wanted parents to be their primary source of information regarding sexuality and sex life [20]. A study developed in the United Kingdom suggested that one-third of the adolescents preferred to receive additional information about sex from parents (33%) and schools (34%) [21].

In general, the scientific literature focused on the opinion of parents about sexuality and sex education in family and school. Diverse studies were conducted in different countries where this topic is a taboo or included a different population where sex education was limited by the national curricula. For example, Iranian parents considered that sexual health-related information must be trained through life and practice and, therefore, education in school is not necessary. The questioned parents stated that sexual health education encouraged children to be rude [22]. In opposition with these results, Reza et al. (2020) pointed out that Indonesian parents agreed that children must be trained by knowing parts of the body that may or may not be touched by others, covering up the genitals, and acknowledging who can hug and kiss the cheek of a child, knowing the abusive behavior and how to reject and report it [23]. Nair et al. (2012) conducted a study on Indian parents. The authors identified that more than half of them were not sure whether information on various reproductive and sexual health topics should be given to adolescents and were not sure about the way to inform their offspring about it [24]. McKibben (2017) identified that sex education in the UK must take into consideration gender risks. The author identified that targeting grooming and problematic sexual behavior is mandatory in children and adolescents, and formal content of the sex education must focus on sexual health, normal sexual development, mutual consent, the minimum age for sexual contact, gender stereotypes, grooming and sexual abuse, pornography, and healthy sexual life [25]. The same ideas were developed by Green and Mason (2002) who also found that girls conflated love and sex, whereas boys constructed sex as a physical conquest. This type of construction made girls extremely vulnerable to sexual exploitation, especially female adolescents with no families to support them or those living in residential children's homes [26].

Jankovic et al. (2013) identified that most Croatian parents found it inappropriate to be talked to about sexual satisfaction and pleasure, masturbation, pornography, and prostitution [27]. On the other hand, Baker (2016) showed that British teachers and professionals in the UK declared that since the Internet made sexually explicit information more accessible to young people, this could have a negative impact on their sexual development and future relationships during their lifetime. The study revealed that young people and teachers considered that there were numerous negative effects of viewing pornography, especially online, and this topic must be discussed during classes at a young age [28].

Some authors counselled that the precise age at which this information should be provided is closely related to the physical, emotional, and intellectual development of the child. Some studies identified that the proper age was differently mentioned by mothers. For example, more than 60% of Nigerian women considered that children had to be informed about sexual-related issues before the age of ten [29].

Opara et al. (2010) identified that whereas almost half of the mothers found out about menstruation from their mothers, only thirteen (8.2%) of the questioned mothers discussed menstruation with their daughters. Educated mothers proved to be more aware of the importance of sexual education among offspring and were more willing to communicate with their children about sexual activity, contraception, and sexually transmitted diseases [29]. Kose et al. (2014) identified significant correlations between the educational status of the mothers and their knowledge about HPV vaccination but no significant correlation in terms of economic conditions [30]. Similar results were provided by a study conducted in nine European countries and revealed that maternal support and the maternal level of knowledge about sexuality are negatively correlated to the early initiation [31]. Genz et al. (2017) identified that 89.2% of the teenage girls were able to properly define the concept of a sexually transmitted disease [32] and Doreto et al. (2007) showed that teenagers knew of five to six sexually transmitted diseases, such as syphilis (35.6%), genital herpes (33.3%), gonorrhea (30.0%), and HPV (27.2%) [33]. Early pregnancy was related to an older partner [18] less interested in contraception. The evidence suggested that much of the adolescent sexual activity is spontaneous, unplanned, and sometimes involuntary [34], and that the most common profile of patients looking for care for sexually transmitted diseases is men with a high level of education, poor use of condoms, and a high number of partners [35].

Mothers' age at which menarche occurred was about 13.50 ± 1.64 and in what their daughters were concerned, the respondents mentioned 12.47 ± 1.29 years old. Our results are congruent with those from the scientific literature. Menarche occurs between the ages of 10 and 16 years in most girls in developed countries. Over the past century, the age at menarche has fallen in industrialized countries, but that trend has stopped and may even be reversing. In 1840, the average age at menarche was 16.5 years but nowadays it is 13 [36]. The same trend was registered in many studies from different countries: in Norway, Gottschalk et al. (2020) developed a study on an extremely large population of women and showed that the mean age at menarche was 13.42 years among women born during 1936–1939, and 13.24 years (95%) among women born during 1960–1964 [37]. A study conducted by Biro et al. (2018) on American female teenagers identified that the median age at menarche overall was 12.25 year [38]. Meng et al. (2017) also found a continuous downward secular trend of age at menarche for Chinese girls in both urban and rural areas, who were born from 1973 to 2004 [39].

Our research showed that the age mothers married at was 21.27 ± 3.51. They also appreciated that the minimum age for marriage should be about $M = 18.62 \pm 2.09$ years old, but in the case of their daughters, the statistical analysis proved that they would prefer an older age (23.56 ± 9.37). Therefore, compared to their own experience, mothers would like their daughters to marry later than they did.

Our survey showed that mothers appreciated that the most frequent risks related to teen pregnancy were school dropout (68.30%) and psychological trauma (59.20%), but a lot of researchers identified that there was a high risk for physical health as for psychological health among teenage mothers. For example, Paul (2018) proved that an early maternal age at marriage substantially increased the risk of adverse pregnancy outcomes (pregnancy and post-natal complications) [40]. These results strongly suggested that the existing laws and policies must be strengthened to decrease the age at pregnancy or marriage among teenagers [41].

We identified that more than two-thirds of the mothers considered that school-based sexual education was useful for their daughters but also suggested that the main sources for education were parents, teachers, and family doctors. Our results are congruent with those from other countries. Shams et al. (2017) conducted a study on Iranian mothers and showed that the respondents believed that limited sexual health education for adolescent girls was necessary. The authors stated that mothers must be trained how to deliver sexual education to their daughters and identified that trained mothers were best equipped to educate their daughters. Special training on communication, sexual health education, and how to develop a good relationship between parent and child were appreciated as being the key to empowering mothers to be ready to educate their daughters regarding sexual life and to answer their children's questions regarding sexual issues at any age [21]. Lefkowitz et al. (2000) showed that a trained mother talked more freely about sexuality to their daughters and acted less judgmental [42].

4.1. Reflections and Planning

The opinion about sexual education is influenced by familial, social, and community norms, peers' influences, religious beliefs, or own experience—the relationship with parents, especially mothers, the level of education for both teenagers and parents, the relationship with the partner (mutual consent or abuse); sexual education must take into consideration a lot of factors. School and family are the most secure environments and many policymakers had to tailor the program for teenagers to satisfy the triad adolescent–family–school. The results of the present study highlighted this idea, investigating mothers from both hypostases: mothers of teenage daughters and those of former teenage daughters.

4.2. Strengths and Limitations of the Study

The most important strength of the study was that the results covered a great gap of scientific information related to the impact of sexual education on adolescent's life and the opinions of mothers, as one of the main important sources of education for girls.

The second strength was due to the study population; Romanian teenagers are among the high-risk populations with continuously increasing rates of unwanted pregnancies and births in girls under the age of 18. Therefore, the present paper focused on what mothers know about their daughters' sexual lives and how they can help them.

Our study presented some limitations. First, the research was conducted in a single-center hospital for children. Even if the University hospital gathers patients from almost one-quarter of the country and the results can be generalized for the Romanian teenage population, it must be treated with precociousness by other countries because it was already proved by the scientific literature that national laws, community rules, and religious aspects must be always taken into consideration when collecting data about sexual activity. Secondly, the results obtained were specific for the Romanian population (considering that race is related to different ages at menarche, for example) or that the present study did not take into consideration other variables (such as high body mass index, poor nutrition, low physical activity or a low financial status that proved to be related to earlier menarche). Additionally, only mothers who had a comfortable literacy level agreed to fill in the questionnaire, limiting the investigated population.

5. Conclusions

A school-based program should rely on parental beliefs and the family–adolescent relationship, considering that parental sexual education and school-based sexual education are not congruent. That is why school, as a creator of values and models, must find the golden ratio to satisfy family, community, and social norms, and to preserve a healthy physical and psychological healthy generation.

Author Contributions: Conceptualization, S.D. and M.I.; Data curation, L.P. and N.G.; Formal analysis, L.-M.P. and M.I.; Investigation, S.D., N.G., L.P. and M.I.; Methodology, L.-M.P., N.G. and M.I.; Supervision, M.I.; Writing—original draft, M.I., S.D. and L.-M.P.; Writing—review and editing, L.-M.P. and M.I. All authors have read and agreed to the published version of the manuscript.

Funding: The research was part of the project Identifying and tackling economic, cultural and social factors that lead to inappropriate sexual education in Romanian teens (P-2015-A-05) funded by the European Society of Contraception and Reproductive Health.

Institutional Review Board Statement: The study was conducted according to the guidelines of the Declaration of Helsinki and approved by the Ethical Committee of "Sf. Maria" Clinical Emergency Hospital for Children no. 23403/30.10.2015.

Informed Consent Statement: Informed consent was obtained from all subjects involved in the study.

Data Availability Statement: Data available upon request from corresponding author.

Conflicts of Interest: The authors declare no conflict of interest.

References

1. World Health Organization. Department of Economic and Social Affairs, United Nations (UN) Population Division. In *Report of the International Conference on Population and Development, Cairo, Egypt, 5–13 September 1994*; United Nations: New York, NY, USA, 1994.
2. Shtarkshall, R.A.; Santelli, J.S.; Hirsch, J.S. Sex education and sexual socialization: Roles for educators and parents. *Perspect. Sex. Reprod. Health* **2007**, *39*, 116–119. [CrossRef] [PubMed]
3. Saarreharju, M.; Uusiautti, S.; Määttä, K. It goes beyond the fundamentals of sex and education. Analysis on the online commenting on the curriculum reform in Ontario. *Int. J. Adolesc. Youth* **2020**, *25*, 609–623. [CrossRef]
4. Steutel, J.; De Ruyter, D.J. What should be the moral aims of compulsory sex education? *Br. J. Educ. Stud.* **2011**, *59*, 75–86. [CrossRef]
5. Hashimoto, N.; Shinohara, H.; Tashiro, M.; Suzuki, S.; Hirose, H.; Ikeya, H.; Ushitora, K.; Komiya, A.; Watanabe, M.; Motegi, T.; et al. Sexuality education in junior high schools in Japan. *Sex Educ.* **2012**, *12*, 25–46. [CrossRef]
6. Greslé-Favier, C. Adult discrimination against children: The case of abstinence-only education in twenty-first-century USA. *Sex Educ.* **2013**, *13*, 715–725. [CrossRef]
7. Ambrosius, M.B. Childhood as Subject of Rights? Children & Adolescents through the Socio-Legal Discourse in Argentina's Sexual Education Act. *Sortuz Oñati J. Emergent Socio-Leg. Stud.* **2019**, *10*, 1–24.
8. Spišák, S. Everywhere they say that it's harmful but they don't say how, so I'm asking here': Young people, pornography and negotiations with notions of risk and harm. *Sex Educ.* **2016**, *16*, 130–142. [CrossRef]
9. Cornelius, J.B.; Whitaker-Brown, C.; Neely, T.; Kennedy, A.; Okoro, F. Mobile phone, social media usage, and perceptions of delivering a social media safer sex intervention for adolescents: Results from two countries. *Adolesc. Health Med. Ther.* **2019**, *10*, 29. [CrossRef]
10. Sorbring, E.; Hallberg, J.; Bohlin, M.; Skoog, T. Parental attitudes and young people's online sexual activities. *Sex Educ.* **2015**, *15*, 129–143. [CrossRef]
11. Lamb, S.; Pagán-Ortiz, M.; Bonilla, S. How to Provide Sexual Education: Lessons from a Pandemic on Masculinity, Individualism, and the Neoliberal Agenda. *Int. J. Environ. Res. Public Health* **2021**, *18*, 4144. [CrossRef]
12. Budu, E.; Ahinkorah, B.O.; Seidu, A.-A.; Hagan, J.E., Jr.; Agbemavi, W.; Frimpong, J.B.; Adu, C.; Dickson, K.S.; Yaya, S. Child Marriage and Sexual Autonomy among Women in Sub-Saharan Africa: Evidence from 31 Demographic and Health Surveys. *Int. J. Environ. Res. Public Health* **2021**, *18*, 3754. [CrossRef] [PubMed]
13. Ivanova, O.; Rai, M.; Michielsen, K.; Dias, S. How Sexuality Education Programs Have Been Evaluated in Low- and Lower-Middle-Income Countries? A Systematic Review. *Int. J. Environ. Res. Public Health* **2020**, *17*, 8183. [CrossRef] [PubMed]
14. Lyu, J.; Shen, X.; Hesketh, T. Sexual Knowledge, Attitudes and Behaviours among Undergraduate Students in China—Implications for Sex Education. *Int. J. Environ. Res. Public Health* **2020**, *17*, 6716. [CrossRef]
15. Sedgh, G.; Finer, L.B.; Bankole, A.; Eilers, M.A.; Singh, S. Adolescent pregnancy, birth, and abortion rates across countries: Levels and recent trends. *J. Adolesc. Health* **2015**, *56*, 223–230. [CrossRef]
16. Socolov, D.G.; Iorga, M.; Carauleanu, A.; Ilea, C.; Blidaru, I.; Boiculese, L.; Socolov, R.V. Pregnancy during adolescence and associated risks: An 8-year hospital-based cohort study (2007–2014) in Romania, the country with the highest rate of teenage pregnancy in Europe. *BioMed Res. Int.* **2017**, *2017*, 9205016. [CrossRef] [PubMed]
17. World Health Organisation. Adolescent Pregnancy. Fact Sheet N°364. 2014. Available online: http://www.who.int/mediacentre/factsheets/fs364/en/ (accessed on 20 April 2021).
18. Iorga, M.; Socolov, R.V.; Socolov, D.G. An 8 Years Analysis of Pregnancies and Births among Teenagers in a University Hospital in North-Eastern Romania. *Rev. Cercet. Interv. Soc.* **2016**, *52*, 55–65.
19. Diaconescu, S.; Ciuhodaru, T.; Cazacu, C.; Sztankovszky, L.Z.; Kantor, C.; Iorga, M. Teenage Mothers, an Increasing Social Phenomenon in Romania. Causes, Consequences and Solutions. *Rev. Cercet. Interv. Soc.* **2015**, *51*, 162–175.
20. Shtarkshall, R.A.; Carmel, S.; Woloski-Wruble, A. Survey on Sexual Knowledge. In *Attitudes and Practices in the General Educational System in Israel*; Israeli Ministry of Health: Jerusalem, Israel, 2002.
21. Macdowall, W.; Wellings, K.; Mercer, C.H.; Nanchahal, K.; Copas, A.J.; McManus, S.; Fenton, K.A.; Erens, B.; Johnson, A.M. Learning about sex: Results from Natsal 2000. *Health Educ. Behav.* **2006**, *33*, 802–811. [CrossRef] [PubMed]
22. Shams, M.; Mousavizadeh, A.; Majdpour, M. Mothers' views about sexual health education for their adolescent daughters: A qualitative study. *Reprod. Health* **2017**, *14*, 24. [CrossRef]
23. Reza, M.; Ningrum, M.A.; Saroinsong, W.P.; Maulidiyah, E.C.; Fitri, R. Trial Design of Sexual Education Module on Children. In *1st International Conference on Early Childhood Care Education and Parenting (ICECCEP 2019)*; Atlantis Press: Amsterdam, The Netherlands, 2020; pp. 108–110. [CrossRef]
24. Nair, M.K.C.; Leena, M.L.; Paul, M.K.; Pillai, H.V.; Babu, G.; Russell, P.S.; Thankachi, Y. Attitude of parents and teachers towards adolescent reproductive and sexual health education. *Indian J. Pediatrics* **2012**, *79*, 60–63. [CrossRef]
25. McKibbin, G. Preventing Harmful Sexual Behaviour and Child Sexual Exploitation for children & young people living in residential care: A scoping review in the Australian context. *Child. Youth Serv. Rev.* **2017**, *82*, 373–382. [CrossRef]
26. Green, L.; Masson, H. Adolescents who sexually abuse and residential accommodation: Issues of risk and vulnerability. *Br. J. Soc. Work* **2002**, *32*, 149–168. [CrossRef]

27. Jankovic, S.; Malatestinic, G.; Bencevic Striehl, H. Parents' Attitudes on Sexual Education–What and When? *Coll. Antropol.* **2013**, *37*, 17–22. [PubMed]
28. Baker, K.E. Online pornography–Should schools be teaching young people about the risks? An exploration of the views of young people and teaching professionals. *Sex Educ.* **2016**, *16*, 213–228. [CrossRef]
29. Opara, P.I.; Eke, G.K.; Akani, N.A. Mothers' perception of sexuality education for children. *Niger. J. Med.* **2010**, *19*, 168–172. [CrossRef] [PubMed]
30. Kose, D.; Erkorkmaz, U.; Cinar, N.; Altinkaynak, S. Mothers' knowledge and attitudes about HPV vaccination to prevent cervical cancers. *Asian Pac. J. Cancer Prev.* **2014**, *15*, 7263–7266. [CrossRef] [PubMed]
31. Madkour, A.S.; Farhat, T.; Halpern, C.T.; Gabhainn, S.N.; Godeau, E. Parents' support and knowledge of their daughters' lives, and females' early sexual initiation in nine European countries. *Perspect. Sex. Reprod. Health* **2012**, *44*, 167–175. [CrossRef]
32. Genz, N.; Meincke, S.M.K.; Carret, M.L.V.; Corrêa, A.C.L.; Alves, C.N. Sexually transmitted diseases: Knowledge and sexual behavior of adolescents. *Texto Contexto Enferm.* **2017**, *26*, e5100015. [CrossRef]
33. Doreto, D.T.; Vieira, E.M. O conhecimento sobre doenças sexualmente transmissíveis entre adolescentes de baixa renda em Ribeirão Preto, São Paulo, Brasil. *Cad. Saúde Publica* **2007**, *23*, 2511–2516. [CrossRef]
34. Charles, J.M.; Rycroft-Malone, J.; Hendry, M.; Pasterfield, D.; Whitaker, R. Reducing repeat pregnancies in adolescence: Applying realist principles as part of a mixed-methods systematic review to explore what works, for whom, how and under what circumstances. *BMC Pregnancy Childbirth* **2016**, *16*, 1–10. [CrossRef]
35. Fasciana, T.; Capra, G.; Di Carlo, P.; Calà, C.; Vella, M.; Pistone, G.; Colomba, C.; Giammanco, A. Socio-Demographic Characteristics and Sexual Behavioral Factors of Patients with Sexually Transmitted Infections Attending a Hospital in Southern Italy. *Int. J. Environ. Res. Public Health* **2021**, *18*, 4722. [CrossRef] [PubMed]
36. Rees, M. The age of menarche. ORGYN Organon's Mag. *Women Health* **1995**, *4*, 2–4.
37. Gottschalk, M.S.; Eskild, A.; Hofvind, S.; Gran, J.M.; Bjelland, E.K. Temporal trends in age at menarche and age at menopause: A population study of 312 656 women in Norway. *Hum. Reprod.* **2020**, *35*, 464–471. [CrossRef]
38. Biro, F.M.; Pajak, A.; Wolff, M.S.; Pinney, S.M.; Windham, G.C.; Galvez, M.P.; Greenspan, L.C.; Kushi, L.H.; Teitelbaum, S.L. Age of menarche in a longitudinal US cohort. *J. Pediatric Adolesc. Gynecol.* **2018**, *31*, 339–345. [CrossRef]
39. Meng, X.; Li, S.; Duan, W.; Sun, Y.; Jia, C. Secular trend of age at menarche in Chinese adolescents born from 1973 to 2004. *Pediatrics* **2017**, *140*, e2017008. [CrossRef] [PubMed]
40. Paul, P. Maternal age at marriage and adverse pregnancy outcomes: Findings from the India human development survey, 2011–2012. *J. Pediatric Adolesc. Gynecol.* **2018**, *31*, 620–624. [CrossRef]
41. Sekine, K.; Hodgkin, M.E. Effect of child marriage on girls' school dropout in Nepal: Analysis of data from the Multiple Indicator Cluster Survey 2014. *PLoS ONE* **2017**, *12*, e0180176. [CrossRef] [PubMed]
42. Lefkowitz, E.S.; Sigman, M.; Au, T.K.F. Helping mothers discuss sexuality and AIDS with adolescents. *Child. Dev.* **2000**, *71*, 1383–1394. [CrossRef] [PubMed]

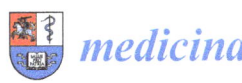

Article

Perspectives and Values of Dental Medicine Students Regarding Domestic Violence

Oana-Maria Isailă [1,2], Sorin Hostiuc [1,2,*] and George-Cristian Curcă [2,3]

1. Department of Legal Medicine and Bioethics, Faculty of Dental Medicine, "Carol Davila" University of Medicine and Pharmacy, RO-020021 Bucharest, Romania; oana_maria.isaila@yahoo.com
2. "Mina Minovici" National Institute of Legal Medicine, RO-042122 Bucharest, Romania; cgcurca@yahoo.com
3. Department of Legal Medicine and Bioethics, Faculty of Medicine, "Carol Davila" University of Medicine and Pharmacy, RO-020021 Bucharest, Romania
* Correspondence: sorin.hostiuc@umfcd.ro

Abstract: *Background and Objectives*: The purpose of this study is to evaluate dental medical students' opinions concerning domestic violence from a social and medical standpoint and from the perspective of the moral values of the physician–patient relationship. *Materials and Methods*: We performed an observational study with 4- and 5-year dental medical students at the UMF "Carol Davila" in Bucharest from October 2020–May 2021, using a questionnaire containing 20 items on domestic violence (DV). The questionnaire was uploaded online on the e-learning platform where the students have access. To collect the data, we used Microsoft Excel 365, and the statistical analysis was performed using Jamovi. *Results*: Of the 600 students enrolled, 415 answered the questionnaire, the answering rate being 69.16%. A total of 215 (53.1%) personally knew victims of DV, 4 (1.0%) considered that violence within a couple is necessary for certain situations, 401 (99.0%) considered that domestic violence is a fundamental problem in today's society, and 170 (41.5%) felt that in domestic violence situations, the blame lies solely with the partner who resorts to physical violence. Regarding the role of the physician, 220 (56%) considered that the physician should breach confidentiality and report cases when patients state they are a victim of DV, 337 (88.2%) thought that free medical treatment should be provided for DV victims who have a dire financial situation, and 212 (56.7%) considered that victims of DV are non-compliant patients. *Conclusions*: Domestic violence is a phenomenon well-known to stomatology students, which creates the premise of an excellent physician–patient relationship with them, aiding in proper management of ethical issues such as a potential need to breach confidentiality or evaluate the potential conflicts between autonomy and beneficence.

Keywords: domestic violence; physician–patient relationship; dental medical students' opinion

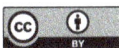

1. Introduction

The United Nations defines domestic violence as "a pattern of behavior in any relationship that is used to gain or maintain power and control over an intimate partner. Abuse is physical, sexual, emotional, economical or psychological actions or threats of actions that influence another person. This includes any behaviors that frighten, intimidate, terrorize, manipulate, hurt, humiliate, blame, injure, or wound someone" [1]. According to the WHO, domestic violence represents "any behavior within an intimate relationship that causes physical, psychological or sexual harm to those in the relationship, including acts of physical aggression, sexual coercion, psychological abuse and controlling behaviors [2]."

Domestic violence can be unidirectional when only one partner is the aggressor, or bidirectional—mutual violence within a couple, a situation in which the victim is also an aggressor [3–5]. According to the study conducted by Melander et al., depressive persons and persons who consume alcohol are more likely to be both a victim and an aggressor within the couple [5]. Previous studies have shown that when the woman is the aggressor, she may act aggressively toward the violent partner to defend herself, thus mimicking bidirectional violence [6–8].

The consequences of domestic violence can be physical, such as traumatic injuries, chronic pain, chronic diseases, sexually transmitted diseases, pregnancy, miscarriage/abortion, sexual dysfunction [9]; psychological, such as depression, suicidal ideation, the decrease in the level of satisfaction with life [10], anxiety, sleep disorders, post-traumatic stress disorder, low self-esteem, somatization [9]; or behavioral [9]. Studies performed on traumatic injuries of dental interest resulting from domestic violence showed fractures of the incisors to have the highest prevalence [11,12]. Additionally, DV victims have poor oral health due to improper hygiene, altered periodontal status, dental loss, and dental fractures [13]. Other lesions recognizable by the dental practitioner potentially suggest domestic violence are face bruises, cervical bruises, and abrasions due to manual/nose compression, bruising of the palatal arch, facial fractures, bitemark injuries, and tears lingual frenulum, or injuries on the upper limbs [14].

The most critical factors for domestic violence include a history of violence during childhood, alcohol use, a low social and professional status of the woman [15], drug abuse, a low education level of either the victim or the perpetrator, or a history of psychiatric disorders [16]. The leading causes of domestic violence, after Worden, can be based on individual factors (substance abuse, history of violence in the family, adultery/jealousy, psychiatric pathology, dominant personality), family factors (communication problems, relationship problems, stress, coming from an abusive family), macro-factors (low economic status, problems in the workplace or lack of employment) and other factors, such as lack of education, social isolation, not respecting the norms of society [17]. Protection factors are the relational and social ones, represented by restrictive legislation, social/community support, resources, and services offered by specialized structures [18] to provide victims with increased self-esteem, social integration, or optimal access to medical care [19].

As dental medicine students, who are future dental practitioners, will have patients who are victims of domestic violence, analyzing their perspectives and attitudes towards this phenomenon helps assure an adequate education and ensure an optimal response to domestic violence cases. The purpose of this study is to evaluate dental medical students' opinions concerning domestic violence from a social and medical standpoint and the perspective of the moral values of the physician–patient relationship.

2. Materials and Methods

We performed an observational study with 4- and 5-year dental medical students at the UMF "Carol Davila" in Bucharest from October 2020–May 2021, using a questionnaire containing 20 items on domestic violence (DV). The questionnaire was uploaded online on the e-learning platform, where the students have access. To collect the data, we used Microsoft Excel 365, and the statistical analysis was performed using Jamovi.

The study IRB outcome code is 972/26.01.2021. The questionnaire was approved by the institutional ethics board, validated, and uploaded online on the e-learning platform, to which all dental students had access to online classes at the discipline. The questionnaire was optional and anonymous, this being the reason for which no demographic data was requested.

The first seven questions (1–7) targeted the quantification of the severity of this phenomenon using case vignettes in which answers were evaluated using a four-point scale, using the following potential answers: it is not a case of domestic violence; it is a case of slight domestic violence; it is a case of moderate domestic violence; it is a case of severe domestic violence. The following 10 questions (8–18) were dichotomous, with yes or no answers and targeted aspects concerning the importance of this phenomenon and the physician's role in the relationship with the patient who is also a DV victim. Finally, the last two questions were multiple-choice and evaluated the media coverage and the potential causes of this phenomenon.

The data extracted from the questionnaire was collected using Excel 365, and the resulting database was processed with Jamovi v 1.2.27 (Topeka, KS, USA). We used descriptive statistics to evaluate the results obtained from the questionnaire.

3. Results

Of the 600 students, 415 answered the questionnaire; thus, the response rate was 69.16%. As there was no mandatory answer, some students only responded partially to the questionnaire. The responses to the case vignettes are summarized in Table 1. Briefly, most respondents correctly identified gross DV cases, even if they were not physical, directed toward the spouse. Bidirectional DV was harder to identify (answer to Q1), as was economic (Q3) or social (Q5).

Table 1. Answers to the first seven questions.

Question (Number & Statement)	It's Not DV	It's a Slight DV	It's a Moderate DV	It's a Severe DV
Q1. It is a case of DV when the partners shout at each other?	133 (32.1%)	183 (44.2%)	86 (20.8%)	12 (2.9%)
Q2 Is cheating a form of DV?	275 (66.4%)	43 (10.4%)	52 (12.6%)	44 (10.6%)
Q3. A husband refusing to give money to his wife to pay the household utilities a type of DV?	189 (45.9%)	107 (26.0%)	86 (20.9%)	30 (7.3%)
Q4. Forgetting the spouse's birthday is a form of DV?	383 (92.3%)	21 (5.1%)	9 (2.2%)	2 (0.5%)
Q5. A woman forbidding her spouse to go to a football match is a form of DV?	183 (44.2%)	166 (40.1%)	55 (13.3%)	10 (2.4%)
Q6. A man being aggressive with pets in the presence of his partner is a form of DV?	111 (26.7%)	70 (16.9%)	127 (30.6%)	107 (25.8%)
Q7. If the man does not pay the bill at a restaurant, is it a form of DV?	384 (92.5%)	20 (4.8%)	7 (1.7%)	4 (1.0%)

DV: domestic violence.

More than half of the respondents personally knew victims of domestic violence (215, 53.1%). Only four respondents (1.0%) considered domestic violence necessary in some instances. Most considered domestic violence a critical problem in today's society (401 respondents, 99.0%).

Almost half of the respondents (170, 41.5%) considered that, in domestic violence, the partner who resorts to physical violence is the only one to blame (see Table 2).

Regarding the physician's role in recognizing this phenomenon, 257 (65.6%) considered that the physician must ask any patient about the existence of eventual conflicts in the family environment when there are physical signs potentially suggesting DV. Most respondents (323, 81.4%) did not consider that the physician should report the case to state authorities without discussing it with the patient first. More than half (212, 56.7%) believed that victims of DV are non-compliant patients, 220 (56%) thought that the physician should breach confidentiality and report the case when the patient affirms they are a victim of DV, 337 (88.2%) thought that free medical treatment should be offered to victims of DV who have low financial status, 182 (49.1%) considered that women who are victims of DV are discriminated on the assumption that their symptoms are imaginary, and 178 (48.1%) feel that men who are victims of DV are believed to exaggerate their symptoms. (see Table 3).

Table 2. The evaluation of the perception of the phenomenon.

Question (Number & Statement)	No	Yes
Q8. Do you personally know victims of domestic violence?	190 (46.9%)	215 (53.1%)
Q9. Do you consider violence within a couple necessary in certain situations?	402 (99.0%)	4 (1.0%)
Q10. Do you consider domestic violence a critical problem in today's society	5 (1.2%)	401 (98.8%)
Q11. Do you consider that in domestic violence, the only responsible person is the one who resorts to physical violence?	222 (56.61%)	170 (43.4%)

Table 3. Perception of the physician's role in the context of the domestic violence phenomenon.

Question (Number & Statement)	No	Yes
Q12. Do you consider that the physician should ask any patient about eventual conflicts within the family?	135 (34.4%)	257 (65.6%)
Q13. Suppose a person with traumatic lesions to the face and upper limbs visits the physician. Should the physician assume that the patient is a victim of domestic violence and breach confidentiality by notifying the competent authorities without discussing beforehand with the patient?	323 (81.4%)	74 (18.6%)
Q14. Do you consider victims of domestic violence non-compliant?	162 (43.3%)	212 (56.7%)
Q15. If a person claiming they were assaulted by their spouse visits the physician, should the physician breach confidentiality and report the case?	173 (44.0%)	220 (56.0%)
Q16. Do you consider that low-income patients who are victims of domestic violence should benefit from free medical treatment?	45 (11.8%)	337 (88.2%)
Q17. Do you consider that women who are victims of domestic violence are discriminated against when they go to the physician because they are simulating their symptoms?	189 (50.9%)	182 (49.1%)
Q18. Do you consider that men who are victims of domestic violence are discriminated against when they go to the physician because they are highly exaggerating their symptoms?	192 (51.9%)	178 (48.1%)

Regarding the attitude of mass media's towards domestic violence, 241 (58.4%) respondents considered that cases of domestic violence are shown with the primary purpose to increase ratings, 104 (25.2%) believed these cases are presented to help raise awareness and to stop the phenomenon, and 68 (16.5%) considered that cases of domestic violence are not frequently showcased.

Regarding the students' answers about the possible causes of domestic violence, they considered them being as follows: poverty, 323 (77.8%); different religions, 221 (53.3%); social status, 267 (64.3%); lack of education, 359 (86.5%); character problems, 353 (85.1%); lack of trust in the partner, 333 (80.2%); substance abuse, 400 (96.4%). See Figure 1 for details.

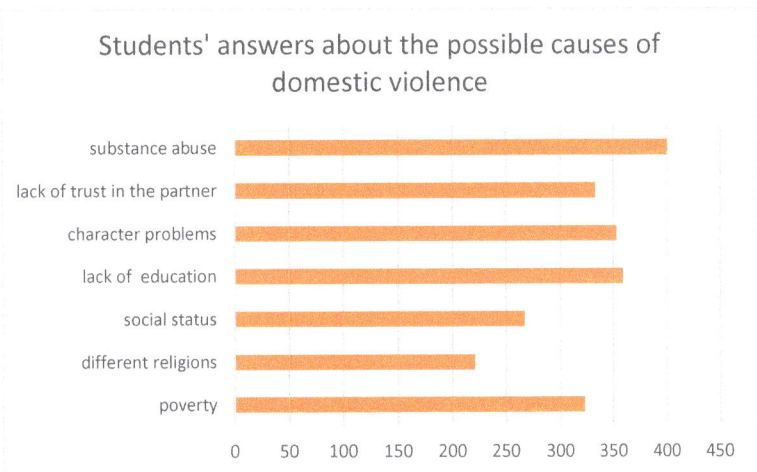

Figure 1. Students' answers about the possible causes of domestic violence.

4. Discussion

Our study evaluated future dental practitioners' perception of domestic violence, emphasizing the severity of its types and the physician's role.

The first seven questions evaluated the recognition and evaluation of the degrees of DV. From the received answers, students understood the clear-cut forms of domestic violence (verbal and physical). Still, they were less aware of the types that can be ambivalent and contextually arguable (social and economical).

The next items from the questionnaire have shown that future physicians know the significance and consequences of this phenomenon at both a micro level (families) and macro-level (societies). Regarding the physician's role in recognizing and managing DV, most respondents considered DV victims non-compliant patients, which emphasizes the need for a personalized approach of the victim within the physician–patient relationship. McCloskey et al. have shown that for women who are victims of domestic violence, especially if they have a lower financial status and a low education level, the abusive partner stopped them from seeking medical assistance and, as a result, it generated deficits regarding proper access to medical care [20]. This can be seen as a significant control, affecting the autonomy of the victim. Seeking medical assistance by DV victims is often completed in secrecy (when the abuser is not home or sleeping). This emphasizes three main aspects that must be taken into account. First, emergency medical and social care for these patients should be given whenever possible, even outside regular hours. This approach is based on the virtues of loyalty—the physician should prioritize their patients, especially those that are particularly vulnerable, whenever the need arises and benevolence—assisting a person in need more than the physician is obligated is within their professional duties. The second aspect is the need for a more personalized approach to confidentiality that must be vigorously enforced with the family and friends of the patient but also breached toward relevant state agents (such as social workers or even the criminal system) whenever the physician believes there is an inherent risk for the patient [21]. The more robust type of confidentiality toward the family and friends is generated by potential (even if unwilling) disclosures about the visit to the medical office directed toward the perpetrator or somebody close to him. Therefore, physicians should not allow the presence of a third party when issues regarding DV are discussed with the patient, nor should they disclose such information to third parties, even if the patient accepts, unless they consider the involvement of these third parties indispensable for the management of the patient. Additionally, physicians should always inform the patient about the need to keep secrecy about the visit to the perpetrator (including issues such as hiding the receipt for the consultation or the medical letter containing details about the medical visit), as they can generate a new aggressive event. If, toward relatives and friends of the family, the disclosure should be minimized (even with the patient's agreement), concerning social workers and other persons potentially helpful in managing acts of domestic violence, disclosure should be allowed, based on the duty to warn. For example, in Romania, a specific law provides anybody who suspects an act of domestic violence (medical workers included) to inform relevant state authorities [22]. The mandatory reporting of DV cases has been a highly controversial topic in the scientific literature throughout the years. For example, Antle et al. found DV victims to prefer disclosure for them and other patients in similar situations [23]. On the other side, Colter and Chez found that DV victims considered mandatory reporting useful only for other DV victims, but not if they were the subject [24]. In our study, most respondents (56.0%) agreed that when the physician is confronted with a DV victim, they should breach confidentiality and report the case. The third issue that has to be considered is the need for a particular type of physician–patient relationship. As the patients are often in shock or show increased anxiety levels, a purely informative model of the physician–patient relationship is not advisable, as the decisional capacity is often temporarily decreased. However, a paternalist model should never be applied in these cases, as it might reinforce some feelings generated by the aggressor (who is often dominant in relation with the victim). From our clinical experience, we recommend an interpretative approach to the professional relationship [25], which allows a translation of the actual wants and needs of the patient while maximizing its autonomy.

Most responders (88.2%) considered that free medical treatment would be helpful for victims of domestic violence who are in a dire financial situation. A lack of financial resources is known to be positively linked with increased DV. Therefore, from a Rawlsian perspective [26], providing free medical care to DV victims is the right act, this measure being able to increase their addressability to medical care but also (indirectly) to social, psychological, and judicial systems that could aid in limiting aggressive behaviors [27].

Regarding the role of mass media, most respondents (58.4%) considered that exposing domestic violence cases has the purpose of increasing ratings. Only 25.2% believed that increased media exposure might raise awareness and prevent this phenomenon. This result shows that mass media does not seem to have a preventive approach to DV but rather uses it for financial purposes.

Similar results regarding the inefficiency of mass media in preventing DV have been shown by Maquibar et al. [28].

Most responders (96.4%) considered substance abuse to be a main factor in generating DV. Alcohol and drug abuse are known to increase aggressive behavior in general [29] and in a domestic context in particular [30].

Dentists are less aware of DV, as shown by other published studies. For example, Love et al. found that most dentists never checked if their patients were victims of domestic violence and, in general, have intervened to a very little extent to help in cases of domestic violence. Among the obstacles they have encountered were the presence of the spouse or the child of the victim during the consultation, the embarrassment to ask, and a lack of instruction in this sense. It has been found that respondents who benefitted from adequate training were more determined to verify this phenomenon and intervene [31], this being one of the main reasons for which we have developed this questionnaire and brought it to the attention of medical dental students (together with a special course regarding the particularities of DV in dentistry, which is taught to 4-year medical dental students, in the legal medicine curriculum). Another study by Skelton et al. on the same subject indicated the need for dental practitioners to have supplemental instruction on the theme of domestic violence [32]. Drigeard et al. showed that most dental practitioners do not look for signs of potential domestic abuse in patients, only 36% declaring they have encountered DV, and 75.9% felt the need for additional training on the subject of domestic violence [33]. AlAlyani and Alshouibi concluded, in a similar study, that for dental practitioners, the following barriers exist in identifying patients as victims of domestic violence: a lack of instruction on this subject and an implicit hesitation of asking questions on this topic [34]. Mythri H. et al.'s study has found a low level of knowledge in dentists about DV and pointed out the need for additional education on this theme [35].

Studies performed on medical workers of other specialties have also shown significant barriers regarding the screening for domestic violence due to a lack of availability or time of the medical staff [36,37] or a lack of training in this respect [38,39].

The limitations of this study were the relatively small number of participants and the lack of their stratification according to demographic variables.

5. Conclusions

Domestic violence is a phenomenon well known to stomatology students, which creates the premise of an excellent physician–patient relationship with them, aiding in proper management of ethical issues such as a potential need to breach confidentiality or evaluate the potential conflicts between autonomy and beneficence.

Author Contributions: Conceptualization, S.H., O.-M.I. and G.-C.C.; methodology, O.-M.I. and S.H.; software, S.H. and O.-M.I.; validation, S.H., O.-M.I. and G.-C.C.; formal analysis, O.-M.I., S.H. and G.-C.C.; investigation, O.-M.I.; resources, S.H. and O.-M.I.; data curation, O.-M.I.; writing—original draft preparation O.-M.I. and S.H.; writing—S.H., G.-C.C. and O.-M.I. All authors have read and agreed to the published version of the manuscript.

Funding: This research received no external funding.

Institutional Review Board Statement: The study was conducted according to the guidelines of the Declaration of Helsinki and approved by the Institutional Ethics Committee "Mina Minovici" Bucharest (headquarters of the discipline of legal medicine and bioethics). The reference number is 972/26.01.2021.

Informed Consent Statement: Informed consent was obtained from all subjects involved in the study.

Data Availability Statement: Data supporting this results can be available online on elearnmed.ro only following an explicit request in this regard.

Conflicts of Interest: The authors declare no conflict of interest.

References

1. United Nations. Domestic Abuse. 2021. Available online: https://www.un.org/en/coronavirus/what-is-domestic-abuse (accessed on 1 June 2021).
2. Krug, E.G.; Dahlberg, L.L.; Mercy, J.A.; Zwi, A.B.; Lozano, R.; World Health Organization. World Report on Violence and Health/Edited by Etienne G. Krug. [et al.]. World Health Organization, Geneva PP—Geneva. 2002. Available online: https://apps.who.int/iris/handle/10665/42495 (accessed on 5 June 2021).
3. Bonnet, F. Intimate Partner Violence, Gender, and Criminalisation. *Rev. Fr. Sociol.* **2015**, *56*, 357–383. [CrossRef]
4. Palmetto, N.; Davidson, L.L.; Rickert, V.I.; Breitbart, V. Predictors of Physical Intimate Partner Violence in the Lives of Young Women: Victimization, Perpetration, and Bidirectional Violence. *Violence Vict.* **2013**, *28*, 103–121. [CrossRef]
5. Melander, L.A.; Noel, H.; Tyler, K.A. Bidirectional, Unidirectional, and Nonviolence: A Comparison of the Predictors among Partnered Young Adults. *Violence Vict.* **2010**, *25*, 617–630. [CrossRef]
6. Swan, S.C.; Gambone, L.J.; Caldwell, J.E.; Sullivan, T.P.; Snow, D.L. A review of research on women's use of vi-olence with male intimate partners. *Violence Vict.* **2008**, *23*, 301–314. Available online: http://www.ncbi.nlm.nih.gov/pubmed/18624096%0Ahttp://www.pubmedcentral.nih.gov/articlerender.fcgi?artid=PMC2968709 (accessed on 5 June 2021). [CrossRef] [PubMed]
7. Swan, S.C.; Snow, D.L. A Typology of Women's Use of Violence in Intimate Relationships. *Violence Women* **2002**, *8*, 286–319. [CrossRef]
8. Holmes, S.C.; Johnson, N.L.; Rojas-Ashe, E.E.; Ceroni, T.L.; Fedele, K.M.; Johnson, D. Prevalence and Predictors of Bidirectional Violence in Survivors of Intimate Partner Violence Residing at Shelters. *J. Interpers. Violence* **2016**, *34*, 3492–3515. [CrossRef]
9. WHO. *Understanding and Addressing Violence against Women Health Consequences*; WHO: Geneva, Switzerland, 2012.
10. Liu, M.; Xue, J.; Zhao, N.; Wang, X.; Jiao, D.; Zhu, T. Using Social Media to Explore the Consequences of Domestic Violence on Mental Health. *J. Interpers. Violence* **2021**, *36*, NP1965–1985NP. [CrossRef] [PubMed]
11. Mythri, H.M. Role of public health dentist towards domestic violence. *Indian J. Public Health* **2013**, *57*, 50. [CrossRef]
12. Garbin, C.; Queiroz, A.P.D.D.G.E.; Rovida, T.A.S.; Garbin, A. Occurrence of traumatic dental injury in cases of domestic violence. *Braz. Dent. J.* **2012**, *23*, 72–76. [CrossRef] [PubMed]

13. Kundu, H.P.B.; Singla, A.; Kote, S.; Singh, S.; Jain, S.; Singh, K.; Vashishtha, V. Domestic Violence and its Effect on Oral Health Behaviour and Oral Health Status. *J. Clin. Diagn. Res.* **2014**, *8*, ZC09–ZC12. [CrossRef]
14. McDowell, J.D. Forensic dentistry. Recognizing the signs and symptoms of domestic violence: A guide for dentists. *J. Okla. Dent. Assoc.* **1997**, *88*, 21–28. [PubMed]
15. Jewkes, R.; Levin, J.; Penn-Kekana, L. Risk factors for domestic violence: Findings from a South African cross-sectional study. *Soc. Sci. Med.* **2002**, *55*, 1603–1617. [CrossRef]
16. Almis, B.H.; Kütük, E.K.; Gümüştaş, F.; Celik, M. Risk Factors for Domestic Violence in Women and Predictors of Development of Mental Disorders in These Women. *Arch. Neuropsychiatry* **2018**, *55*, 67–72. [CrossRef]
17. Worden, A.P.; Carlson, B.E. Attitudes and Beliefs About Domestic Violence: Results of a Public Opinion Survey. *J. Interpers. Violence* **2005**, *20*, 1219–1243. [CrossRef]
18. Spiranovic, C.; Hudson, N.; Winter, R.; Stanford, S.; Norris, K.; Bartkowiak-Theron, I.; Cashman, K. Navigating risk and protective factors for family violence during and after the COVID-19 'perfect storm'. *Curr. Issues Crim. Justice* **2021**, *33*, 5–18. [CrossRef]
19. Carlson, B.E.; McNutt, L.-A.; Choi, D.Y.; Rose, I.M. Intimate Partner Abuse and Mental Health. *Violence Women* **2002**, *8*, 720–745. [CrossRef]
20. McCloskey, L.A.; Williams, C.M.; Lichter, E.; Gerber, M.; Ganz, M.L.; Sege, R. Abused Women Disclose Partner Interference with Health Care: An Unrecognized Form of Battering. *J. Gen. Intern. Med.* **2007**, *22*, 1067–1072. [CrossRef]
21. Hostiuc, S.; Curca, C.G.; Dermengiu, D. Consent and Confidentiality in Medical Assistance for Women Victims of Domestic Violence. *Rev. Romana Bioet.* **2011**, *9*, 1.
22. Hostiuc, S.; Teodoru-Răghină, D.-V.; Isailă, O.; Buda, O.; Costescu, M. *Tratat de Medicină Legală Odontostomatologică*; Editura All: București, Romania, 2020.
23. Antle, B.; Barbee, A.; Yankeelov, P.; Bledsoe, L. A Qualitative Evaluation of the Effects of Mandatory Reporting of Domestic Violence on Victims and Their Children. *J. Fam. Soc. Work* **2010**, *13*, 56–73. [CrossRef]
24. Coulter, M.L.; Chez, R.A. Domestic Violence Victims Support Mandatory Reporting: For Others Domestic Violence Victims Support Mandatory Reporting: For Others. *J. Fam. Violence* **1997**, *12*, 349–355. [CrossRef]
25. Emanuel, E.J.; Emanuel, L.L. Four models of the physician-patient relationship. *JAMA* **1992**, *267*, 2221–2226. [CrossRef]
26. Rawls, J. *A Theory of Justice*; Belknap Press: Cambridge, MA, USA, 1999.
27. Curca, G.C.; Buda, O.; Capatina, C.; Marinescu, M.V.; Hostiuc, S.; Dermengiu, D.; Cartina, C.; A Cretoiu, V.; A Stoica, N.; Bădescu, I.; et al. Study on domestic violence: A legal medicine perspective. *Romanian J. Leg. Med.* **2008**, *16*, 226–242. [CrossRef]
28. Maquibar, A.; Vives-Cases, C.; Hurtig, A.-K.; Goicolea, I. Professionals' perception of intimate partner violence in young people: A qualitative study in northern Spain. *Reprod. Health* **2017**, *14*, 86. [CrossRef] [PubMed]
29. Fishbein, D. Neuropsychological Function, Drug Abuse, and Violence. *Crim. Justice Behav.* **2000**, *27*, 139–159. [CrossRef]
30. Kraanen, F.L.; Scholing, A.; Emmelkamp, P.M.G. Substance Use Disorders in Perpetrators of Intimate Partner Violence in a Forensic Setting. *Int. J. Offender Ther. Comp. Criminol.* **2009**, *54*, 430–440. [CrossRef] [PubMed]
31. Love, C.; Gerbert, B.; Caspers, N.; Bronstone, A.; Perry, D.; Bird, W. Dentists' attitudes and behaviors regarding domestic violence. *J. Am. Dent. Assoc.* **2001**, *132*, 85–93. [CrossRef] [PubMed]
32. Skelton, J.; Herren, C.; Cunningham, L.L.; West, K.P. Knowledge, attitudes, practices, and training needs of Kentucky dentists regarding violence against women. *Gen. Dent.* **2007**, *55*, 581–588.
33. Drigeard, C.; Nicolas, E.; Hansjacob, A.; Roger-Leroi, V. Educational needs in the field of detection of domestic violence and neglect: The opinion of a population of French dentists. *Eur. J. Dent. Educ.* **2012**, *16*, 156–165. [CrossRef]
34. AlAlyani, W.S.; Alshouibi, E.N. Dentists awareness and action towards domestic violence patients. *Saudi Med J.* **2017**, *38*, 82–88. [CrossRef]
35. Mythri, H.; Kashinath, K.R.; Raju, A.S.; Suresh, K.V.; Bharateesh, J.V. Enhancing the Dental Professional's Responsiveness Towards Domestic Violence; A Cross-Sectional Study. *J. Clin. Diagn. Res.* **2015**, *9*, ZC51–ZC53. [CrossRef]
36. Yonaka, L.; Yoder, M.K.; Darrow, J.B.; Sherck, J.P. Barriers to Screening for Domestic Violence in the Emergency Department. *J. Contin. Educ. Nurs.* **2007**, *38*, 37–45. [CrossRef] [PubMed]
37. Elliott, L.; Nerney, M.; Jones, T.; Friedmann, P.D. Barriers to screening for domestic violence. *J. Gen. Intern. Med.* **2002**, *17*, 112–116. [CrossRef]
38. Kirk, L.; Bezzant, K. What barriers prevent health professionals screening women for domestic abuse? A literature review. *Br. J. Nurs.* **2020**, *29*, 754–760. [CrossRef] [PubMed]
39. Hoke, N. Barriers to Screening for Domestic Violence in the Emergency Department. *J. Trauma Nurs.* **2008**, *15*, 79. [CrossRef]

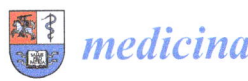

Article

Gender Differences in Healthy Lifestyle, Body Consciousness, and the Use of Social Networks among Medical Students

Lavinia-Maria Pop [1], Magdalena Iorga [2,*], Lucian-Roman Șipoș [3] and Raluca Iurcov [3]

1. Faculty of Psychology and Education Sciences, "Alexandru Ioan Cuza" University, 700111 Iasi, Romania; lavinia.pop@student.uaic.ro
2. Behavioral Sciences Department, "Grigore T. Popa" University of Medicine and Pharmacy, 700115 Iasi, Romania
3. Dentistry Department, Faculty of Medicine, University of Oradea, 410073 Oradea, Romania; lsipos@uoradea.ro (L.-R.Ș.); riurcov@uoradea.ro (R.I.)
* Correspondence: magdalena.iorga@umfiasi.ro

Abstract: *Background and Objectives*: The goal of this survey was to identify the relationship between the level of satisfaction with body image, perceived health, and the usage of social media among freshmen medical university students. The influence of social media and peers was also related to body image. *Materials and Methods*: An online survey was distributed among freshmen healthcare students. The questionnaire collected sociodemographic, anthropometric data, and information about students' perception about healthy lifestyle using open-ended questions, as well as their opinion about the importance of perfect body image and the level of satisfaction with their physical appearance. Questions focusing on the use of social media and the relationship with body image collected data on the use of social networks and how they affect students' opinion about their own body image. Psychometric data were also gathered using the Body Consciousness Scale. For the statistical analysis, QSR NUD*IST (Non-numerical Unstructured Data Indexing Searching and Theorizing) Vivo 12 was used for qualitative data and IBM Statistical Package for Social Sciences (SPSS) Statistics for Windows, version 23 (SPSS Inc., Chicago, IL, USA) was used for descriptive and comparative results. *Results*: In total, 77 students aged 20.09 ± 2.47 years, of which the majority were women (75.30%), were included in the survey. The use of social network was about 4.81 ± 3.60 h/day. Facebook was the most used social networking site (94.80%), followed by Instagram (92.20%), Snapchat (16.90%), WhatsApp (15.60%), and TikTok (10.40%). The most common reason for using these sites was socialization. We found that 64.90% of healthcare students were normal weight. The main barriers for having a healthy lifestyle, as they were perceived by students, were the busy schedule and the lack of time needed to prepare healthy meals, lack of motivation, and lack of money. Women scored higher for the Private Body Consciousness and Public Body Consciousness scales. The main aspects related to a healthy lifestyle referred to physical activity, consumption of fruit and vegetables, water consumption, and a good quality of sleep. Gender differences were discussed as well. *Conclusions*: The results illustrated the complexity of the relationship between social media and body image and the need to prevent body image concerns, especially in young women.

Keywords: students; medicine; healthcare; lifestyle; body image; social network; self-esteem; body mass index; physical health

Citation: Pop, L.-M.; Iorga, M.; Șipoș, L.-R.; Iurcov, R. Gender Differences in Healthy Lifestyle, Body Consciousness, and the Use of Social Networks among Medical Students. *Medicina* 2021, 57, 648. https://doi.org/10.3390/medicina57070648

Academic Editor: Janina Petkevičienė

Received: 10 May 2021
Accepted: 22 June 2021
Published: 24 June 2021

Publisher's Note: MDPI stays neutral with regard to jurisdictional claims in published maps and institutional affiliations.

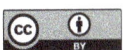

Copyright: © 2021 by the authors. Licensee MDPI, Basel, Switzerland. This article is an open access article distributed under the terms and conditions of the Creative Commons Attribution (CC BY) license (https://creativecommons.org/licenses/by/4.0/).

1. Introduction

Lifestyle is defined as a pattern of behavior, the attempt to ensure optimal health, or the sum of health-related habits that have a positive effect on overweight and obesity [1,2]. In the current study, lifestyle was considered by the researchers as a key factor in health status, owing to the statement by the World Health Organization (WHO) that 60% of factors related to individual health and quality of life are correlated with lifestyle [3].

According to current data, lifestyle is based on personal choices and identities and has a significant influence on the physical and mental health of the people [3]. At the micro level, the personality, biological, and psychological characteristics of the individual, family, friends, school, and society affect the daily life and lifestyle of the individual. At the macro level, the city and the environment in which the individual lives, the media, and the cultural climate of the individual's society all affect the lifestyle and changes in the life of the individual [4].

According to the WHO, late adolescence (from 19 to 24 years) is an important stage in a person's development and is defined as a period in which the individual prepares for work and assumes adult responsibilities [5]. The basis of a healthy lifestyle is built during youth, when eating habits develop intensively and body weight and body image become correlated [6]. Lifestyle, weight, body image, and satisfaction define the physical and mental health status during adulthood. An unhealthy diet during the period of intense growth can affect the development of young people, triggering the body's nonacceptance and causing diet-related diseases in adulthood [7].

During the period of their academic studies (late youth), students should be physically and mentally healthy, practicing an active life and having healthy eating behaviors to maintain their health status. They need a good physical and mental condition to cope with the effort required during their academic years and to have a satisfactory body image [5,8]. A poor perception of well-being can lead to less involvement in good self-care practices or poor adherence to interventional programs, while a perceived good or excellent level of well-being is associated with good personal care [9].

Body image has several components, which can be divided into two dimensions: (a) Perceptual (how we see our size, shape, weight, face, movement, and actions) and (b) attitudinal (how we feel about these traits and how these feelings affect our behaviors) [10]. Body image includes the thoughts, beliefs, and evaluation of emotions and behaviors about the physical appearance of an individual, all of which are affected by multiple factors. To improve their mental body image, people resort to different methods, including various diets that promise weight loss, exercise, or even cosmetic surgery [11].

Researchers have identified that healthcare students have an increased focus on their own health, practice a better lifestyle compared to other student populations, and have a favorable perception of their own health and body [12,13]. The strong relationship between healthy lifestyle, body image, and healthy behaviors is interrelated with mental health [9]. Body image and beauty are some of the main causes of stress among young people [10]. However, on the other hand, healthcare students have also been shown to experience high levels of stress related to their academic tasks, which is a causative factor in eating disorders [14]. The sedentary lifestyle and stressful nature of medical student activity seems to prevent them from maintaining a positive perception of body image [15].

Body dissatisfaction and exposure to the thin-ideal image are major predictors of the development of an eating disorder, the latter having significant health implications. Students experience psychological and social changes, which are more pronounced in subjects experiencing considerable social pressures [11]. Thus, the standards of cultural beauty, as communicated by the media, become messages with a strong impact both for women and men, leading to the development of unhealthy weight control practices [16].

In the Western European countries, body image has become increasingly important, with images of movie stars and fashion models having a strong impact on girls' body shape and image perception. Such means of mass communication and various sociocultural pressures are considered to cause an increased awareness of being thin as an ideal and contribute to the misperception of body weight [17]. Media has a significant impact on body image as a powerful force that uses various aspects, including the internet, television, magazines, video games, and smartphones to present the ideal of beauty [8]. Currently, media promotes a slim figure model among women and muscular/athletic figure among men, promoting foods and diets with inadequate nutritional value, which can also lead to unwanted nutritional and health behaviors and the nonacceptance of body weight [7]. Both women and men often choose to expose themselves to idealized body images as presented in the media. There is a two-way relationship between exposure to a thin-ideal environment and body dissatisfaction: People who are dissatisfied with their appearance address the media that present thin and beautiful models, possibly for advice or information or to see advertising products designed to bring the aspects of the appearance closer to the perceived ideal [16].

The influence of advertising on social networks and its effect on young people's self-image has been studied [18,19]. Social platforms are often used by students for communication (social life), as well as for academic tasks [20]. Social platforms such as Instagram, Pinterest, and Facebook are extremely popular. Some social media platforms—such as Instagram—are more visual/image-based compared to others—such as Facebook [21]—and have great impact on body consciousness (awareness of observable aspects of body). A person's awareness of her/his failure to meet these standards leads to dissatisfaction, and media is seen as particularly important promotor of the ideal body image.

In the last decade, social networks have become the most common form of sociocultural interaction for young people due to various factors such as communicating with peers, maintaining contact with friends and family, and sharing information. On social networks, people often present an idealized version of themselves by uploading only the most attractive images of them (which can be edited and enhanced) in their profile and removing any images they find unattractive. Although social networks contain images of several different types of people (e.g., friends, family, strangers, celebrities), these are generally used to interact with colleagues. Finally, in addition to images, people often post other content related to appearance and comments on social networks, which could also impact users' feelings about their appearance [22].

However, among students, it has been shown that comparison to other colleagues' pictures and posting on social media influences self-satisfaction with the body image considerably. Body dissatisfaction and exposure to thin-ideal images are major predictors for eating disorders. Social networks have a strong influence on young people, even changing their habits and lifestyles [23,24]. Some studies conducted on students have shown that body worship currently prevails among college students, and it is impossible to deny the influence of many factors such as food habits, social pressure, the aesthetic of thinness, and the popular models on social media and social networks [25,26].

The goal of the present study was to explore health-related beliefs, body image perception, and influence of social networks on the ideal body image among freshmen healthcare students enrolled in kinesiotherapy studies with a focus on gender differences. The study is part of a larger one focusing on health status, body image, and the impact of social media on the ideal body among healthcare students in Romania.

2. Materials and Methods

2.1. Study Population

The questionnaire was sent to 90 freshmen students enrolled in Balneo-Physio-Kinesiotherapy specialization. The respondents were informed about the purpose of the study and the confidentiality of data. No incentive was given to the participants. Students were informed that they could withdraw from the study whenever they wanted without consequences. The inclusion criteria were students enrolled in their first year of study and surveys returned before deadline. Criteria for excluding surveys from the research were incomplete questionnaires or questionnaires submitted after the deadline. Finally, 77 questionnaires were included in the research.

2.2. Data Collection

The questionnaire was created using Google Docs and was distributed online during March–April 2021. The qualitative research design was developed to obtain detailed information about students' perceptions of the following aspects, namely healthy eating, body image, and the influence of social media.

This study used a triangular research method which included drawing, free association method, and open-ended question surveys. The study collected information regarding the following issues:

- The first part of the questionnaire gathered sociodemographic and anthropometric data (age, gender, marital status, environment, members of the household, average monthly financial income, weight, height, body mass index).
- The second section contained items evaluating students' perception about healthy lifestyle. The items were constructed as an open-ended question (such as changes considered necessary in students' eating behavior, reasons why a healthy lifestyle is needed, reasons why they practice/would like to practice physical activity, aspects that prevent them from maintaining a healthy lifestyle). One item referred to the free association method and asked students to write the first 5 words that came to their mind when they thought of a healthy lifestyle.
- The third part of the questionnaire addressed the Body Consciousness Scale developed by Miller, Murphy, and Buss in 1981 [27]. This instrument is a self-report tool that includes 3 subscales related to private body consciousness (awareness of internal sensations), public body consciousness (awareness of observable aspects of body), and body competence. Respondents had to indicate their level of correspondence with the 15 statements using a 5-item Likert-type scale. Answers included "extremely uncharacteristic", "uncharacteristic", "neutral", "characteristic", and "extremely characteristic". The minimum score possible for each question is 0 and the maximum is 4. Subjects' scores were calculated on each separate scale by adding each item's score and forming 3 subscale composites.
- The fourth section included items related to body image and aimed to identify the main characteristics that students associated with their body, the opinion about the importance of body image today, and the level of satisfaction with their body image. The answers were rated on a Likert-type scale from 1 to 10, where 1 = very dissatisfied and 10 = very satisfied.
- The fifth section comprised questions focusing on the use of social media and the relationship with body image (the use of social networks, the frequency, the reason why these were used, the impact these had on students, the emotional state created by following the posts of colleagues or celebrities, the influence of social networks in students' tendency to compare themselves with other people, the influence of social networks in the way students perceived their own body, etc.).
- In the sixth section, students were asked to open a separate document, draw the first thing that came into their mind when they thought of a healthy lifestyle, and upload that document in the space provided within the questionnaire.

2.3. Statistical Analysis

The data were analyzed using a qualitative data analysis program, QSR NUD*IST (Non-numerical Unstructured Data Indexing Searching and Theorizing) Vivo 12, also called NVivo. To present the sociodemographic characteristics of the samples, we performed analyses using IBM Statistical Package for Social Sciences (SPSS) Statistics for Windows, version 23 (SPSS Inc., Chicago, IL, USA). Results for descriptive statistics were expressed as means and standard deviations (SD), frequencies, and percentages. The same library was used to report the results of the Body Consciousness Scale. A qualitative analysis (word cloud) of the students' personal perception of a healthy lifestyle was created using the Orange software [28]. Using the same software, a hierarchical clustering analysis was used to compute the similarity of the images sent by the participants regarding their perception of a healthy lifestyle. The Body Mass Index (BMI) calculation was carried out according to WHO guidelines, using standards for the European population: A BMI < 18.5 kg/m^2 was categorized as underweight, 18.5–24.9 kg/m^2 as normal weight, 25.0–29.9 kg/m^2 as pre-obese, 30–34.9 kg/m^2 as obese class I, 35.0–39.9 kg/m^2 as obese class II, and $\geq$40 kg/m^2 as obese class III [29].

2.4. Ethical Approval

The present study was conducted in accordance with the Declaration of Helsinki, and the protocol was approved by the Ethical Committee of Faculty of Medicine, University of Oradea, Romania, with the registration number No. 26214/18.11.2020.

3. Results

3.1. Sociodemographic and Anthropometric Data

The respondents were students enrolled in the first year and studying kinesiotherapy specialty. Students came from rural and urban areas, aged M = 20.09 ± 2.47 (with a minimum of 18 and a maximum of 39 years old). Most of them were female students (75.30%). Body Mass Index (BMI) was also calculated, conforming to WHO guidelines. The detailed information about sociodemographic and anthropometric data are presented in Table 1.

Table 1. Sociodemographic and anthropometric data [1].

Sociodemographic and Anthropometric Characteristics	M ± S.D and %
Age	20.09 ± 2.47
Gender	
Male	19 (24.7%)
Female	58 (75.3%)
Environment of origin	
Urban	42 (54.5%)
Rural	35 (45.5%)
Marital status	
Married	4 (5.2%)
Unmarried	73 (94.8%)
Members of the household	
Single	12 (15.6%)
Colleagues/friends	41 (53.2%)
Partner	9 (11.7%)
Parents	15 (19.5%)
Average monthly financial income	
20–100 €	28 (36.4%)
100–200 €	26 (33.8%)
200–400 €	15 (19.5%)
>400 €	8 (10.4%)
Weight	64.58 ± 14.75
Body mass index	22.14 ± 3.50
Nutritional status	
Underweight	11 (14.3%)
Normal weight	50 (64.9%)
Overweight	12 (15.6%)
Obese class I	4 (5.2%)

[1] Means and standard deviations (M ± S.D), frequency, and percentages (%).

3.2. Overview of the Questionnaire Results

The results of this survey present findings concerning different aspects of students' life, perceptions about health and body image, and the use of social networks. The themes that emerged from the present research are presented below as headings and supported by quotes from the participants. Each quote is accompanied by the identification number assigned to the participant (participant ID), sex, and age of the participant in parentheses.

3.2.1. Theme 1: Personal Reflections of a Healthy Lifestyle

The first question in the second section of the survey invited students to reflect. They were asked to mention, in a few words, what their perception of a healthy lifestyle was. The results obtained are shown in Figure 1.

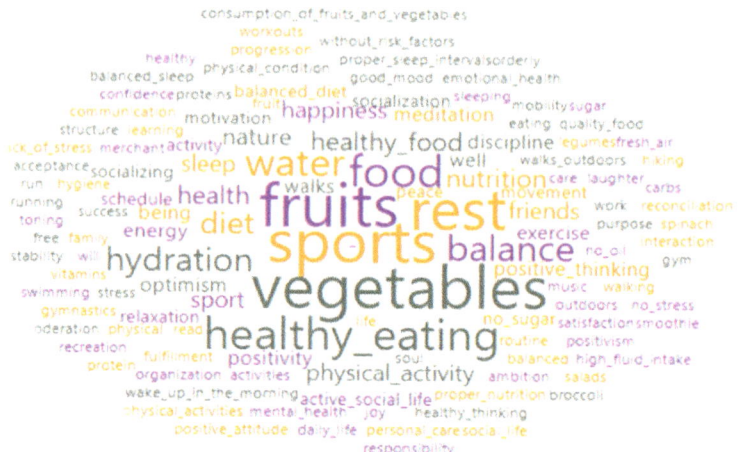

Figure 1. Word cloud of the students' reflections on the healthy lifestyle.

As shown in the word cloud visualization, where the size of the word indicates the frequency of its use, the most used words were "sports", "vegetables", "fruits", "healthy eating", "balance", "healthy food", "nutrition", and "diet". The importance of hydration, sleep, and rest are highlighted as the main components of a healthy lifestyle through words such as "water", "hydration", "sleep", "rest", "relaxation", "proper sleep", "balanced sleep", and "high fluid intake". The students also focused on mental and social health, mentioning various words that refer to these components of a healthy lifestyle, such as "happiness", "friends", "optimism", "positive thinking", "positive attitude", "positivity", "meditation", "motivation", "active social life", "socialization", "healthy thinking", "walks", "outdoors walks", "nature", "mental health", and "soul".

Regarding the reasons why a healthy lifestyle is necessary, most students scored an increased quality of life, physical, mental, and social well-being and lack of diseases: *A healthy lifestyle is necessary starting with the health of the physical body, to the mental, emotional, spiritual well-being* (participant ID 9: Female, age 20); *Through a healthy lifestyle we stay in shape, we will have a longer and happier life* (participant ID 23: Male, age 20); *The main reason why I consider it is necessary to have a healthy lifestyle is to avoid certain diseases, to maintain a general state of well-being* (participant ID 72: Female, age 20).

Some of the students highlighted the relationship between a healthy lifestyle and physical appearance or body shape: *A healthy lifestyle is necessary because in this way we can maintain both physical and mental balance of the body. Moreover, a healthy lifestyle gives us the opportunity to have a pleasant physical appearance* (participant ID 8: Male, age 19); *For physical appearance, implicit self-esteem and health* (participant ID 71: Female, age 20); *You feel much better in your body, it helps to have a better physical and mental condition* (participant ID 41: Male, age 23); *Because it helps us look better, but in addition our body will feel much better, and this can also help us in emotional states* (participant ID 50: Female, age 21).

At the same time, practicing sports, as another important component of lifestyle, helps to maintain a good physical condition, a harmonious body, to lose weight, and to increase muscle mass, as evidenced by the participants' answers: *To lose weight, to keep fit, for immunity* (participant ID 10: Female, age 19); *To develop muscle mass* (participant ID 25: Male, age 19); *For better physical condition, optimal body weight, better mood* (participant ID 68: Female, age 19).

3.2.2. Theme 2: Changes in Lifestyle

Most students acknowledged that they had an unhealthy eating behavior, characterized by high consumption of fast food, high carbohydrate intake, low consumption of fruits and vegetables, and other unhealthy behaviors: *I should eat fewer sweets, I should quit smoking, I should practice more sports* (participant ID 70: Female, age 19); *I should reduce sedentary lifestyle, eat a lot more fruits and vegetables, be more organized with the time I eat, and drink less coffee* (participant ID 46: Female, age 19).

Some students mentioned that they would change these things in their lifestyle but face certain obstacles, most often highlighted by the lack of time, busy schedule, lack of motivation, and sometimes money: *Lack of motivation and will, laziness, insufficient time* (participant ID 27: Female, age 20); *The busy schedule and the responsibilities of some days, job and college* (participant ID 60: Female, age 23); *Time, money* (participant ID 73: Female, age 19).

3.2.3. Theme 3: Perception of Body Image

The students were asked to mention three characteristics that they considered most important when thinking about their body and the way it looked. Thus, the most used words were "fit" ($N = 14$), "slender" ($N = 13$), "sensitive" ($N = 9$), "beautiful" ($N = 9$), "small" ($N = 12$), "acceptable" ($N = 12$), "healthy" ($N = 11$), or "cared" ($N = 6$).

The level of satisfaction with body image measured on a Likert-like scale from 1 to 10 (1 = very dissatisfied and 10 = very satisfied) showed that most students were satisfied with the way they looked ($M = 7.61 \pm 1.57$). The Spearman correlation analysis showed that the level of body satisfaction correlated negatively with BMI: The higher the BMI, the lower the satisfaction related to body shape ($r = -0.395$ **, $p < 0.001$).

Students were also asked to express their opinion about the importance of body image in today's society and culture. Most believe that beauty standards have been created by culture and imposed by social media: *The body image is important for having success in business, personal and social life* (participant ID 52: Female, age 19); *This is what people see for the first time, plus the media promotes so-called perfection and people tend to frame people in those patterns* (participant ID 65: Female, age 20); *Body image is important only for that person and not for those around them, however it influences relationships between people* (participant ID 37: Female, age 19).

Some other male students considered that the body image is not important: *The body image steals glances, as it were. If you do not have an attractive body image, people will look at you differently, at least that is what I realized and saw in my case, but that is another story. I have been satisfied with myself for many years and people's opinions no longer matter* (participant ID 28: Male, age 21); *I do not necessarily think that body image is important, for me everyone must feel good in their body no matter what the world says* (participant ID 19: Male, age 20).

3.2.4. Theme 4: Use of Social Media

Although the participants mentioned the use of several social networks, the results show that Facebook was the most used among students (94.8%, $N = 73$), followed by Instagram (92.2%, $N = 71$), Snapchat (16.9%, $N = 13$), WhatsApp (15.6%, $N = 12$), TikTok (10.4%, $N = 8$), YouTube (13%, $N = 10$), Pinterest (5.2%, $N = 4$), and Discord (1.3%, $N = 1$), with students spending an average of $M = 4.81 \pm 3.60$ h/day on these networks. The most common reasons why students used social networks were for socialization (54.6%, $N = 42$), entertainment (26%, $N = 20$), an information source ($N = 16.9\%$, $N = 13$), or a way to relax (2.6%, $N = 2$).

For the most part, students stated that social media and peer posts did not influence how they felt about their own body and did not influence the tendency to compare themselves with others. Some of the female students stated that they were affected by these posts in a negative way, leading them to feel insecure and uncomfortable in their own body or becoming envious, while others felt motivated to make a change about the way they looked: *It does not affect me at all. I know my value.* (participant ID 1: Female, age 20); *Sometimes it makes me feel uncomfortable in my body, but most of the time it does not affect me* (participant ID 47: Female, age 19); *Sometimes it motivates me to reach the stage where I am satisfied with my body* (participant ID 68: Female, age 19); *I don't compare myself to anyone, I'm my only competition* (participant ID 2: Female, age 18); *After I started maturing, they didn't influence me at all. When I was younger, they had an extremely great influence* (participant ID 61: Female, age 20).

The impact of social networks on body image was found to be seen differently by the respondents. Students considered that social networks had a negative consequence on their psychological status, while some others mentioned that the body-image standard imposed by the social media helped them motivate themselves to become more careful with their weight. Many students agreed that significant time was invested in social networks to the detriment of the individual study program, of the physical activity, or of the effective face-to-face socialization: *It increases the desire to socialize and the need to express yourself freely* (participant ID 8: Male, age 19); *Some people think that it is not a very positive impact, because many people are disrespectful when they see such people, but many of these stars should motivate us to become our best version* (participant ID 22: Female, age 20); *It helped me develop my level of knowledge, I found information that I would not have found* (participant ID 57: Male, age 19); *At least, sedentary lifestyle occurs because we keep looking on social networks and physical activity remains forgotten* (participant ID 28: Male, age 21); *The impact may be different for each person. It may not affect me at all while other people are trying to change because they want to be appreciated and integrate into the standards that are being promoted* (participant ID 37: Female, age 19); *As for me, these social networks kidnap a lot of my life* (participant ID 72: Female, age 20).

3.3. Body Consciousness Scale (BCQ)

A three-factor structure of BCQ indicates three dimensions of this scale:

- Private body (representing the disposition to focus on internal bodily sensations)—M = 13.19 ± 2.89,
- Public body (which involves a chronic tendency to focus on and be concerned with the external appearance of the body)—M = 17.68 ± 3.22,
- Body competence (which refers to effective body functioning)—M = 9.83 ± 2.13.

The correlation analysis showed that there was a negative correlation between students' age and public body subscale ($r = -0.380$ **, $p = 0.001$): The older the students, the lower their desire to be concerned on with the external appearance of the body.

For the present research, the Cronbach Alpha score was 0.75.

Table 2 presents the results according to gender for the three BCQ subscales.

Table 2. Gender differences for BCQ Scale [1].

Subscales	Men	Women	Differences
Private Body Consciousness	11.00 ± 3.16	13.91 ± 2.42	$p = 0.000$
Public Body Consciousness	15.31 ± 3.36	18.46 ± 2.79	$p = 0.000$
Body Competence	9.26 ± 2.49	$10.01 + 1.99$	$p = 0.183$

[1] Means and standard deviations (M ± S.D), frequency, and percentages (%).

3.4. Drawings

The last item of the survey asked students to open a separate document and draw a picture that came to mind when thinking about a healthy lifestyle. This requirement was doubled by a previous item that asked students to mention, in a few words, what their point of view about a healthy lifestyle was. Thus, analyzing the previous Figure 1, which reflects the themes used by the students to represent a healthy life, we can see that the main aspects related to the positive lifestyle were used (physical activity, fruit and vegetable consumption, water consumption, quality of sleep).

A hierarchical clustering analysis was used to compute the similarity of the images and is presented in Figure 2.

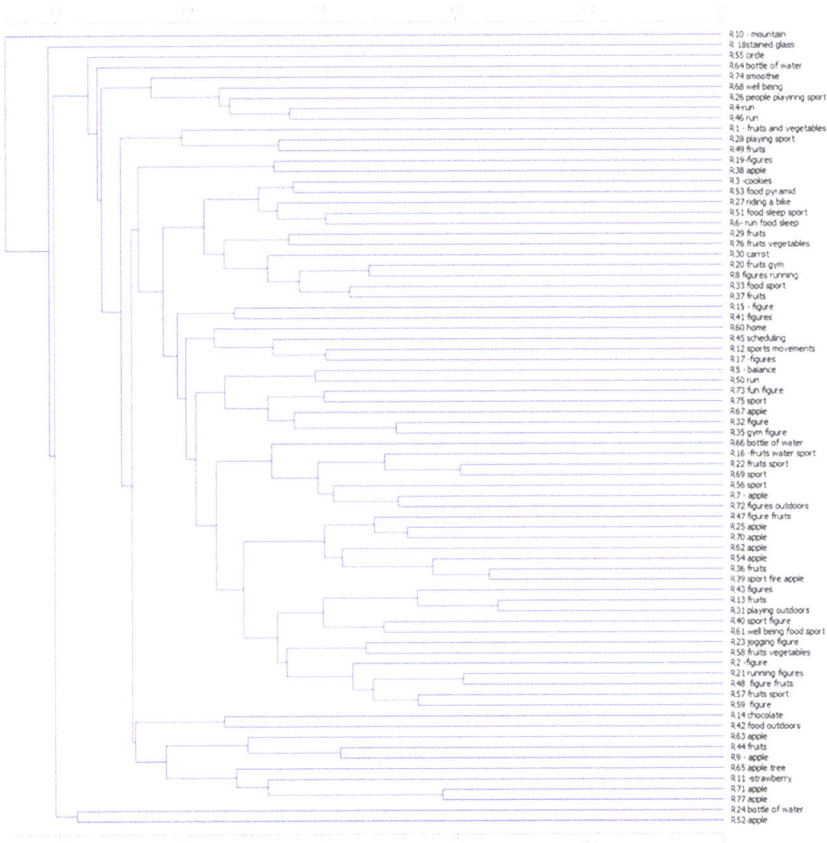

Figure 2. Hierarchical clustering on images that present a healthy lifestyle (R = respondent).

4. Discussion

This study presents a qualitative approach with a significant contribution to the inherent aspects of body image, perceived health, and the usage of social media among freshmen medical university students. At the same time, this study provides updated data on the association between self-image and students' opinions related to the relationship between body-image and social ideals, showing how social media and peers may influence this relationship.

The relationship between body image and healthy lifestyles has been identified in many studies [30–32], which have shown that young people dissatisfied with their body might also have poorer health habits. However, few qualitative designs have identified this relationship among medical students.

In our study, we identified a direct relationship between the importance of maintaining a healthy lifestyle and physical appearance. We found that students considered that a healthy lifestyle was necessary because it offered the possibility to have a pleasant physical appearance, to look better, and, implicitly, to have a high self-esteem. A positive association between healthy eating habits and normal body image perception has also been observed in other studies [33,34], which have shown that body image is an important factor for healthy body weight [35].

Students associated a healthy lifestyle with physical activity, eating behavior (which includes eating fruits and vegetables and having a balanced diet), as well as rest and hydration. Although, in theory, they knew the guidelines for following a healthy lifestyle, many of them acknowledged that they would have to improve many aspects to reach a positive lifestyle (namely, reducing the consumption of fast food, carbonated beverages, increasing the consumption of fruits and vegetables, increasing the level of physical activity, etc.). Our results are different from others conducted on students, in general, showing that they failed to achieve a healthy lifestyle due to the practice of diets, lack of physical activity, consumption of cigarettes, and high level of stress [36]. In addition to the results reported by Sogari et al. [37], which showed that students considered "healthy eating" as something related to a lifestyle with positive consequences on the general mentality of the individual, and the concept of "being healthy" as referring to physical and mental health, the questioned students stated that following a healthy lifestyle was necessary for well-being, social health, lack of disease, and overall, an increased quality of life.

The results of the present survey show that the most important barriers for a heathy lifestyle perceived by students were the busy schedule and lack of time needed to prepare healthy meals, lack of motivation, and lack of money. Some studies have reported similar findings, showing that the most common factors perceived as barriers to a healthy diet were time constraints, high food prices, and availability, followed by a lack of motivation in food preparation, which is intricately linked to intention, the main factor in predicting behavior regarding the consumption of healthy foods, such as fruits and vegetables [38–41]. As the main barriers to a healthy lifestyle that students mentioned, Hilger et al. [42] reported the short time for cooking meals due to academic schedule, some hedonic behaviors (taste of healthy food perceived as unpleasant), the lack of healthy food on campus, and the high cost of healthy food.

BMI values are useful predictors for the risk of bodily dissatisfaction, as some authors have identified [11,43], with younger women being more affected than men [44]. Our results are consistent with these findings, as we identified a negative correlation between BMI and level of body satisfaction among students for both sexes. Most students in this study had a normal BMI (64.9%, $N = 50$), while the rest of the participants were underweight (14.3%, $N = 11$), overweight (15.6%, $N = 12$), or fell into the first class of obesity (5.2%, $N = 4$). However, on a Likert scale from 1 to 10, most participants in our study were quite satisfied with the way they looked. Similar to our results, some other studies conducted on students showed that, in general, most students had a normal weight [45,46], although recent studies on young Europeans have shown increasing trends in overweight and obesity [47,48]. However, contradictory with our results, scientific evidence showed that body image was negatively perceived by most of the women [43]. As comparative results, the study of Aparicio-Martínez [49] identified a higher degree of body satisfaction in men than in women. Aparicio-Martínez also found that body image was focused on obtaining a similar image to that presented by social networks, with analogous findings identified in both men and women subjects.

The scores for the three BCQ subscales proved that women had high scores on the Private Body Consciousness and Public Body Consciousness scales, similar to another study showing that women scored higher on Public Body Consciousness [27] and were more prone to be vulnerable to body image concerns. In our study, a negative correlation was identified between age and public body subscale, which is not consistent with the findings of another study which showed that healthy older people are more aware of external physical appearance and are more positive in self-assessment of body competence than young subjects [50].

The students in our survey mentioned Facebook as the most used social networking site (94.8%, $N = 73$), followed by Instagram (92.2%, $N = 71$), Snapchat (16.9%, $N = 13$), WhatsApp (15.6%, $N = 12$), and TikTok (10.4%, $N = 8$), with the most common reason for using these sites being socialization. There is evidence that social media and internet use are associated with concerns about body image and eating disorders, especially in women, but the causal direction between specific social media and body dissatisfaction cannot be clearly highlighted [51]. A particular type of social media is represented by social networking sites (SNS) such as Facebook, Snapchat, and Instagram that allow users to create public or private profiles and form a network of "friends" or "followers" [52]. Of these networks, Facebook is the most popular social networking site, with over two billion monthly users worldwide in 2017. In addition, in 2016, about 98% of Western students reported having a Facebook account [53]. Instagram (a social networking service exclusively for sharing photos and videos) has grown dramatically in popularity, with over 600 million active users sharing over 95 million photos per day. Instagram is the second most used SNS in Western countries after Facebook [54].

We identified that students spent M = 4.81 ± 3.60 h/day on these networks. Consistent with our finding, another recent study showed that most respondents used social media for 4–6 h a day [55]. Moreover, most medical students (55%) spent 1–4 h a day on social media, and 23% of them spent more than 4 h daily [56]. Moreover, women accessed social networking sites between 6–10 h a day, more than men who spent between 1–5 h on social networking sites every day [57].

The large number of images posted on some social platforms provides regular opportunities for users to make social comparisons related to appearance, with research showing that regular comparison of appearance with others (especially with those seen as more attractive than oneself) can lead to a negative image of one's own body [58]. Thus, physical aspect comparisons seem to play an important role in the relationship between the use of social networks and concerns about body image [59]. Our results do not fully confirm the findings of these studies related to the influence of social media on the students' body. Some participants said they knew their own value or were mature enough not to be influenced by posts about the perfect body promoted by social media, while others felt motivated to make the change they wanted in the shape of their body, or on the contrary, they felt uncomfortable in their own body.

However, the participants of this study stated that social networks had both a positive impact on their lives. Social networks increased the desire for free expression and helped students develop knowledge or even motivation by overcoming their own condition regarding physical appearance. However, social networks also had a negative impact by creating addiction, wasting time, or negatively affecting self-image.

Alperstein [60] showed that sharing idealized female images on networks such as Pinterest can contribute to feelings of inadequacy or upward social comparison. Another study among female college students specifically examined the maladaptive use of Facebook (which included seeking negative social assessments from others and generalizing social comparisons), and found that this type of use was associated with increased body dissatisfaction at 4 weeks later [61]. Congruent with these results, Wang et al. [24] identified that individuals presenting a need for social network popularity were more likely to be affected by selfie-viewing behavior in terms of life satisfaction and self-esteem compared with individuals presenting a low need for popularity. According to our results, Heiman and Olenik-Shemesh [62] identified that more women reported higher dissatisfaction with their body appearance, and their parents' remarks about bodies had an ongoing effect and significant influence on their body self-perceptions.

Social media has the potential to allow more fluidity in gender expression but it also has the potential to perpetuate stereotypes, including beauty standards and body ideals [63]. Social networks that students prefer effectively support their education, for example, YouTube can be an education support channel where teachers find interesting and useful videos or upload ones, and information can be shared on Instagram [64].

The relationship between the promoted image about thinness on social networks and eating disorders and dissatisfaction with body-image has been identified by several studies. For example, Jiotsa et al. [65] revealed that the widespread use of social media in adolescents and young adults was associated with an increase level of dissatisfaction as well as the drive for thinness, therefore rendering subjects more vulnerable to eating disorders. Apacio-Martienz et al. [49] showed that disordered eating attitudes were strongly linked to self-esteem, body image, the desired body, and the use of social media, especially among female subjects. Baceviciene et al. [66] identified the relationship between satisfaction with body image and quality of life among college students. Ansari et al. [67] pointed out that high BMI and depressive symptoms were found more often among students dissatisfied with their weight.

5. Strengths and Limitations of the Study

This study brings important results regarding body image, body satisfaction, and the impact on social media on contentment with body image among healthcare students from their first year of study. Another strength is represented by the fact that quantitative and qualitative results are presented, covering a gap of information about students enrolled in kinesiotherapy studies. Third, the results reveal gender differences in perception about body image.

The limitations of the study are represented by the small number of subjects involved in the research and the fact that results cannot be generalized for all categories of students enrolled in different medical specialties. Also, the alpha Cronbach score for the BCQ scale must be evaluated with precociousness, as multiple studies have obtained, in general, a low alpha Cronbach score between 0.59–0.78 [50,68,69].

6. Reflections and Planning

The results of the present study highlight the relationship between body image, the influence of social networks, and the importance of a healthy lifestyle on students' quality of life. Due to the utility of the findings, such information should be disseminated among students, especially to those from medical sciences who are the promoters of a healthy lifestyle and those who will work on providing healthcare to people in need. The impact of these relationships on the satisfaction with body image and the impact on both physical and mental health are important, especially on subjects at this age. In addition, because healthcare students will work with teenagers and young adults, it is useful consider factors such as satisfaction with physical appearance, ideal body image, and the impact of media and social media on health status. The relevant relationship between the perception of one's physical appearance and depression [70], stress [71], intimate relationship [72], eating disorders [73], food addiction, body mass index [46,74], mental health [75], orthorexia nervosa [76], perfectionism dimensions and physical appearance [77], body image distortions [78], and loneliness [72] are important for both the personal and professional lives of healthcare students.

7. Conclusions

The results of the present study illustrate the complexity of the relationship between social media and body image among healthcare students. Furthermore, they emphasize the need to prevent the concerns on the individual's concept of one's body, especially in young women. Because of the important impact on physical and psychological health, as well as on practices related to healthy lifestyle, these findings are useful for students, healthcare workers, and university staff to provide better assistance to students and to encourage a high quality of life and satisfaction during academic years.

Author Contributions: Conceptualization, L.-M.P. and M.I.; methodology, L.-M.P. and M.I.; investigation, L.-M.P., R.I. and M.I.; resources, L.-M.P. and M.I.; data curation, L.-M.P.; R.I. and M.I.; writing—original draft preparation, L.-M.P. and M.I.; writing—review and editing, L.-M.P. and M.I.; visualization, R.I.; L.-R.Ș.; supervision, M.I. All authors equally contributed to the article. All authors have read and agreed to the published version of the manuscript.

Funding: This research received no external funding.

Institutional Review Board Statement: The study was conducted according to the guidelines of the Declaration of Helsinki and approved by the Ethics Committee of University of Oradea, No. 26214/18.11.2020.

Informed Consent Statement: Informed consent was obtained from all subjects involved in the study.

Data Availability Statement: The data presented in this study are available on request from the corresponding author.

Conflicts of Interest: The authors declare no conflict of interest.

References

1. Tapia-Serrano, M.A.; Jorge, M.-L.; David, S.-O.; Mikel, V.-S.; Sánchez-Miguel, P.A. Mediating effect of fitness and fatness on the association between lifestyle and body dissatisfaction in Spanish youth. *Physiol. Behav.* **2021**, *232*, 113340. [CrossRef]
2. Divine, R.L.; Lepisto, L. Analysis of the healthy lifestyle consumer. *J. Consum. Mark.* **2005**, *22*, 275–283. [CrossRef]
3. Farhud, D.D. Impact of Lifestyle on Health. *Iran. J. Public Health* **2015**, *44*, 1442–1444.
4. Farhud, D.; Aryan, Z. Circadian Rhythm, Lifestyle and Health: A Narrative Review. *Iran. J. Public Health* **2018**, *47*, 1068–1076. [PubMed]
5. Sánchez-Ojeda, M.A.; De Luna-Bertos, E. Healthy lifestyles of the university population. *Nutr. Hosp.* **2015**, *31*, 1910–1919.
6. Kelly, S.A.; Melnyk, B.M.; Jacobson, D.L.; O'Haver, J.A. Correlates among Healthy Lifestyle Cognitive Beliefs, Healthy Lifestyle Choices, Social Support, and Healthy Behaviors in Adolescents: Implications for Behavioral Change Strategies and Future Research. *J. Pediatr. Health Care* **2011**, *25*, 216–223. [CrossRef]
7. Wawrzyniak, A.; Myszkowska-Ryciak, J.; Harton, A.; Lange, E.; Laskowski, W.; Hamulka, J.; Gajewska, D. Dissatisfaction with Body Weight among Polish Adolescents Is Related to Unhealthy Dietary Behaviors. *Nutrients* **2020**, *12*, 2658. [CrossRef]
8. Önder, Ö.Ö.; Öztürk, M.; Yildiz, Ş.; Çaylan, A. Evaluation of the Attitudes of the Students of the Faculty of Health Sciences Towards Healthy Nutrition and Physical Activity. *Konuralp Tıp Derg.* **2020**, *12*, 400–405. [CrossRef]
9. Amattayakong, C.; Klunklin, A.; Kunawiktikul, W.; Kuntaruksa, K.; Turale, S. Wellness among nursing students: A qualitative study. *Nurse Educ. Pract.* **2020**, *48*, 102867. [CrossRef]
10. Yarmohammadi, S.; Ghaffari, M.; Yarmohammadi, H.; Koukamari, P.H.; Ramezankhani, A. Relationship between Quality of Life and Body Image Perception in Iranian Medical Students: Structural Equation Modeling. *Int. J. Prev. Med.* **2020**, *11*, 11.
11. Kasmaei, P.; Hassankiade, R.F.; Karimy, M.; Kazemi, S.; Morsali, F.; Nasollahzadeh, S. Role of Attitude, Body Image, Satisfaction and Socio-Demographic Variables in Cosmetic Surgeries of Iranian Students. *World J. Plast. Surg.* **2020**, *9*, 186–193. [CrossRef]
12. Iorga, M.; Pop, L.; Muraru, I.D.; Alwan, S.; Ioan, B.G. Dietary habits and health-related behaviors among medical dentistry students-a cross-sectional study. *Rom. J. Oral Rehabil.* **2018**, *10*, 32–40.
13. Pop, L.-M.; Iorga, M.; Muraru, I.-D.; Petrariu, F.-D. Assessment of Dietary Habits, Physical Activity and Lifestyle in Medical University Students. *Sustainability* **2021**, *13*, 3572. [CrossRef]
14. Vijayalakshmi, P.; Thimmaiah, R.; Gandhi, S.; Math, S.B. Eating Attitudes, Weight Control Behaviors, Body Image Satisfaction and Depression Level Among Indian Medical and Nursing Undergraduate Students. *Commun. Ment. Health J.* **2018**, *54*, 1266–1273. [CrossRef] [PubMed]
15. Prathiba, T.; Rajkumar, G.; Anbarasi, M. Self-perception of Body Weight and Physical Activity with its Relationship to Actual Body Weight among Students in a Medical College: An Analytical Cross-sectional Study. *J. Clin. Diagn. Res.* **2021**, *15*. [CrossRef]
16. Mills, J.S.; Shannon, A.; Hogue, J. Beauty, Body Image, and the Media. In *Perception of Beauty*; InTech: London, UK, 2017; pp. 145–157.
17. El Ansari, W.; Clausen, S.V.; Mabhala, M.A.; Stockton, C. How Do I Look? Body Image Perceptions among University Students from England and Denmark. *Int. J. Environ. Res. Public Health* **2010**, *7*, 583–595. [CrossRef] [PubMed]
18. Barlett, C.P.; Vowels, C.L.; Saucier, D.A. Meta-Analyses of the Effects of Media Images on Men's Body-image Concerns. *J. Soc. Clin. Psychol.* **2008**, *27*, 279–310. [CrossRef]
19. Grabe, S.; Ward, L.M.; Hyde, J.S. The role of the media in body image concerns among women: A meta-analysis of experimental and correlational studies. *Psychol. Bull.* **2008**, *134*, 460–476. [CrossRef]
20. Kircaburun, K.; Alhabash, S.; Tosuntas, S.B.; Griffiths, M.D. Uses and Gratifications of Problematic Social Media Use Among University Students: A Simultaneous Examination of the Big Five of Personality Traits, Social Media Platforms, and Social Media Use Motives. *Int. J. Ment. Health Addict.* **2020**, *18*, 525–547. [CrossRef]
21. Index, G.W. GlobalWebIndex's Quarterly Report on the Latest Trends in Social Networking. Available online: https://www.globalwebindex.com/reports/social?__hssc=237476959.1.1438834573571&__hstc=237476959.a42fc84f05cdfdea98ac026ac9f39bf1.1438831258631.1438831258631.1438834573571.2&hsCtaTracking=83b791bc-3f59-457b-8ad4-%207d6d0cde3896ja6a79ee4-64dc-4a90-b247-4f (accessed on 13 August 2015).
22. Fardouly, J.; Vartanian, L. Social Media and Body Image Concerns: Current Research and Future Directions. *Curr. Opin. Psychol.* **2016**, *9*, 1–5. [CrossRef]
23. Dhir, A.; Tsai, C.-C. Understanding the relationship between intensity and gratifications of Facebook use among adolescents and young adults. *Telemat. Inf.* **2017**, *34*, 350–364. [CrossRef]
24. Wang, R.; Yang, F.; Haigh, M.M. Let me take a selfie: Exploring the psychological effects of posting and viewing selfies and groupies on social media. *Telemat. Inf.* **2017**, *34*, 274–283. [CrossRef]
25. Aparicio-Martínez, P.; Perea-Moreno, A.; Martinez-Jimenez, M.; Varo, I.S.-V.; Abellan, M.V. Social networks' unnoticed influence on body image in Spanish university students. *Telemat. Inf.* **2017**, *34*, 1685–1692. [CrossRef]
26. Rodgers, R.; Chabrol, H. The impact of exposure to images of ideally thin models on body dissatisfaction in young French and Italian women. *L'encephale* **2008**, *35*, 262–268. [CrossRef] [PubMed]

27. Miller, L.; Murphy, R.; Buss, A.H. Consciousness of body: Private and public. *J. Pers. Soc. Psychol.* **1981**, *41*, 397–406. [CrossRef]
28. Demšar, J.; Curk, T.; Erjavec, A.; Gorup, Č.; Hočevar, T.; Milutinovič, M.; Zupan, B. Orange: Data mining toolbox in Python. *J. Mach. Learn. Res.* **2013**, *14*, 2349–2353.
29. WHO. Body Mass Index—BMI. Available online: https://www.euro.who.int/en/health-topics/disease-prevention/nutrition/ahealthy-lifestyle/body-mass-index-bmi (accessed on 20 March 2021).
30. Wilkosz, M.E.; Chen, J.-L.; Kenndey, C.; Rankin, S. Body dissatisfaction in California adolescents. *J. Am. Acad. Nurse Pract.* **2011**, *23*, 101–109. [CrossRef] [PubMed]
31. Eaton, D.K.; Kann, L.; Kinchen, S.; Shanklin, S.; Flint, K.H.; Hawkins, J.; Wechsler, H. Youth risk behavior surveil-lance—United States, Morbidity and mortality weekly report: Surveillance summaries. *Center Dis. Control Prevent.* **2012**, *61*, 1.
32. Bednarzyk, M.S.; Wright, T.L.; Bloom, K.C. Body image and healthy lifestyle behaviors of university students. *Int. J. Adv. Nurs. Stud.* **2013**, *2*, 107. [CrossRef]
33. Kargarnovin, Z.; Asadi, Z.; Rashidkhani, B.; Azar, M. Assessing Body Image and Its Relation with Body Mass Index, Food Group Consumption and Physical Activity among the University of Economic Sciences. *Iran. J. Endocrinol. Metab.* **2013**, *14*, 455–463.
34. Alipour, B.; Farhangi, M.A.; Dehghan, P.; Alipour, M. Body image perception and its association with body mass index and nutrient intakes among female college students aged 18–35 years from Tabriz, Iran. *Eat. Weight Disord. Stud. Anorex. Bulim. Obes.* **2015**, *20*, 465–471. [CrossRef]
35. Shirasawa, T.; Ochiai, H.; Nanri, H.; Nishimura, R.; Ohtsu, T.; Hoshino, H.; Tajima, N.; Kokaze, A. The relationship between distorted body image and lifestyle among Japanese adolescents: A population-based study. *Arch. Public Health* **2015**, *73*, 32. [CrossRef]
36. Hanawi, S.A.; Saat, N.Z.M.; Zulkafly, M.; Hazlenah, H.; Taibukahn, N.H.; Yoganathan, D.; Low, F.J. Impact of a Healthy Lifestyle on the Psychological Well-being of University Students. *Int. J. Pharmac. Res. All. Sci.* **2020**, *9*, 1–7.
37. Sogari, G.; Velez-Argumedo, C.; Gómez, M.I.; Mora, C. College Students and Eating Habits: A Study Using an Ecological Model for Healthy Behavior. *Nutrients* **2018**, *10*, 1823. [CrossRef] [PubMed]
38. Lacaille, L.J.; Dauner, K.N.; Bas, R.J.K.; Pedersen, J. Psychosocial and Environmental Determinants of Eating Behaviors, Physical Activity, and Weight Change Among College Students: A Qualitative Analysis. *J. Am. Coll. Health* **2011**, *59*, 531–538. [CrossRef] [PubMed]
39. Allom, V.; Mullan, B. Maintaining healthy eating behaviour: Experiences and perceptions of young adults. *Nutr. Food Sci.* **2014**, *44*, 156–167. [CrossRef]
40. Ashton, L.; Hutchesson, M.J.; Rollo, M.E.; Morgan, P.J.; Collins, C.E. Motivators and Barriers to Engaging in Healthy Eating and Physical Activity. *Am. J. Men's Health* **2017**, *11*, 330–343. [CrossRef] [PubMed]
41. Menozzi, D.; Sogari, G.; Mora, C. Explaining Vegetable Consumption among Young Adults: An Application of the Theory of Planned Behaviour. *Nutrients* **2015**, *7*, 7633–7650. [CrossRef] [PubMed]
42. Hilger, J.; Loerbroks, A.; Diehl, K. Eating behaviour of university students in Germany: Dietary intake, barriers to healthy eating and changes in eating behaviour since the time of matriculation. *Appetite* **2017**, *109*, 100–107. [CrossRef]
43. Pop, C. Self-Esteem and Body Image Perception in a Sample of University Students. *Euras. J. Educ. Res.* **2016**, *16*, 31–44. [CrossRef]
44. Pop, C.L. Body Mass Index and Body Image Anxiety in a Sample of Undergraduate Students. *Phys. Educ. Stud.* **2018**, *22*, 77–82. [CrossRef]
45. Cena, H.; Porri, D.; De Giuseppe, R.; Kalmpourtzidou, A.; Salvatore, F.; El Ghoch, M.; Itani, L.; Kreidieh, D.; Brytek-Matera, A.; Pocol, C.; et al. How Healthy Are Health-Related Behaviors in University Students: The HOLISTic Study. *Nutrients* **2021**, *13*, 675. [CrossRef]
46. Radwan, H.; Hasan, H.A.; Ismat, H.; Hakim, H.; Khalid, H.; Al-Fityani, L.; Mohammed, R.; Ayman, A. Body Mass Index Perception, Body Image Dissatisfaction and Their Relations with Weight-Related Behaviors among University Students. *Int. J. Environ. Res. Public Health* **2019**, *16*, 1541. [CrossRef] [PubMed]
47. Drosopoulou, G.; Sergentanis, T.N.; Mastorakos, G.; Vlachopapadopoulou, E.; Michalacos, S.; Tzavara, C.; Bacopoulou, F.; Psaltopoulou, T.; Tsitsika, A. Psychosocial health of adolescents in relation to underweight, overweight/obese status: The EU NET ADB survey. *Eur. J. Public Health* **2021**, *31*, 379–384. [CrossRef]
48. NCD Risk Factor Collaboration (NCD-RisC). Worldwide trends in body-mass index, underweight, overweight, and obesity from 1975 to 2016: A pooled analysis of 2416 population-based measurement studies in 128 9 million children, adolescents, and adults. *Lancet* **2017**, *390*, 2627–2642. [CrossRef]
49. Aparicio-Martinez, P.; Perea-Moreno, A.-J.; Martinez-Jimenez, M.P.; Redel-Macías, M.D.; Pagliari, C.; Vaquero-Abellan, M.; Martinez, A.; Moreno, P.; Jimenez, M.; Macías, R.; et al. Social Media, Thin-Ideal, Body Dissatisfaction and Disordered Eating Attitudes: An Exploratory Analysis. *Int. J. Environ. Res. Public Health* **2019**, *16*, 4177. [CrossRef] [PubMed]
50. Ross, M.J.; Tait, R.C.; Grossberg, G.T.; Handal, P.J.; Brandeberry, L.; Nakra, R. Age Differences in Body Consciousness. *J. Gerontol.* **1989**, *44*, P23–P24. [CrossRef]
51. Franchina, V.; Coco, G.L. The influence of social media use on body image concerns. *Int. J. Psychoanal. Edu.* **2018**, *10*, 5–14.
52. Perloff, R.M. Social Media Effects on Young Women's Body Image Concerns: Theoretical Perspectives and an Agenda for Research. *Sex. Roles* **2014**, *71*, 363–377. [CrossRef]
53. Wilson, R.E.; Gosling, S.D.; Graham, L.T. A Review of Facebook Research in the Social Sciences. *Perspect. Psychol. Sci.* **2012**, *7*, 203–220. [CrossRef]

54. Coco, G.L.; Maiorana, A.; Mirisola, A.; Salerno, L.; Boca, S.; Profita, G. Empirically-derived subgroups of Facebook users and their association with personality characteristics: A Latent Class Analysis. *Comput. Hum. Behav.* **2018**, *86*, 190–198. [CrossRef]
55. Talaue, G.M.; Alsaad, A.; AlRushaidan, N.; Alhugail, A.; Alfahhad, S. The Impact of Social Media on Academic Performance of Selected College Students. *Int. J. Adv. Inf. Technol.* **2018**, *8*, 27–35. [CrossRef]
56. AlFaris, E.; Irfan, F.; Ponnamperuma, G.; Jamal, A.; Van Der Vleuten, C.; Al Maflehi, N.; Al-Qeas, S.; Alenezi, A.; Alrowaished, M.; Alsalman, R.; et al. The pattern of social media use and its association with academic performance among medical students. *Med. Teach.* **2018**, *40*, S77–S82. [CrossRef]
57. Knight-McCord, J.; Cleary, D.; Grant, N.; Herron, A.; Lacey, T.; Livingston, T.; Emanuel, R. What social media sites do college students use most. *J. Undergrad. Ethnic Minor. Psychol.* **2016**, *2*, 21–26.
58. Myers, T.A.; Crowther, J.H. Social comparison as a predictor of body dissatisfaction: A meta-analytic review. *J. Abnorm. Psychol.* **2009**, *118*, 683–698. [CrossRef] [PubMed]
59. Kim, J.W.; Chock, T.M. Body image 2.0: Associations between social grooming on Facebook and body image concerns. *Comput. Hum. Behav.* **2015**, *48*, 331–339. [CrossRef]
60. Alperstein, N. Social comparison of idealized female images and the curation of self on Pinterest. *J. Soc. Med. Soc.* **2015**, *4*, 5.
61. Smith, A.R.; Hames, J.L.; Joiner, T.E. Status Update: Maladaptive Facebook usage predicts increases in body dissatisfaction and bulimic symptoms. *J. Affect. Disord.* **2013**, *149*, 235–240. [CrossRef] [PubMed]
62. Heiman, T.; Olenik-Shemesh, D. Perceived Body Appearance and Eating Habits: The Voice of Young and Adult Students Attending Higher Education. *Int. J. Environ. Res. Public Health* **2019**, *16*, 451. [CrossRef]
63. Lewallen, J.; Behm-Morawitz, E. Pinterest or Thinterest? Social Comparison and Body Image on Social Media. *Soc. Media Soc.* **2016**, *2*, 1–9. [CrossRef]
64. Kaya, T.; Bicen, H. The effects of social media on students' behaviors; Facebook as a case study. *Comput. Hum. Behav.* **2016**, *59*, 374–379. [CrossRef]
65. Jiotsa, B.; Naccache, B.; Duval, M.; Rocher, B.; Grall-Bronnec, M. Social Media Use and Body Image Disorders: Association between Frequency of Comparing One's Own Physical Appearance to That of People Being Followed on Social Media and Body Dissatisfaction and Drive for Thinness. *Int. J. Environ. Res. Public Health* **2021**, *18*, 2880. [CrossRef] [PubMed]
66. Baceviciene, M.; Jankauskiene, R.; Balciuniene, V. The Role of Body Image, Disordered Eating and Lifestyle on the Quality of Life in Lithuanian University Students. *Int. J. Environ. Res. Public Health* **2020**, *17*, 1593. [CrossRef]
67. El Ansari, W.; Berg-Beckhoff, G.; Ansari, E.; Beckhoff, B. Association of Health Status and Health Behaviors with Weight Satisfaction vs. Body Image Concern: Analysis of 5888 Undergraduates in Egypt, Palestine, and Finland. *Nutrients* **2019**, *11*, 2860. [CrossRef] [PubMed]
68. Goldsmith, E.; Frewer, L.; Risvik, E. Food, People and Society: A European Perspective of Consumers' Food Choices. *J. Consum. Mark.* **2003**, *20*, 175–177. [CrossRef]
69. Yilmaz, T. Turkish adaptation of the Objectified Body Consciousness Scale and the Self-Objectification Questionnaire. *Dusunen Adam: J. Psychiatry Neurol. Sci.* **2020**, *32*, 214. [CrossRef]
70. Chin, Y.S.; Appukutty, M.; Kagawa, M.; Gan, W.Y.; Wong, J.E.; Poh, B.K.; Shariff, Z.M.; Taib, M.N.M. Comparison of Factors Associated with Disordered Eating between Male and Female Malaysian University Students. *Nutients* **2020**, *12*, 318. [CrossRef]
71. Kato, Y.; Greimel, E.; Hu, C.; Müller-Gartner, M.; Salchinger, B.; Freidl, W.; Saito, S.; Roth, R. The Relationship between Sense of Coherence, Stress, Body Image Satisfaction and Eating Behavior in Japanese and Austrian Students. *Psychology* **2019**, *1*, 39. [CrossRef]
72. Diehl, K.; Jansen, C.; Ishchanova, K.; Hilger-Kolb, J. Loneliness at Universities: Determinants of Emotional and Social Loneliness among Students. *Int. J. Environ. Res. Public Health* **2018**, *15*, 1865. [CrossRef] [PubMed]
73. Radwan, H.; Hasan, H.A.; Najm, L.; Zaurub, S.; Jami, F.; Javadi, F.; Deeb, L.A.; Iskandarani, A. Eating disorders and body image concerns as influenced by family and media among university students in Sharjah, UAE. *Asia Pac. J. Clin. Nutr.* **2018**, *27*, 695–700.
74. Argyrides, M.; Anastasiades, E.; Alexiou, E. Risk and Protective Factors of Disordered Eating in Adolescents Based on Gender and Body Mass Index. *Int. J. Environ. Res. Public Health* **2020**, *17*, 9238. [CrossRef] [PubMed]
75. Zhang, L.; Qian, H.; Fu, H. To be thin but not healthy—The body-image dilemma may affect health among female university students in China. *PLoS ONE* **2018**, *13*, e0205282. [CrossRef]
76. Brytek-Matera, A.; Onieva-Zafra, M.D.; Parra-Fernández, M.L.; Staniszewska, A.; Modrzejewska, J.; Fernández-Martínez, E. Evaluation of Orthorexia Nervosa and Symptomatology Associated with Eating Disorders among European University Students: A Multicentre Cross-Sectional Study. *Nutrients* **2020**, *12*, 3716. [CrossRef]
77. Sherry, S.B.; Vriend, J.L.; Hewitt, P.L.; Sherry, D.L.; Flett, G.L.; Wardrop, A.A. Perfectionism dimensions, appearance schemas, and body image disturbance in community members and university students. *Body Image* **2009**, *6*, 83–89. [CrossRef] [PubMed]
78. Myers, J.P.N.; Biocca, F.A. The Elastic Body Image: The Effect of Television Advertising and Programming on Body Image Distortions in Young Women. *J. Commun.* **1992**, *42*, 108–133. [CrossRef]

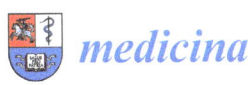

Article

Metabolic Syndrome Prevalence and Cardiovascular Risk Assessment in HIV-Positive Men with and without Antiretroviral Therapy

Win-Long Lu [1], Yuan-Ti Lee [2,3,*] and Gwo-Tarng Sheu [1,4,*]

[1] Institute of Medicine, Chung Shan Medical University, No. 110, Section 1, Jianguo N. Road, Taichung City 402, Taiwan; winlonglu@gmail.com
[2] School of Medicine, Chung Shan Medical University, No. 110, Section 1, Jianguo N. Road, Taichung City 402, Taiwan
[3] Division of Infectious Diseases, Department of Internal Medicine, Chung Shan Medical University Hospital, No. 110, Section 1, Jianguo N. Road, Taichung City 402, Taiwan
[4] Department of Medical Oncology and Chest Medicine, Chung Shan Medical University Hospital, No. 110, Section 1, Jianguo N. Road, Taichung City 402, Taiwan
* Correspondence: leey521@yahoo.com.tw (Y.-T.L.); gtsheu@csmu.edu.tw (G.-T.S.)

Abstract: Treatment of HIV infection is a lifelong process and associated with chronic diseases. We evaluated the prevalence and predictors of metabolic syndrome (MetS) and cardiovascular diseases (CVDs) with individual antiretroviral drugs exposure among HIV-infected men in Taiwan. A total of 200 patients' data were collected with a mean age of 32.9. Among them, those who had CD4 positive cell number less than 350/mL were eligible to have highly active antiretroviral therapy (HAART). Patients were divided into group-1 that contains 45 treatment-naïve participants, and group-2 that includes 155 HAART treatment-experienced participants. MetS prevalence between group-1 and group-2 was 18% and 31%, respectively. The Framingham Risk Score (FRS) for the naïve and experienced groups were 4.7 ± 4.2 and 3.87 ± 5.92, respectively. High triglyceride (TG > 150 mg/dL) in group-1 and group-2 were 15.6% and 36.6% ($p < 0.05$), whereas, lower high-density lipoprotein (HDL < 39 mg/dL) in group-1 and group-2 presented as 76.7% versus 51% ($p < 0.05$), respectively. In group-2, treatment with protease inhibitors (PIs) resulted in higher TG levels when compared with non-nucleotide reverse transcriptase inhibitors (NNRTIs) and integrase inhibitors (InSTIs). The prevalence of MetS in the treatment-naïve group was lower than that of the treatment-experienced group; high TG level resulted in higher MetS prevalence in the treatment-experienced group. In contrast, the cardiovascular risk of FRS in the treatment-naïve group was higher than that of the treatment-experienced group, which may result from the low HDL level. Although group-1 participants have a higher risk of developing CVDs, in group-2, an increasing TG level in PIs user indicated higher CVDs risk. TG and HDL are two significant biofactors that required regular evaluation in HIV-positive individuals.

Keywords: HIV; cardiovascular disease; metabolic syndrome; HAART; Framingham risk score

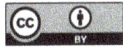

1. Introduction

According to the WORLD AIDS DAY 2020 fact sheet, in 2019, 38.0 million [31.6–44.5 million] people globally were living with human immunodeficiency virus (HIV). A total of 75.7 million [55.9–100 million] people have become infected with HIV since the start of the epidemic. HIV infection is a lethal disease, and approximately 32.7 million people have died from acquired immune deficiency syndrome (AIDS)-related illnesses since the start of the epidemic [1]. Fortunately, combined antiretroviral therapy (ART) improves health, prolongs life and substantially reduces the risk of HIV transmission with spectacular success [2]. The survival time of the HIV/AIDS individuals became longer by 10 years in the past 20 odd years [3]. People nowadays believe the end of AIDS is possible [4]. However, a new set of

HIV-associated complications have emerged, such as cardiomyopathy, heart failure [5–8] and diabetes mellitus [9–12] resulting in a chronic disease that spans several decades of life, and has become an important health issue.

Among HIV-infected individuals, the mortality due to cardiovascular diseases (CVDs) ranges between 6% and 15%, and the incidence of CVD is higher than that among noninfected individuals; moreover, HIV-infected individuals are usually affected at a younger age [13,14]. Irrespective of HIV-1 status, infants with vertically transmitted HIV have significantly worse cardiac function than other infants have recorded [15]. A retrospective cohort study of the HIV-infected patients residing in the Local Health Authority of Brescia, northern Italy, from 2000 to 2012, reported that overall cardiovascular event (CVE) risk in HIV-positive patients was twice as high as CVE risk in the general population [16].

With the application of effective highly active antiretroviral therapy (HAART), people living with HIV are ageing, but the most frequent complications are metabolic abnormalities related to the chronicity of the infection, including metabolic syndrome (MetS) [17–19], lipodystrophy [20] and mitochondrial toxicity [21–23].

The U.S. National Cholesterol Education Program Adult Treatment Panel III (ATPIII) report identified MetS as a multifaceted risk factor for CVDs [24]. An international cross-sectional study that used a well-characterized cohort of 788 HIV-infected adults recruited at 32 centers reported that the prevalence of MetS was 14% according to the International Diabetes Federation (IDF) criteria and 18% by the U.S. ATPIII criteria [25]. In addition, the prevalence of MetS among those HIV-infected patients (17%) was similar to that previously reported in uninfected individuals [26]. Furthermore, the overall prevalence of MetS was reported to be similar among an HIV-infected group and HIV-seronegative group (25.5% vs. 26.5%, respectively) from the US outpatient population [27]. Although high prevalence of CVDs is associated with HIV infection, the above-mentioned reports found no significant differences in MetS prevalence among HIV-infected and noninfected groups.

Interestingly, a higher prevalence of MetS was observed in the HAART group (ATPIII—33.3%; IDF—36.4%) than in the HAART-naïve group (ATPIII—2%; IDF—12%) in a cross-sectional study carried out in a teaching hospital in North India [28] Furthermore, another study found that the prevalence of MetS among HAART-exposed patients was 19.3%, while it was 5.3% among HAART naïve patients, within African populations with a majority of female patients (64%) [29]. The above reports indicated that HAART is associated with a higher prevalence of MetS. Therefore, analyzing the prevalence of MetS among HIV-infected patients from different ethnic populations and HAART patients is still an important issue.

HIV infection itself and HAART can both modify the risk of CVDs [14]. HAART regimes inhibit viral replication by acting at different stages with different combinations of drugs, as reported previously [2,30]. HAART regimes have been classified in different therapeutic groups according to their mechanisms of action: nucleoside reverse transcriptase inhibitors (NRTIs), nonnucleoside reverse transcriptase inhibitors (NNRTIs), protease inhibitors (PIs), fusion inhibitors, entry inhibitors and integrase strand transfer inhibitors (InSTIs) [30]. The role of HAART in promoting atherosclerosis and CVDs has been extensively reviewed [31]; HAART is associated with increase of total cholesterol (CHO), low-density lipoprotein (LDL) and triglycerides (TG) and reduced values of high-density lipoprotein (HDL) [32]. Therefore, the present study focuses on MetS prevalence, CVD risk and characteristics of the possible related factors, including individual antiretroviral drug exposure in HIV-infected men.

2. Materials and Methods
2.1. Study Design

This was a prospective cross-sectional study of metabolic syndrome and cardiovascular disease risk factors in HIV-positive men attending a tertiary care hospital in central Taiwan. The study protocol was reviewed and approved by the Hospital's Research and Ethics Committee (IRB approval number CS14034).

2.2. Study Population

The study population was made up of male adult patients and was diagnosed as HIV-1 positive by Western blot or polymerase chain reaction analysis at the hospital.

2.3. Data Collection

In this study, a survey was used to collect 200 copies of case reports from the HIV-infected patients between 2014 and 2016. The research analyzed the compliance of medication, metabolic syndrome, cardiovascular disease, and treatment of viral resistance through systematic follow-up of medical guidance cases. The inclusion criteria were: (1) age greater than or equal to 20 years old; (2) diagnosis of AIDS confirmed (ICD9 042); (3) only cases in this hospital and patients who have been treated for more than 6 months; (4) cases of HIV-infected patients taking either HAART (Experienced) or not taking cocktail therapy (naïve) who are willing to accept the investigation and service. The exclusion criteria were: (1) male patient younger than 20 years old; (2) when the subject, legal representative or person with consent is unable to read; (3) incomplete data, or unable to assess efficacy; (4) patient is tracked for less than 6 months in the hospital. This is a noninvasive treatment plan, so no withdrawal or rescue treatment conditions were included. Questionnaires were introduced to the subjects to obtain basic demographic data and history of education, occupation, HAART type and duration, cigarette smoking, alcohol drinking, exercise, antihypertensive and diabetic medication. Thereafter, blood pressure was taken in the sitting position after five minutes of rest. Weight, height and waist circumference were measured to calculate body mass index (BMI). MetS was defined as the presence of 3 or more of the following 5 abnormalities for men: (1) waist ≥ 90 cm, (2) systolic blood pressure (SBP) ≥ 131 mmHg or diastolic blood pressure (DBP) ≥ 81 mmHg, (3) HDL < 40 mg/dL, (4) fasting glucose ≥ 100 mg/dL, and (5) triglyceride (TG) ≥ 150 mg/dL. The HAART backbone is NRTIs (Zidovudine; Lamivudine; Abacavir; Tenofovir/Emtricitabine) that was combined with PIs (Atazanavir; Lopinavir/Ritonavir; Darunavir) or NNRTIs (Nevirapine; Efavirenz; Rilpivirine; Efavirenz/Tenofovir/Emtricitabine) or InSTIs (Raltegravir).

2.4. Statistical Analysis

Data from the completed questionnaires and laboratory results were categorized as HIV-positive treatment-naïve (group-1) and HIV-positive treatment-experienced (group-2). Ten-year risk assessments for CVD was performed by the Framingham risk score (FRS) calculator [33] using age, diabetes, smoking, SBP, CHO, LDL, and HDL as predictors. Statistical analyses were performed using SPSS version 18 (Chicago, IL, USA). Continuous variables were compared using the Mann–Whitney U test for non-normally distributed variables. The chi-squared test was used to determine whether there is a significant difference between one or more categories with numbers indicated. The level of statistical significance was established at the p value of <0.05. One-way ANOVA was used to compare the mean values between the three subgroups and calculated by the Tukey honest significant difference test (HSD).

3. Results

3.1. Epidemiology of Participants

During the period from June 2014 to April 2016, a total of 200 HIV infected men in the hospital signed the consent form. Before 2016, patients of Taiwan who had CD4 positive cell number less than 350/mL were eligible to have HAART therapy. After evaluating their anti-HIV therapy, patients were divided into group-1 ($n = 45$) those not taking cocktail therapy (Naïve), and group-2 ($n = 155$) those taking HAART (Experienced), respectively (Table 1). After 2015, the HAART was applied to every HIV positive patient without restriction of CD4 positive cell number. The overall mean ($\pm$SD) age was 32.9 ($\pm$8.2) years; the group-1 mean ($\pm$SD) age was 30.5 ($\pm$7.6) years old and the group-2 mean ($\pm$SD) age was 33.6 ($\pm$8.2) years old; group-1 was significantly younger than group-2. Our data showed that the mean of HAART treatment period was 3.3 y ($\pm$2.1) that may reflect why group-1 was younger than group-2. Among them, only 10 individuals were married. A total of 66% of participants had received college education and the student status in group-1 (17.8%) was significantly higher than that in group-2 (7.1%). A total of 77.5% participants had a full-time job, 51% were smokers and 41% of participants drank alcohol. We found no significant difference in regular excise habits between the two groups.

Table 1. Characteristics of HIV-infected patients ($n = 200$).

Demographics		Total $n = 200$	Group-1 $n = 45$	Group-2 $n = 155$	p Value
Gender	Male	200 (100%)	45 (22.5%)	155 (77.5%)	
Age (yr) ± SD		32.9 ± 8.2	30.5 ± 7.6	33.6 ± 8.2	0.024 *
	20–30	81 (40.5%)	24 (53.3%)	57 (36.8%)	0.134
	31–40	94 (47.0%)	17 (37.8%)	77 (49.7%)	
	≧41	25 (12.5%)	4 (8.9%)	21 (13.5%)	
Marital status	No	190 (95.0%)	44 (97.8%)	146 (94.2%)	0.331
	Yes	10 (5.0%)	1 (2.2%)	9 (5.8%)	
Education	High school	68 (34.0%)	15 (33.3%)	53 (34.2%)	0.915
	College	132 (66.0%)	30 (66.7%)	102 (65.8%)	
Occupation	Full-time	155 (77.5%)	32 (71.1%)	123 (79.4%)	0.379
	Part-time	21 (10.5%)	5 (11.1%)	16 (10.3%)	
	Jobless	24 (12.0%)	8 (17.8%)	16 (10.3%)	
Student	No	181 (90.5%)	37 (82.2%)	144 (92.9%)	0.031 *
	Yes	19 (9.5%)	8 (17.8%)	11 (7.1%)	
Smoking	No	102 (51.0)	20 (44.4)	82 (52.9)	0.159
	Quit	23 (11.5)	3 (6.7)	20 (12.9)	
	Yes	75 (37.5)	22 (48.9)	53 (34.2)	
Drinking	No	82 (41.0)	15 (33.3)	67 (43.2)	0.421
	Quit	32 (16.0)	7 (15.6)	25 (16.1)	
	Yes	86 (42.0)	23 (51.1)	63 (40.6)	
Regular exercise	No	108 (54.0)	24 (53.3)	84 (54.2)	0.919
	Yes	92 (46.0)	21 (46.7)	71 (45.8)	

SD, standard deviation. * Statistically significant, p value of <0.05. Group-1: naïve; group-2: HAART-treated.

3.2. Basic Physiological Data of the Participants

The overall mean (±SD) waist circumference was 80.9 cm (±6.1), height was 171.8 cm (±6.1) and weight was 67.5 kg (±12.6) for all participants (Table 2). The calculated mean BMI for all participants was 22.8 (±3.8), with no significant difference in BMI in group-1 (23.1 ± 4.3) and group-2 (22.7 ± 3.7). There were also no significant differences in average SBP, DBP and heartbeat in the two groups.

3.3. Laboratory Variables of the Participants

The TG analysis data were 92 (median) and 115 mg/dL in group-1 and group-2, respectively. In group-1, 15.6% of participants had a high TG level (≧151 mg/dL), whereas, in group-2, 36.6% of patients presented a high level, resulting in a significant difference (Table 3). Although no significant differences were found in CHO, LDL and fasting blood glucose (glucose), there was a significant difference in the HDL levels between the two groups. The HDL level in group-1 was 34.3 mg/dL (median) and it was 39.8 mg/dL in group-2 ($p < 0.05$). The median number of CD4+ cells in both groups showed no significant difference, but the median plasma HIV-RNA viral load (VL) was significantly different, with 20,535 copies/mL in group-1 and 20 copies/mL in group-2. In group-2, 63.2% of patients have less than 20 copies/mL of VL, 20.6% had 21–1000 copies/mL of VL and 16.1% had more than 1000 copies/mL of VL. Two participants lacked TG and CHO data and four participants had no HDL, LDL and glucose data.

Table 2. Basic physiological data of the participants ($n = 200$).

Variables		Total $n = 200$	Group-1 $n = 45$	Group-2 $n = 155$	p Value
Mean waist circumference	(cm)	80.9 ± 6.1	80.3 ± 10.2	81.1 ± 10.0	0.635
Mean height	(cm)	171.8 ± 6.1	172.3 ± 4.7	171.6 ± 6.5	0.427
Mean weight	(kg)	67.5 ± 12.6	68.7 ± 13.0	67.2 ± 12.5	0.502
BMI	≤17	12 (6.0%)	3 (6.7%)	9 (5.8%)	0.903
	18–24	125 (62.5%)	29 (64.4%)	96 (61.9%)	
	≥25	63 (31.5%)	13 (28.9%)	50 (32.3%)	
Mean BMI		22.8 ± 3.8	23.1 ± 4.3	22.7 ± 3.7	0.539
Systolic blood pressure	≤130 mmHg	146 (73.0%)	31 (68.9%)	115 (74.2%)	0.480
	≥131 mmHg	54 (27.0%)	14 (31.1%)	40 (25.8%)	
Mean SBP	(mmHg)	122.4 ± 17.8	122.4 ± 14.3	122.3 ± 13.6	0.980
Diastolic blood pressure	≤80 mmHg	122 (61.0%)	25 (55.6%)	97 (62.6%)	0.395
	≥81 mmHg	78 (39.0%)	20 (44.4%)	58 (37.4%)	
Mean DBP	(mmHg)	78.7 ± 10.0	79.0 ± 10.7	78.6 ± 9.8	0.839
Mean heartbeat	(beat/min)	82.5 ± 12.2	84.8 ± 12.0	81.8 ± 12.3	0.148

BMI, body mass index. DBP, diastolic blood pressure. SBP, systolic blood pressure. Group-1: naïve; group-2: HAART-treated.

Table 3. Laboratory variables of the participants ($n = 200$).

Variables		Total	Group-1	Group-2	p Value
TG median	mg/dL	108.5	92.0	115.0	0.078
	95% C.I.	(69.8, 165.3)	(67.0, 132.5)	(70.0, 181.0)	
TG level ($n = 198$)	≤150 mg/dL	135 (68.2%)	38 (84.4%)	97 (63.4%)	0.008 *
	≥151 mg/dL	63 (31.8%)	7 (15.6%)	56 (36.6%)	
CHO median	mg/dL	164.0	167.0	164.0	0.892
	95% C.I.	(140. 8185.0)	(143.5, 186.0)	(140.0, 184.0)	
CHO level ($n = 198$)	≤200 mg/dL	169 (85.4%)	39 (86.7%)	130 (85.0%)	0.777
	≥201 mg/dL	29 (14.6%)	6 (13.3%)	23 (15.0%)	
HDL median	mg/dL	38.4	34.3	39.8	0.005 *
	95% C.I.	(31.8, 45.2)	(28.6, 39.8)	(32.5, 47.1)	
HDL level ($n = 196$)	<39 mg/dL	111 (56.6%)	33 (76.7%)	78 (51.0%)	0.003 *
	≥40 mg/dL	85 (43.4%)	10 (23.3%)	75 (49.0%)	
LDL median	mg/dL	96.0	101.0	93.0	0.074
	95% C.I.	(79.3, 116.0)	(78.0, 127.0)	(79.5, 114.0)	
LDL level ($n = 196$)	≤100 mg/dL	114 (58.2%)	20 (46.5%)	94 (61.4%)	0.080
	≥101 mg/dL	82 (41.8%)	23 (53.5%)	59 (38.6%)	
Glucose median ($n = 196$)	mg/dL	98	97	99	0.471
	95% C.I.	(73,325)	(77,135)	(73,325)	
CD4+ median	Cells/mm^3	472.5	442.0	479.0	0.391
	95% C.I.	(342.0, 633.8)	(338.5, 601.0)	(351.0, 642.0)	
CD4+ level	<200 cells/mm^3	15 (7.5%)	2 (4.4%)	13 (8.4%)	
	200–500 cells/mm^3	96 (48.0%)	26 (57.8%)	70 (45.2%)	0.291
	>500 cells/mm^3	89 (44.5%)	17 (37.8%)	72 (46.5%)	
VL median	Copies/mL	22.0	20,535.0	20	0.000 *
	95% C.I.	(20. 9156)	(7813, 50,567)	(20, 96)	0.000 *
VL level	≤20 copies/mL	98 (49.0%)	0	98 (63.2%)	
	21–1000 copies/mL	36 (18.0%)	4 (8.9%)	32 (20.6%)	
	>1000 copies/mL	66 (33.0%)	41 (91.1%)	25 (16.1%)	

C.I., confidence intervals. CHO, cholesterol. HDL, high-density lipoprotein. LDL, low-density lipoprotein. TG, triglyceride. VL, plasma HIV-RNA viral load. * Statistically significant, p value of <0.05. Group-1: naïve; group-2: HAART-treated.

3.4. Prevalence of Metabolic Syndrome in HIV-Positive Patients

The numbers of all participants with MetS were analyzed (Table 4). In total, 56 individuals (28%) had MetS and the positive percentage was correlated with older age. When the MetS was analyzed in group-1 and group-2 (Table 4), 18% of participants in group-1 had MetS and the prevalence was 31% in group-2. The correlation of aging and MetS in naïve and HAART participants was further analyzed as listed in Table 4 with p value. HAART significantly increased metabolic syndrome prevalence in men over 50 years of age.

Table 4. Metabolic syndrome among naïve and HAART patients by age (n = 199).

Range of Age	Group-1	MetS	%	Group-2	MetS	%	p Value	Total (G-1 + G-2)	MetS	%
20–30	24	2	8%	57	15	26%	0.0810	81	17	21%
31–40	15	5	33%	78	20	26%	0.5373	93	25	27%
41–50	3	1	33%	14	7	50%	1.0000	17	8	47%
>50	2	0	0%	6	6	100%	0.0357 *	8	6	75%
Total	44	8	18%	155	48	31%	0.1281	199	56	28%

Group-1: naïve; group-2: HAART-treated. MetS was defined as the presence of 3 or more of the following 5 abnormalities for men: (1) waist $\geq$ 90 cm, (2) systolic blood pressure (SBP) $\geq$ 131 mmHg or diastolic blood pressure (DBP) $\geq$ 81 mmHg, (3) HDL < 40 mg/dL, (4) fasting glucose $\geq$ 100 mg/dL, and (5) triglyceride (TG) $\geq$ 150 mg/dL. * Statistically significant, p value of <0.05 was estimated by Fisher's exact test.

3.5. Association of Cardiovascular Risk in HIV Therapy

Sufficient data were available for 42 participants in group-1 and 154 participants in group-2 to evaluate cardiovascular risk by FRS (Table 5). The percentage of 10-year estimated coronary heart disease (CHD) risk among all of the HIV-infected participants was 4.53. Percentage of cardiovascular risk by group was 4.70 and 3.87 for group-1 and group-2, respectively. The calculated heart age/vascular age was 38 years old, which was higher than average age (32.9 yr.) of all of the HIV-infected participants. For ages 20–30, FRS results were 1.64 and 1.43 for group-1 and group-2, respectively. For ages 31–40, FRS results were 5.32 and 4.18 for group-1 and group-2, respectively (Supplemental Table S1). The results indicate that group-1 participants without HAART treatment have a higher risk of developing CVDs. Although, only "Age" was significantly associated with cardiovascular risk but not FRS; the possible explanation is that only HDL significantly elevated by HAART, whereas other FRS factors of smoking, BMI, sugar, and cholesterol were not significantly different between these two groups as data listed in Tables 1–3.

Table 5. Cardiovascular risk among naïve and HAART participants (n = 196).

Items	Total	Group-1 ($\pm$SD)	Group-2 ($\pm$SD)	p Value
Numbers	196	42	154	
FRS (%)	4.53	4.70 ($\pm$4.20)	3.87 ($\pm$5.92)	0.3956
Age (mean)	32.9	29.95 ($\pm$7.18)	33.70 ($\pm$8.32)	0.0084 *
Heart age/vascular age (mean)	38	36.00 ($\pm$12.14)	38.00 ($\pm$13.80)	0.3946

Group-1: naïve; group-2: HAART-treated. * Statistically significant, p value of <0.05 was estimated by Fisher's exact test.

3.6. Analysis of the Lipid Profile Association with HAART Drugs

Since TG level was significantly higher in group-2 who had received HAART (Table 3), the data of TG, CHO, HDL and LDL were collected from 153 HAART-treated participants (Supplemental Table S2). Sixty-two participants were treated with PIs, 72 participants were treated with NNRTIs, and 19 participants were treated with InSTIs. The TG (mean) level was 162.95 mg/dL for users of PIs, 121.75 mg/dL for users of NNRTIs and 110.32 mg/dL for users of InSTIs. An ANOVA test was conducted to test the significance of TG level among groups as listed in Supplemental Table S3. To further analyze the statistical significance for pairwise comparison of multiple treatments, post-hoc Tukey HSD method was applied, and the results are listed in Table 6. The TG was significantly higher among users of PIs than among users of NNRTIs ($p=0.010$); whereas TG was significantly lower among NNRTIs users than among users of PIs ($p = 0.010$) according to Tukey HSD calculation (Table 6). Analyses of CHO, HDL and LDL showed no statistical differences from calculation.

Table 6. Multiple comparison between every two HAART regimens based on lipid profiles by the Tukey honest significant difference (HSD) test.

Variable		(I) Drug	(J) Drug	Average Difference (I-J)	SE	Sig.	95% C.I. Low	95% C.I. High
TG	Tukey HSD (TG)	PIs	NNRTIs	41.202 *	13.953	0.010 *	8.17	74.23
			InSTIs	52.636 *	21.118	0.036 *	2.64	102.63
		NNRTIs	PIs	−41.202 *	13.953	0.010 *	−74.23	−8.17
			InSTIs	11.434	20.772	0.846	−37.74	60.60
		InSTIs	PIs	−52.636 *	21.118	0.036 *	−102.63	−2.64
			NNRTIs	−11.434	20.772	0.846	−60.60	37.74
CHO	Tukey HSD (CHO)	PIs	NNRTIs	5.361	6.001	0.645	−8.85	19.57
			InSTIs	16.834	9.083	0.156	−4.67	38.33
		NNRTIs	PIs	−5.361	6.001	0.645	−19.57	8.85
			InSTIs	11.473	8.933	0.406	−9.67	32.62
		InSTIs	PIs	−16.834	9.083	0.156	−38.33	4.67
			NNRTIs	−11.473	8.933	0.406	−32.62	9.67
	Tukey HSD (HDL)	PIs	NNRTIs	−1.898	1.841	0.559	−6.26	2.46
			InSTIs	2.063	2.787	0.740	−4.53	8.66
		NNRTIs	PIs	1.898	1.841	0.559	−2.46	6.26
			InSTIs	3.961	2.741	0.321	−2.53	10.45
		InSTIs	PIs	−2.063	2.787	0.740	−8.66	4.53
			NNRTIs	−3.961	2.741	0.321	−10.45	2.53
	Tukey HSD (LDL)	PIs	NNRTIs	3.823	5.124	0.736	−8.31	15.95
			InSTIs	11.296	7.755	0.315	−7.06	29.65
		NNRTIs	PIs	−3.823	5.124	0.736	−15.95	8.31
			InSTIs	7.474	7.628	0.591	−10.58	25.53
		InSTIs	PIs	−11.296	7.755	0.315	−29.65	7.06
			NNRTIs	−7.474	7.628	0.591	−25.53	10.58

CHO, cholesterol. HDL, high-density lipoprotein. HSD, honest significant difference test. InSTIs, entry inhibitors and integrase strand transfer inhibitors. LDL, low-density lipoprotein. NNRTIs, nonnucleoside reverse transcriptase inhibitors. NRTIs, nucleoside reverse transcriptase inhibitors. PIs, protease inhibitors. TG, triglyceride. * Statistically significant, p value of <0.05.

4. Discussion

In this study, we evaluated the prevalence of MetS and analyzed the associated factors among HIV-infected young men (n = 200) who are ethnic Chinese. The overall MetS prevalence of HIV-infected men was 28% (Table 4). We also found that 31% (48/155) of HIV-infected Taiwanese men in the HAART group had MetS; the MetS prevalence in the naïve group was 18% (Table 4). Our data were similar to those of recently reported study from North India that collected a total of 116 HIV positive male and female patients in contrast to our study group of male only patients; the prevalence of MetS was also higher in the HAART group than in the naïve group [28]. Furthermore, a previous report estimated the prevalence of MetS in Taiwan and found the age-standardized prevalence of MetS was 15.7% according to modified ATP III criteria from a nationwide cross-sectional population-based survey [34]. The prevalence of MetS in the general population was similar to that in the naïve group. Although, the group-1 (treatment-naïve) participants were significantly younger than the group-2 participants (Table 1) that might be due to higher CD4-positve count with recent HIV infection. Therefore, we further analyzed the same range of ages to reduce the bias and found higher MetS prevalence was observed in the group-2 participants

(Table 4). Although aging is a factor tightly associated with metabolic syndrome in general population, our data suggest that HAART significantly increased metabolic syndrome prevalence in men over 50 years of age. According to both results, we can conclude that HAART is associated with a higher prevalence of MetS in HIV-positive Asian patients.

Other significant differences were also detected in our two groups of participants. The viral loads in group-2 were significantly lower than those of the group-1 HAART-naïve participants (Table 3). Apparently, HAART effectively reduced HIV replication. Furthermore, significantly higher TG and HDL levels were observed in group-2 (Table 3). No significant differences in smoking, SBP, CHO and blood glucose levels were found in both groups (Tables 2 and 3), which are factors analyzed by FRS. Therefore, when CVD risk was analyzed by FRS, it was found that group-2 had lower CVD risk than group-1 (Table 5); this could be because HDL is one of the predictors but TG is not. As MetS is positively associated with CVDs, therefore, it should be noted that FRS modified with TG but not CHO may be more appropriate to evaluate CVD risk among HIV-positive patients.

HAART-associated dyslipidemia is characterized by hypertriglyceridemia, hypercholesterolemia, and decreased serum levels of HDL, either accompanied or not accompanied by increased levels of LDL [14,21]. Although our data show that only hypertriglyceridemia was observed in HAART-treated group-2, statistical comparison by Tukey HSD (Table 6) showed TG levels were higher among users of PIs than among users of NNRTIs and InSTIs. Although PIs is highly associated with hypertriglyceridemia, more drug-resistance mutations in the viral protease gene are required for PIs-resistance to develop that make PIs therapy in demand [35]. Since HIV-positive patients usually need to take HAART regularly and even for their whole lives [2], personalized medicine would provide better health management for HIV-positive patients.

This study has several limitations. First, the prospective cross-sectional study design was still composed of several uncontrolled factors, which may affect our results. For instance, the study has missing data such as glycohemoglobin (HbA1c). The HbA1c is important information for long-term blood sugar control among HIV-infected patients [12], but the aim of the study was to evaluate the prevalence and predictors of MetS and CVDs. Second, the 2015 WHO guideline has recommended antiretroviral therapy should be initiated in everyone who living with HIV at any CD4 cell count. However, this study was conducted between 2014 and 2016. Therefore, we had the data for comparing the difference between treatment-naïve and treatment-experienced HIV-positive patients.

5. Conclusions

The prevalence of MetS in the treatment-naïve group was lower than that of the treatment-experienced group. In contrast, the cardiovascular risk in the naïve group was higher than that of the experienced group, which may result from the low HDL level. In the treatment-experienced group, an increasing triglyceride level of PIs indicated higher CVDs risk when compared with NNRTIs and InSTIs. We suggest that FRS modified with TG but not CHO may be more appropriate to evaluate CVD risk among HIV-positive patients.

Supplementary Materials: The following are available online at https://www.mdpi.com/article/10.3390/medicina57060578/s1, Supplemental Table S1. Cardiovascular risk among the naïve and HAART patients by age (n = 196); Table S2. Lipid profiles among the three HAART regimens; Table S3. ANOVA test of TG, CHO, HDL and LDL significance among the three HAART regimens.

Author Contributions: Y.-T.L. and G.-T.S.: designed and implemented the study protocol. W.-L.L. performed statistical analysis and interpreted the results. G.-T.S. and W.-L.L.: drafted the manuscript. G.-T.S. and Y.-T.L. have contributed equally to the work as corresponding authors. All authors have read and agreed to the published version of the manuscript.

Funding: This research received no external funding.

Institutional Review Board Statement: The study was conducted according to the guidelines of the Declaration of Helsinki and approved by the Institutional Review Board of Chung Shan Medical University Hospital (CSMUH No. CS14034, approved May 2014).

Informed Consent Statement: Informed consent was obtained from all subjects involved in the study.

Data Availability Statement: The datasets generated during and/or analyzed during the current study are available from the corresponding authors on reasonable request.

Acknowledgments: We would like to thank the staff of Chung Shan Medical University Hospital for their technical support.

Conflicts of Interest: The authors declare no conflict of interest, financial or otherwise.

References

1. Joint United Nations Programme on HIV/AIDS (UNAIDS). Fact Sheet—World AIDS Day 2020. Available online: https://www.unaids.org/sites/default/files/media_asset/UNAIDS_FactSheet_en.pdf (accessed on 25 June 2020).
2. Lu, D.Y.; Wu, H.Y.; Yarla, N.S.; Xu, B.; Ding, J.; Lu, T.R. HAART in HIV/AIDS Treatments: Future Trends. *Infect. Disord. Drug Targets* **2018**, *18*, 15–22. [CrossRef]
3. Yoshikura, H. Age Distribution of People Dying of HIV/AIDS that Shifted toward Older Ages by 10 Years in the Past 20 Odd Years. *Jpn. J. Infect. Dis.* **2019**, *72*, 31–37. [CrossRef] [PubMed]
4. Deeks, S.G.; Lewin, S.R.; Havlir, D.V. The end of AIDS: HIV infection as a chronic disease. *Lancet* **2013**, *382*, 1525–1533. [CrossRef]
5. Savvoulidis, P.; Butler, J.; Kalogeropoulos, A. Cardiomyopathy and Heart Failure in Patients with HIV Infection. *Can. J. Cardiol.* **2019**, *35*, 299–309. [CrossRef] [PubMed]
6. Belkin, M.N.; Uriel, N. Heart health in the age of highly active antiretroviral therapy: A review of HIV cardiomyopathy. *Curr. Opin. Cardiol.* **2018**, *33*, 317–324. [CrossRef] [PubMed]
7. Dorjee, K.; Baxi, S.M.; Reingold, A.L. Risk of cardiovascular events from current, recent, and cumulative exposure to abacavir among persons living with HIV who were receiving antiretroviral therapy in the United States: A cohort study. *BMC Infect. Dis.* **2017**, *17*, 1–12. [CrossRef] [PubMed]
8. Masiá, M.; Padilla, S.; García, J.A.; García-Abellán, J.; Fernández, M.; Bernardino, I.; Montero, M.; Peraire, J.; Pernas, B.; Gutierrez, F. Evolving understanding of cardiovascular, cerebrovascular and peripheral arterial disease in people living with HIV and role of novel biomarkers: A study of the Spanish CoRIS cohort, 2004–2015. *PLoS ONE* **2019**, *14*, e0215507. [CrossRef] [PubMed]
9. Lin, S.P.; Wu, C.Y.; Wang, C.B.; Li, T.C.; Ko, N.Y.; Shi, Z.Y. Risk of diabetes mellitus in HIV-infected patients receiving highly active antiretroviral therapy: A nationwide population-based study. *Medicine* **2018**, *97*, e12268. [CrossRef] [PubMed]
10. Ataro, Z.; Ashenafi, W.; Fayera, J.; Abdosh, T. Magnitude and associated factors of diabetes mellitus and hypertension among adult HIV-positive individuals receiving highly active antiretroviral therapy at Jugal Hospital, Harar, Ethiopia. *HIV AIDS* **2018**, *10*, 181–192. [CrossRef] [PubMed]
11. Arafath, S.; Campbell, T.; Yusuff, J.; Sharma, R. Prevalence of and Risk Factors for Prediabetes in Patients Infected with HIV. *Diabetes Spectr.* **2018**, *31*, 139–143. [CrossRef] [PubMed]
12. Jeremiah, K.; Filteau, S.; Faurholt-Jepsen, D.; Kitilya, B.; Kavishe, B.B.; Krogh-Madsen, R.; Olsen, M.F.; Changalucha, J.; Rehman, A.; Range, N.; et al. Diabetes prevalence by HbA1c and oral glucose tolerance test among HIV-infected and uninfected Tanzanian adults. *PLoS ONE* **2020**, *15*, e0230723. [CrossRef] [PubMed]
13. Antiretroviral Therapy Cohort Collaboration. Causes of death in HIV-1-infected patients treated with antiretroviral therapy, 1996–2006: Collaborative analysis of 13 HIV cohort studies. *Clin. Infect. Dis.* **2010**, *50*, 1387–1396. [CrossRef] [PubMed]
14. Dominick, L.; Midgley, N.; Swart, L.M.; Sprake, D.; Deshpande, G.; Laher, I.; Joseph, D.; Teer, E.; Essop, M.F. HIV-related cardiovascular diseases: The search for a unifying hypothesis. *Am. J. Physiol. Heart Circ. Physiol.* **2020**, *318*, H731–H746. [CrossRef] [PubMed]
15. Lipshultz, S.E.; Easley, K.A.; Orav, E.J.; Kaplan, S.; Starc, T.J.; Bricker, J.T.; Lai, W.W.; Moodie, D.S.; Sopko, G.; Schluchter, M.D.; et al. Cardiovascular status of infants and children of women infected with HIV-1 (P^2C^2 HIV): A cohort study. *Lancet* **2002**, *360*, 368–373. [CrossRef]
16. Quiros-Roldan, E.; Raffetti, E.; Foca, E.; Brianese, N.; Ferraresi, A.; Paraninfo, G.; Pezzoli, M.C.; Bonito, A.; Magoni, M.; Scarcella, C.; et al. Incidence of cardiovascular events in HIV-positive patients compared to general population over the last decade: A population-based study from 2000 to 2012. *AIDS Care* **2016**, *28*, 1551–1558. [CrossRef]
17. Li Vecchi, V.; Maggi, P.; Rizzo, M.; Montalto, G. The metabolic syndrome and HIV infection. *Curr. Pharm. Des.* **2014**, *20*, 4975–5003. [CrossRef]
18. Alencastro, P.R.; Wolff, F.H.; Oliveira, R.R.; Ikeda, M.L.; Barcellos, N.T.; Brandao, A.B. Metabolic syndrome and population attributable risk among HIV/AIDS patients: Comparison between NCEP-ATPIII, IDF and AHA/NHLBI definitions. *AIDS Res. Ther.* **2012**, *9*, 29. [CrossRef] [PubMed]
19. Paula, A.A.; Falcao, M.C.; Pacheco, A.G. Metabolic syndrome in HIV-infected individuals: Underlying mechanisms and epidemiological aspects. *AIDS Res. Ther.* **2013**, *10*, 32. [CrossRef]
20. Njelekela, M.; Mpembeni, R.; Muhihi, A.; Ulenga, N.; Aris, E.; Kakoko, D. Lipodystrophy among HIV-Infected Patients Attending Care and Treatment Clinics in Dar es Salaam. *AIDS Res. Treat.* **2017**, *2017*, 3896539. [CrossRef] [PubMed]
21. Feeney, E.R.; Mallon, P.W. HIV and HAART-Associated Dyslipidemia. *Open Cardiovasc. Med. J.* **2011**, *5*, 49–63. [CrossRef]

22. Villarroya, F.; Domingo, P.; Giralt, M. Lipodystrophy associated with highly active anti-retroviral therapy for HIV infection: The adipocyte as a target of anti-retroviral-induced mitochondrial toxicity. *Trends Pharmacol. Sci.* **2005**, *26*, 88–93. [CrossRef]
23. Gerschenson, M.; Shiramizu, B.; LiButti, D.E.; Shikuma, C.M. Mitochondrial DNA levels of peripheral blood mononuclear cells and subcutaneous adipose tissue from thigh, fat and abdomen of HIV-1 seropositive and negative individuals. *Antivir. Ther.* **2005**, *10*, M83–M89. [PubMed]
24. National Cholesterol Education Program Expert Panel on Detection Evaluation and Treatment of High Blood Cholesterol in Adults (Adult Treatment Panel III). Third Report of the National Cholesterol Education Program (NCEP) Expert Panel on Detection, Evaluation, and Treatment of High Blood Cholesterol in Adults (Adult Treatment Panel III)—Final Report. *Circulation* **2002**, *106*, 3143–3421. [CrossRef]
25. Samaras, K.; Wand, H.; Law, M.; Emery, S.; Cooper, D.; Carr, A. Prevalence of metabolic syndrome in HIV-infected patients receiving highly active antiretroviral therapy using International Diabetes Foundation and Adult Treatment Panel III criteria: Associations with insulin resistance, disturbed body fat compartmentalization, elevated C-reactive protein, and [corrected] hypoadiponectinemia. *Diabetes Care* **2007**, *30*, 13–119.
26. Jerico, C.; Knobel, H.; Montero, M.; Ordonez-Llanos, J.; Guelar, A.; Gimeno, J.L.; Saballs, P.; Lopez-Comoles, J.L.; Pedro-Botet, J. Metabolic syndrome among HIV-infected patients: Prevalence, characteristics, and related factors. *Diabetes Care* **2005**, *28*, 132–137. [CrossRef] [PubMed]
27. Mondy, K.; Overton, E.T.; Grubb, J.; Tong, S.; Seyfried, W.; Powderly, W.; Yarasheski, K. Metabolic syndrome in HIV-infected patients from an urban, midwestern US outpatient population. *Clin. Infect. Dis.* **2007**, *44*, 726–734. [CrossRef] [PubMed]
28. Theengh, D.P.; Yadav, P.; Jain, A.K.; Nandy, P. Assessment of metabolic syndrome in HIV-infected individuals. *Indian J. Sex. Transm. Dis. AIDS* **2017**, *38*, 152–156.
29. Muhammad, F.Y.; Gezawa, I.D.; Uloko, A.; Yakasai, A.M.; Habib, A.G.; Iliyasu, G. Metabolic syndrome among HIV infected patients: A comparative cross sectional study in northwestern Nigeria. *Diabetes Metab. Syndr.* **2017**, *11*, S523–S529. [CrossRef]
30. Da Cunha, J.; Maselli, L.M.; Stern, A.C.; Spada, C.; Bydlowski, S.P. Impact of antiretroviral therapy on lipid metabolism of human immunodeficiency virus-infected patients: Old and new drugs. *World J. Virol.* **2015**, *4*, 56–77. [CrossRef] [PubMed]
31. Garg, H.; Joshi, A.; Mukherjee, D. Cardiovascular complications of HIV infection and treatment. *Cardiovasc. Hematol. Agents Med. Chem.* **2013**, *11*, 58–66. [CrossRef]
32. Ballocca, F.; D'Ascenzo, F.; Gili, S.; Grosso Marra, W.; Gaita, F. Cardiovascular disease in patients with HIV. *Trends Cardiovasc. Med.* **2017**, *27*, 558–563. [CrossRef] [PubMed]
33. D'Agostino, R.B., Sr.; Vasan, R.S.; Pencina, M.J.; Wolf, P.A.; Cobain, M.; Massaro, J.M.; Kannel, W.B. General cardiovascular risk profile for use in primary care: The Framingham Heart Study. *Circulation* **2008**, *117*, 743–753. [CrossRef]
34. Hwang, L.C.; Bai, C.H.; Chen, C.J. Prevalence of obesity and metabolic syndrome in Taiwan. *J. Formos. Med. Assoc.* **2006**, *105*, 626–635. [CrossRef]
35. Martinez-Cajas, J.L.; Wainberg, M.A. Protease inhibitor resistance in HIV-infected patients: Molecular and clinical perspectives. *Antivir. Res.* **2007**, *76*, 203–212. [CrossRef] [PubMed]

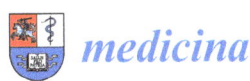

Article

How the SARS-CoV-2 Pandemic Period Influenced the Health Status and Determined Changes in Professional Practice among Obstetrics and Gynecology Doctors in Romania

Magdalena Iorga [1,2], Camelia Soponaru [2,*], Răzvan-Vladimir Socolov [3], Alexandru Cărăuleanu [4,*] and Demetra-Gabriela Socolov [4]

1. Department of Behavioral Sciences, Faculty of Medicine, "Grigore T. Popa" University of Medicine and Pharmacy Iasi, 700115 Iasi, Romania; magdalena.iorga@umfiasi.ro
2. Department of Psychology, Faculty of Psychology and Education Sciences, "Alexandru Ioan Cuza" University, 700111 Iasi, Romania
3. Obstetrics and Gynecology Department, Faculty of Medicine, "Grigore T. Popa" University of Medicine and Pharmacy Iasi, "Elena-Doamna" Obstetrics and Gynecology University Hospital, 700115 Iasi, Romania; razvan.socolov@umfiasi.ro
4. Obstetrics and Gynecology Department, Faculty of Medicine, "Grigore T. Popa" University of Medicine and Pharmacy Iasi, "Cuza-Voda" Obstetrics and Gynecology University Hospital, 700115 Iasi, Romania; demetra.socolov@umfiasi.ro
* Correspondence: camelia.soponaru@uaic.ro (C.S.); alexandru.carauleanu@umfiasi.ro (A.C.)

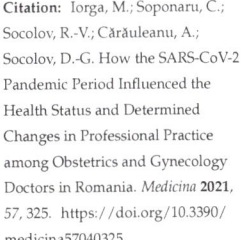

Citation: Iorga, M.; Soponaru, C.; Socolov, R.-V.; Cărăuleanu, A.; Socolov, D.-G. How the SARS-CoV-2 Pandemic Period Influenced the Health Status and Determined Changes in Professional Practice among Obstetrics and Gynecology Doctors in Romania. *Medicina* 2021, 57, 325. https://doi.org/10.3390/medicina57040325

Academic Editor: Nicola Luigi Bragazzi

Received: 1 March 2021
Accepted: 25 March 2021
Published: 1 April 2021

Publisher's Note: MDPI stays neutral with regard to jurisdictional claims in published maps and institutional affiliations.

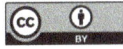

Copyright: © 2021 by the authors. Licensee MDPI, Basel, Switzerland. This article is an open access article distributed under the terms and conditions of the Creative Commons Attribution (CC BY) license (https://creativecommons.org/licenses/by/4.0/).

Abstract: *Background and Objectives*: The beginning of the SARS-Cov-2 pandemic period has had a strong impact on patients' life, but also on doctors. The main goal of this research is to identify the difficulties related to the professional activity and personal life of obstetrics and gynecology doctors. *Material and Methods*: In total, 94 physicians from a single university center answered to an online questionnaire. Socio-demographic, health, family, and job-related data were collected. Data were processed using SPSS (v.25). *Results*: 7.4% of the doctors were confirmed infected with SARS-Cov-2 during the first 6 months of the pandemic, and 48.94% treated infected patients. Due to the large number of patients, 10.64% of the doctors have had no days-off during the last 6 months, and 22.34% of them have had new medical problems that led them to see a specialist. Seventeen to nineteen percent mentioned an increasing number of working hours and shifts per month due to the pandemic period, more than 10% used pills to cope with work-stress, and 25% of them had sleep disorders along with appetite loss. Extra-protection rules and negative consequences of wearing special equipment were identified: thermal discomfort that caused decreasing resistance and concentration during the surgery (52%), reduced mobility and accuracy of surgical or medical gestures (40%), and intraoperative visibility (47%). Doctors who were working with confirmed pregnant women preferred caesarean section. *Conclusions*: Working under the stress of an infection with SARS-Cov-2 is causing a lot of pressure and determines changes in personal, familial, social, and professional life. Understanding the challenges that ob-gyn doctors are facing will help institutions to better provide support.

Keywords: obstetrics and gynecology; physicians; stress; medical practice; psychosomatic symptoms; continuing education; SARS-CoV-2; pandemics; fear of COVID 19

1. Introduction

Coronaviruses are single-stranded RNA viruses that cause illness ranging in severity from common cold-like symptoms to severe complications that may lead to the death of an individual. The novel coronavirus, SARS-CoV-2, shares common features to two other coronaviruses: severe acute respiratory syndrome coronavirus (SARS-CoV) and the Middle East respiratory syndrome coronavirus (MERS-CoV), but it has caused more cases of illness than were reported for the other two combined [1].

The effects of the SARS-CoV-2 pandemic are complex, with multiple reverberations on social, economic, and psychological levels. In this context, it is important to think about the effects on both mental health and quality of life for the vulnerable categories. Healthcare providers are in the first line of defense for this disease, and every day comes with biological and psychological risks, so a careful evaluation of this parameters is necessary to characterize the overall impact of the new pandemic, and to create effective strategies of management, coping, or protection.

During a pandemic, those with pre-existing mental disorders could experience exacerbations or, regardless of their psychiatric background, individuals may become anxious, helpless, or have a mental breakdown [2]. The most significant psychiatric manifestations range from anxiety, depression, panic attacks, somatic symptoms, and post-traumatic stress disorder (PTSD) to delirium, psychosis, and even suicidality, especially for younger persons, or for those with increased feelings of self-blame [3,4].

Any new disorder induces fear of the unknown, and the lack of information, fake news, or conflicting data can increase the perceived amount of stress by healthcare providers. It is necessary to adapt and to embrace polices that focus on correct dissemination of information, reciprocal support, and community-hospital relationships [5–7].

As for the healthcare providers that operate in the field of obstetrics and gynecology, they face numerous daily challenges that may be represented by maternal or fetal complications, material shortcomings, or obstetrical emergencies, which all constitute important stress factors. Even if, theoretically, the risk of contamination from COVID-19 positive patients is lower than for other specialties, they face greater stress, related to the medico-legal responsibility of the medical act in this specialty. For this reason, we consider that the acute stress induced by the COVID-19 pandemic among ob-gyn doctors could have particularities compared to other specialties.

The World Health Organization (WHO) declared 2020 the "Year of the Nurse and the Midwife", and this action outlined the importance of these health professionals, especially during the COVID-19 pandemic [8].

Bahat et al. [9] evaluated the effects of the COVID-19 pandemic on the physical and mental wellbeing of obstetricians and gynecologists in Turkey through a prospective survey-based study and found that the majority of the respondents (76.7%) reported that they were afraid of coming into contact with pregnant women with confirmed COVID-19, and more than half of them (56.1%) thought that vertical transmission from mother to new-born could be possible. Moreover, in this study, most of obstetricians (82.3%) did not initiate labor earlier during this period, and 51.8% reported that they did not opt for more caesarean deliveries, despite their fear of exposure.

Even prior to the COVID-19 pandemic, depression, distress, and burnout were higher among ob-gyn physician [10–12]. Fear of infection and safety measures determine a shorter and more distant contact with patients and their family members, which has a great negative impact on doctor-patient relationships, communication bond, and the trustful link between doctor and patient [13]. Apart from professionally new experiences, physicians must face personal and family challenges: extra working hours with less physical contact with family members, fear of being infected, fear of passing on the infection to family members, isolation, and less physical activity [14].

In a cross-sectional multicenter study by Vafaei et al. [15], the depression score among obstetrics health care providers was negatively associated with quality of life, while social support had a reinforcing effect during the new pandemic.

Since the first reported case of SARS-CoV-2 infection in Wuhan, China, on 31 December 2019 [16], the world has encountered more than 32 million cases, and almost one million deaths [17]. While the first case of COVID-19 was declared in Wuhan on 31 December 2019, in Romania, the first cases of COVID-19 were reported in the second half of March, followed by the first public health measures and social distance limiting rules.

The Romanian health care system had already faced major material and personal shortcomings before the rise of the new pandemic, so the government, community leaders, and healthcare facilities put in their best efforts to manage this situation. The statistics for the SARS-CoV-2 pandemic in Romania indicate a total of almost 122,000 confirmed cases and 4700 deaths [18,19], which reflects the severity of the situation.

Given the developing circumstances with the new coronavirus, evidence synthesis about mental health outcomes is needed to produce guidance for health care facilities and professionals. The level of risk for healthcare workers from obstetrics and gynecology departments remains unclear. The present study evaluated the opinion of ob-gyn doctors working in Romanian hospitals. And it had several aims: to assess general mental and physical health, to identify changes in clinical practice, to evaluate opinions about the pandemic and the fear about COVID-19 and to identify changes regarding personal, familial, and social behavior. This prospective survey-based study is the first one that evaluates the effects of the SARS-CoV-2 pandemic on Romanian obstetricians.

2. Materials and Methods

2.1. Participants and Data Collection

The study was conducted between 1 and 30 September 2020. An online test with non-validated items was distributed to obstetrics and gynecology doctors working in two maternities in Iasi. The city of Iasi is the second largest in Romania and is an important university center. One of the two maternity hospitals was designated to accept female patients with a confirmed diagnostic of infection with SARSCoV-2.

At the time of the research, 133 ob-gyn doctors (80 residents, 8 specialists and 45 consultants) were registered in the two university hospitals. The online questionnaire was distributed to all of them. Doctors were informed that they could withdraw from the study whenever they wanted, without consequences. No incentive was given to participants. The inclusion criteria were doctors who had been active in the last six months in one of the maternity hospitals (regardless of gender, age, length of employment, or medical experience) and who returned questionnaires that were fully filled-in and returned before the deadline.

From the total of 133 ob-gyn physicians, 101 respondents filled in the questionnaire; 7 questionnaires were excluded from the research for being incomplete or submitted after 30 September. Finally, 94 questionnaires were included for the analysis of data. Figure 1 provides details of the response rate.

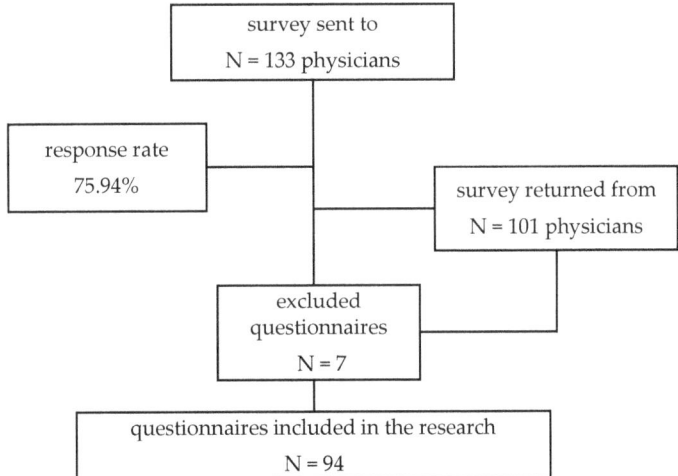

Figure 1. Study profile.

2.2. Questionnaire

The questionnaire was constructed especially for this research and was divided into three parts:

- The first part gathered sociodemographic, medical, and family-related data (age, gender, professional level, length of experience, marital status, chronic disease, medication, sleep and appetite self-declared trouble, depressive symptoms, panic attack, self-administration of pills in order to cope with stress, relation with family members and friends during pandemic period, activities during spare time, etc.;
- The second part had several items investigating the aspects related to their professional life during the pandemic period: number of shifts, supplementary measures in order to protect themselves from infection, relationship with patients and their families, practicing caesarean section/natural delivery, dealing with suspected or confirmed patients infected with SARSCoV-2, professional activity changes imposed by the pandemic restrictions, relationship with colleagues, using special equipment when being in contact with a confirmed patient;
- The third part contained items that investigated the opinion of ob-gyn doctors regarding self-perception about the possibility of being infected with SARSCoV-2, fear of infection, and consequences, etc.

2.3. Statistical Analysis

All analyses were performed using IBM SPSS Statistics for Windows, version 25. Results for descriptive statistics were expressed as means and standard deviations (SD). Correlation analysis was done using *Spearman* correlation, and for comparative analysis we used the *Independent Sample T-Test*. A *p*-value <0.05 was considered statistically significant.

2.4. Ethical Approval

The study was conducted in accordance with the Declaration of Helsinki, and the protocol was approved by "Elena Doamna" University Hospital of Iasi, Romania, with the registration number No. 6843/26.08.2020. Before starting the survey, the participants were informed about the purpose of the research and confidentiality of data. Those who agreed could fill in the on-line questionnaire, and no separate informed consents were obtained or signed.

3. Results

3.1. Sociodemographic Data

A total of 94 obstetrics and gynecology physicians from two university maternity hospitals participated to the survey. The majority of them were female, and the average age was 36.79 ± 10.81 (with a minimum of 25 and a maximum of 61 years old). Fifty-two of the doctors (55.32%) were married or in a relationship, and 54 (51.06%) were parents. The length of experience was 11.46 ± 10.84 years (with a minimum of 8 months and a maximum of 35 years of experience in the medical field). The distribution of respondents, considering socio-demographic variables, is presented in Table 1.

3.2. Health Status and Chronic Disease

Doctors were vey exposed to COVID-19 during pandemic period. Among the questioned ob-gyn physicians, it was revealed that 37 doctors (39.4%) were suspected of being infected and 7 (7.4%) were confirmed.

Most doctors performed the COVID-19 test at the institution (N = 77, 81.93%), and a few others (N = 9, 9.57%) did their tests in private labs (on personal request). During the first 6 months of the pandemic period, only 8 doctors (8.51%) were not verified for SARS CoV2 infection.

Table 1. The distribution of respondents considering the gender and professional level

Socio-Demographic Variables	N(%)/M± [1]
Age	36.79 ± 10.81
Length of employment (years)	11.46 ± 10.84
Gender	
Male	65 (69.15%)
Female	29 (30.85%)
Marital status	
Single	42 (44.68%)
In relationship	52 (55.32%)
Having children	
yes	54 (51.06%)
no	40 (48.94%)
Level of specialization	
Resident	49 (52.13%)
Male	11 (11.70%)
Female	38 (40.43%)
Specialist	13 (13.83%)
Male	3 (3.10%)
Female	10 (10.64%)
Consultant	32 (24.04%)
Male	15 (15.96%)
Female	17 (18.09%)
Working institution	
COVID-19 maternal services	25 (26.60%)
Non- COVID-19 maternal services	69 (73.40%)

[1] Number of answers (N) and percentage (%), Means and standard deviations (M±).

Regarding their health status, 14 (14.89%) presented at least one chronic disease as medical diagnostic. Among the conditions, they mentioned asthma (N = 3), hypertension (N = 5), diabetes (N = 2), autoimmune thyroiditis (N = 2), autoimmune hepatitis (N = 1), chronic rhinitis (N = 1), glaucoma (N = 1), multiple sclerosis (N = 1), chronic migraine (N = 1), vestibular syndrome (N = 1), and liver transplant (N = 1), and 13 (13.83%) were under medical treatment for a chronic disease.

Doctors were asked about consumption of pills for their chronic disease or self-administrated medicines: energy drinks (including caffeine) (N = 35, 37.23%), antalgic/inflammatories (N = 18, 19.15%), antihypertensives (N = 4, 4.26%), immunosuppressives (N = 3, 3.19%), hypnotic/sedatives at bedtime (N = 3, 3.19%), and 32.98% had not used medicines in the last six months.

We identified that more than one third of respondents used energy drinks (including caffeine. The majority (77.1%) of consumers were women; residents were more prone to this kind of drinks (62.9% of residents, 20% of specialists, and 17.1% of consultants were using caffeine-based drinks)

Physicians were questioned if they had been taking medication to cope with work-related stress in the last 6 months. The answer was positive in 10.64% of respondents.

Doctors were asked about psychosomatic symptoms identified in the last six months. The frequency of answers related to sleep and appetite disorders, medical problems, or even thoughts about changing the job in the health services. Results are presented in Table 2.

We identified that more than half of the respondents self-declared that they had sleep disorders. Among them, 80% were women and 54% were residents. Almost one third of them (30%) use to drink energy drinks, including caffeine).

Table 2. The frequency of answers considering the psychosomatic symptoms in the last 6 months.

Items	Yes (N, %) [1]	Women	Men
Have you had any medical problems in the last 6 months that would lead you to see a doctor?	21 (22.34%)	18 (85.7%)	3 (14.3%)
Have you had any sleep disorders in the last 6 months?	50 (53.19%)	40 (80%)	10 (20%)
Have you had any appetite disorders in the last 6 months?	32 (34.04%)	26 (81.30%)	6 (18.80%)
Have you had depressive disorders in the last 6 months?	17 (18.09%)	15 (88.20%)	2 (11.80%)
Have you had panic attacks in the last 6 months?	21 (22.34%)	21 (100%)	0 (0%)
Have you used the psychological services of the unit in the last 6 months?	0 (0%)	0 (0%)	0 (0%)

[1] Number of answers (N) and percentage (%).

3.3. Work-Related and Clinical Practice Data

More than a quarter of doctors (26.60%) worked in a support-COVID-19 hospital. Most of them (91.49%) were in contact with patients suspected of being infected, and almost half of doctors (N = 46, 48.94%) had treated infected patients.

Almost two thirds of the doctors declared that their clinical activity had not changed due to the pandemic period, but almost 20% maintained that their activity in the hospital had changed in the last 6 months; 17% mentioned the increasing number of working hours and 19% mentioned the number of shifts per month.

During the pandemic period, in Romania, medical professionals were not allowed to have free days. One item investigated the number of days off in the case of ob-gyn doctors from both hospitals. We identified that 22.30% of doctors had no free days between 31st March and 1st September. The average was 7.29 ± 6.00 free days during the last 6 months. Strong positive correlations were identified between the number of days off and age (r = 0.270, p = 0.008), number of children (r = 0.347, p = 0.001), and length of experience in the medical field (r = 0.331, p = 0.002).

Doctors were asked if they had thought about changing their job in the last six months. For 22 (23.40%), the answer was affirmative (17 women (77.3%) and 5 men (22.70%)). The distribution of answers considering this item is presented in Table 3.

Table 3. Distribution of answer regarding changing job, considering the level of specialization.

Item Have You Thought about Changing Your Job in the Last 6 Months?	Yes [1]	No [1]
Residents (N = 49)	10 (20.40%)	39 (79.60%)
Specialists (N = 13)	5 (38.47%)	8 (61.53%)
Consultants (N = 32)	7 (21.87%)	25 (78.13%)

[1] Number of answers (N) and percentage (%).

Several items investigated the changes in clinical practice that were imposed by the pandemic situation. Most doctors (89.36%) believed that the pandemic had changed the view of patient interactions and led them to apply new rules and to be more cautious. Items were rated on a 5-point Likert-like scale from 1 to 5 (*never, rarely, sometimes, often, and always*). The frequency of answers is presented in Table 4.

Table 4. The frequency of items investigating the changes in clinical practice.

Items	N (%) [1]
During the pandemic, we followed up pregnant women who missed mandatory tests in the prenatal consultation (double genetic test, 12–14 weeks; TTGO, 24–28 weeks; morphological ultrasound, 19–24 weeks, etc.) due to fear of infection with COVID-19.	2.85 ± 0.91
never	7 (7.40%)
rarely	26 (27.70%)
sometimes	35 (37.20%)
often	26 (27.70%)
always	0
During the pandemic, we changed the way of tracking pregnant women and childbirth assistance by increasing the percentage of private follow-up due to the decrease in outpatient activity in the hospital.	2.79 ± 1.07
never	15 (16.0%)
rarely	21 (22.30%)
sometimes	27 (28.70%)
often	30 (31.90%)
always	1 (1.10%)
During the pandemic, caesarean section was preferred for pregnant women suspected or confirmed with COVID-19 to ensure the protection of staff, by reducing the duration of exposure (4–12h, natural birth vs. 1–2h, caesarean section).	3.65 ± 1.10
never	6 (6.40%)
rarely	9 (9.60%)
sometimes	16 (17.0%)
often	44 (46.80%)
always	19 (20.20%)
During the pandemic, caesarean section was preferred in pregnant women suspected or confirmed with COVID-19 due to the specific maternal risk associated with it (dyspnoea due to maternal respiratory phenomena that would make expulsion difficult).	3.65 ± 1.10
never	15 (16.0%)
rarely	16 (17.0%)
sometimes	18 19.10%)
often	33 (35.10%)
always	12 (12.80%)
During the pandemic, caesarean section was preferred in pregnant women suspected or confirmed with COVID-19 because there are serious cases in which the pregnancy had to be completed immediately.	2.79 ± 1.30
never	21 (22.30%)
rarely	18 (19.10%)
sometimes	25 (26.60%)
often	20 (21.30%)
always	10 (10.60%)
During the pandemic, caesarean section was preferred in pregnant women suspected or confirmed with COVID-19 due to the patient's stress related to childbirth.	2.27 ± 1.15
never	33 (35.10%)
rarely	22 (23.40%)
sometimes	21 (22.30%)
often	17 (18.10%)
always	1 (1.10%)
In the conditions in which communication with the relatives was reduced (compared to the non-COVID-19 period), additional stress was identified in the patient (with panic phenomena, lack of cooperation, aggression).	2.99 ± 0.88
never	5 (5.30%)
rarely	20 (21.3%0)
sometimes	42 (44.7%0)
often	25 (26.6%0)
always	2 (2.10%)

Table 4. Cont.

Items	N (%) [1]
Given the reduced communication with the relatives (compared to the non-COVID-19 period), additional stress of the relatives was identified (with panic phenomena, lack of cooperation, aggression).	2.16 ± 0.67
never	4 (4.30%)
rarely	20 (21.3%)
sometimes	32 (34.0%)
often	35 (37.20%)
always	3 (3.20%)

[1] Number of answers (N) and percentage (%).

We identified significant statistical differences between doctors who treated (M = 3.09) or did not treat (M = 2.49) confirmed patients. We identified that doctors who were working with confirmed pregnant women preferred caesarean section ($t = -2.266$, $p = 0.026$).

The comparative analysis proved that there were significant differences between genders, category of doctors, and type of institution (COVID-19/non COVID 19 hospitals) regarding pregnant women and childbirth assistance. We identified significant differences on the items that determined if there was any change in the way of tracking pregnant women and childbirth assistance by increasing the percentage of private follow-ups due to the decrease in outpatient activity in the hospital between:

- male (M = 2.45) and female (M = 2.95) doctors ($t = -2.042$, $p = 0.046$), meaning that women, more than men, thought that, during the pandemic, they changed the way of tracking pregnant women and childbirth assistance by increasing the percentage of private follow-up due to the decrease in outpatient activity in the hospital;
- residents (M = 2.84) and specialists (M = 3.38), meaning that specialists, more than residents, directed pregnant women to private clinics for medical services ($t = -2.145$, $p = 0.042$). Additionally, specialists dirrected more patients to private services, compared to consultants ($t = 2.836$, $p = 0.009$, Mspecialists = 3.38, Mconsultants = 2.66);
- doctors who worked in hospital providing care for confirmed patients (M = 3.20) directed patients to private medical clinics more than doctors who were practicing in a non-Covid-19 support hospital, M = 2.72 ($t = -2.246$, $p = 0.030$).

Regarding the preference for caesarean section in order to assure the protection of healthworkers, significant differences were identified ($t = -2.904$, $p = 0.005$) between men (M = 3.17) and women (M = 3.86), and there were also significant differences ($t = -3.793$, $p = 0.000$) between non-Covid hospital physicians (M = 3.41) and those who worked in a Covid-19 support hospital (M = 4.32). So, our results showed that there is a significant difference between genders when it comes to caesarean intervention with the purpose of maximizing protection against coronavirus. We identified that women (M = 3.86), more than men (M = 3.7), preferred to provide C-sections ($t = -2.904$, $p = 0.005$). We also found that there is a significant difference ($t = -3.793$, $p = 0.000$) between doctors working in a hospital that provide medical services for patients infected with COVID-19 (M = 4.32) and those who preferred more to have C-sections in confirmed pregnant women compared to those who worked in a hospital that does not accept confirmed pregnant women (M = 3.41).

We identified a negative correlation with age ($t = -0.216$, $p = 0.036$); the older the doctor, the more caesarean section was preferred in pregnant women suspected or confirmed with COVID-19, due to the patients' stress related to birth.

Given the fact that communication with the relatives of patients has decreased compared to the previous period before the pandemic, the doctors were asked to what extent they considered that the stress of the medical staff had changed because of this. More than half (N = 48, 51.06%) maintained that there was an increased level of job-related stress, one third of them (N = 30, 31.91%) considered that there was no change regarding the level of job stress, and the rest (N = 16, 17.02%) felt that stress at work had diminished in the last 6 months.

3.4. Protection Measures and New Behaviours against Infection

Doctors were asked about the effect of the new rules applied to diminish the risk of infection, and they were asked to self-rate their level of fear regarding certain aspects. The answers were distributed on a 5-points Likert scale, from 1 (*never*) to 5 (*always*), and the results are presented in Table 5.

Table 5. The distribution of answers to the items investigating the protection measures against infection.

Items	M ± st.dev/ N (%) [1]
I used the anti-Covid suit for consultations/pregnant ultrasounds/suspicious/COVID-19 positive postpartum women	3.90 ± 1.31
never	7 (7.40%)
rarely	9 (9.60%)
sometimes	16 (17.0%)
often	16 (17.0%)
always	46 (48.90%)
I used anti-Covid clothing during surgery/birth assistance/ICU manoeuvers/resuscitation manoeuvers in the new-born	3.54 ± 1.43
never	14 (14.90%)
rarely	9 (9.60%)
sometimes	16 (17.0%)
often	22 (23.40%)
always	33 (35.10%)
I consider that wearing a protective suit reduces my intraoperative visibility	4.21 ± 0.94
Never agree	−2.1
Rarely agree	3 (3.20%)
Sometimes agree	16 (17.0%)
Often agree	29 (30.90%)
Always agree	44 (46.80%)
I consider that wearing a protective suit reduces my mobility and the accuracy of surgical or medical gestures.	3.94 ± 1.15
Never agree	4 (4.30%)
Rarely agree	9 (9.60%)
Sometimes agree	16 (17.0%)
Often agree	28 (29.80%)
Always agree	37 (39.40%)
I consider that wearing a protective suit warms me too much, and the thermal discomfort decreases my resistance and concentration during surgery.	4.19 ± 1.05
Never agree	3 (3.2%)
Rarely agree	3 (3.2%)
Sometimes agree	15 (16.0%)
Often agree	24 (25.5%)
Always agree	49 (52.1%)
I consider that wearing the FP2/3 mask causes hypoxia, reducing the power of concentration during the surgical gesture/intervention.	3.28 ± 1.21
Never agree	10 1(0.6%)
Rarely agree	13 (13.8%)
Sometimes agree	29 (30.9%)
Often agree	27 (28.7%)
Always agree	15 (16.0%)
I consider that wearing the suit produces unpleasant effects for me: fainting, etc.	3.19 ± 1.37
Never agree	13 (13.8%)
Rarely agree	22 (23.4%)
Sometimes agree	19 (20.2%)
Often agree	20 (21.3%)
Always agree	20 (21.3%)

Table 5. Cont.

Items	M ± st.dev/ N (%) [1]
I consider that wearing the suit causes me difficulties related to physiological needs that must be repressed until the end of the intervention.	3.11 ± 1.34
Never agree	13 (13.8%)
Rarely agree	23 (24.5%)
Sometimes agree	23 (24.5%)
Often agree	17 (18.1%)
Always agree	18 (19.1%)
I am afraid that the protective equipment provided does not protect me enough.	2.51 ± 1.08
never	18 (19.1%)
rarely	32 (34.0%)
sometimes	28 (29.8%)
often	10 (10.6%)
always	6 (6.4%)
I am afraid of contamination when undressing, even if we have the appropriate protective equipment.	3.14 ± 1.23
never	8 (8.5%)
rarely	25 (26.6%)
sometimes	27 (28.7%)
often	19 (20.2%)
always	15 (16.0%)
I am scared because we do not have complete equipment.	2.37 ± 1.164
never	25 (26.6%)
rarely	30 (31.9%)
sometimes	24 (25.5%)
often	7 (7.4%)
always	8 (8.5%)
I am afraid because we have complete equipment, but it is not adequate, although it is complete.	2.33 ± 1.15
never	28 (29.80%)
rarely	28 (29.80%)
sometimes	22 (23.40%)
often	10 (10.60%)
always	6 (6.40%)

[1] Number of answers (N) and percentage (%), Means (M) and standard deviations (±).

More than half of the doctors (65.96%) declared that they had short periods in which they had not lived at home or had not visited their families in order to protect them from possible infection.

Additionally, 87.23% of respondents maintained that they applied additional protection measures when getting home in order to secure their home (they undressed at the door, took a shower immediately, disinfected themselves etc.).

3.5. Daily Life, Social and Leisure Activities

We found that, in the last 6 months, more than a third of the ob-gyn physicians (N = 34, 36.17%) spent more time with their family, and a quarter of them (N = 25, 26.60%) had increased their physical activity during the previous 6 months. Among the most frequent activities that doctors spent their free time doing during previous 6 months were: watching TV (28.72%), reading (11.7%), jogging, and cooking (12%).

Three quarters of doctors (73.40%) declared that the pandemic had changed the view of the profession rules; for 71.28%, the pandemic had changed the hierarchy of their priorities in life, and 65.96% maintained that this last period had changed their vision about life and the world.

Socializing had been another problem from the beginning of the pandemic. Respondents were questioned about changes in their relationships with family members, colleagues, and friends. The most affected relationships were those with friends, and the less affected were relationships with colleagues at work. The distribution of answers for these items is presented in Table 6.

Table 6. Relationship with family members, friends, and colleagues—in the last 6 months [1].

Items	Developed in the Same Way N (%)	Have Deteriorated N (%)	Have Improved N (%)	I Do Not Know N (%)
In the last 6 months, family relationships:	63 (67)	10 (10.6)	11 (11.7)	10 (10.6)
In the last 6 months, relationships with friends:	45 (47.9)	31 (33)	8 (8.5)	10 (10.6)
In the last 6 months, relations with colleagues:	70 (74.5)	13 (13.8)	5 (5.3)	6 (6.4)

[1] Number of answers (N) and percentage (%).

3.6. Impact of the Pandemic Period on ongoing Education, Organization Rules

Ongoing medical education was also affected by the restrictions imposed by the pandemic; all courses were provided online. Almost three quarters of the doctors (74.47%) maintained that they had online lectures, and 68.09% stated that it was exceedingly difficult to adjust to ongoing online medical development.

Subjects also appreciated what the advantages of online education were, compared to onsite education. Among the advantages, doctors mentioned that online course reduced related costs (18.09% of respondents), it streamlined the integration of online medical education into their daily schedule (40.43%), the course content was always available (34.04%), it helped to improve practical ability by respecting social distancing (2.1%), and it was considered much better than onsite courses because it allowed socializing with colleagues from other hospitals and counties (5.32%).

A series of items were formulated to identify the changes in clinical activity, protocol, and organizational rules. Some others pointed out the changes regarding relationships with colleagues and how clinical activity was affected by social distance rules. Answers were credited using a 5-points Likert scale, from 1 (*never*) to 5 (*always*). The frequency of answers is presented in Table 7.

Table 7. Relationship with superiors and colleagues—in the last 6 months.

Items	M ± St.dev. [1]
I noticed that, during the pandemic, socializing with colleagues changed.	3.16 ± 1.26
never	13 (13.80%)
rarely	15 (16.0%)
sometimes	24 (25.50%)
often	28 (29.80%)
always	14 (14.90%)
I noticed that, during the pandemic, the morning handovers were cancelled.	4.47 ± 1.17
never	7 (7.40%)
rarely	2 (2.10%)
sometimes	4 (4.30%)
often	7 (7.40%)
always	74 (78.70%)
I noticed that, during the pandemic, the morning handovers were kept online.	2.52 ± 1.78
never	49 (52.1%)
rarely	7 (7.40%)
sometimes	6 (6.40%)
often	4 (4.30%)
always	28 (29.80%)

Table 7. Cont.

Items	M ± St.dev. [1]
I noticed that, during the pandemic, extra professional discussions in the locker rooms/hospital lobby/cafe were rarer.	3.29 ± 1.26
never	10 (10.60%)
rarely	14 (14.90%)
sometimes	29 (30.90%)
often	20 (21.30%)
always	21 (22.30%)
I noticed that, during the pandemic, the visits to the sector were made with a smaller number of colleagues or residents.	3.80 ± 1.20
never	5 (5.30%)
rarely	10 (10.60%)
sometimes	18 (19.10%)
often	26 (27.70%)
always	35 (37.20%)
I noticed that, during the pandemic, professional online communication groups/networks were created at hospital, clinic, by residents, and in ward.	4.36 ± 1.02
never	3 (3.20%)
rarely	3 (3.20%)
sometimes	11 (11.70%)
often	17 (18.10%)
always	60 (63.80%)
I noticed that, during the pandemic, there were professional discussions over the phone or online rather than face to face.	3.76 ± 0.97
never	2 (2.10%)
rarely	6 (6.40%)
sometimes	28 (29.80%)
often	34 (36.20%)
always	24 (25.50%)
I believe that the reduction in hospital activity means that residents have fewer cases to deal with personally.	4.28 ± 1.00
never	1 (1.10%)
rarely	6 (6.40%)
sometimes	13 (13.80%)
often	19 (20.20%)
always	55 (58.50%)

[1] Means, number of answers (N) and percentage (%).

Working in a hospital that provided medical care to women who had been confirmed with COVID-19 needed more rules to protect medical professionals. The results showed a significant difference between COVID-19 and non-COVID-19 maternity hospitals, in the sense that doctors working in non-COVID-19 hospitals noticed, to a greater extent, the fact that, starting from the beginning of pandemic period:

- on-call reports were cancelled (M = 4.87, t = 5.137, p = 0.000) compared to subjects working in COVID-19 hospitals (M = 3.56);
- on-call reports were kept online (M = 3, t = 4.974, p = 0.000) compared to subjects working in COVID-19 hospitals (M = 1.20);
- more professional online communication groups/networks were created at the hospital, clinic, residents, and ward level (M = 4.54, t = 3.052, p = 0.004) compared to subjects working in COVID-19 hospitals (M = 3.88);
- there were more professional discussions on the phone or online than face-to-face meetings (M = 3.91, t = 2.295, p = 0.028) compared to subjects working in COVID-19 hospitals (M = 3.36);
- more medical education was conducted online (M = 4.28, t = 2.494, p = 0.014)) compared to subjects working in COVID-19 hospitals (M = 3.60).

3.7. Ethical Concerns and Malpractice

Obstetricians were asked if they thought their specialty could be adapted to online consultations due to pandemic restrictions. More than one third of them (32.96%) did not agree to have online medical consultations with pregnant patients. Out of all questioned doctors, only a quarter (N = 23, 24.47%) maintained that they offered online advice to their patients.

Among the reasons why they did not give online consultations, ob-gyn doctors mentioned risk of malpractice–misdiagnosis (N = 48, 51.06%), lack of legal or professional regulation (N = 41, 43.61%), lack of access to the online system (N = 10, 9.4%), and lack of remuneration (N = 6, 6.38%).

3.8. Fear of Infection, Hospitalization, and Disease Side-Effects

Participants were asked about their fear of being infected by their patients and passing on the disease to their family members. Additionally, due to the paucity of scientific information regarding the recovery, side-effects, and impact on healthy people, some items focused on identifying their fear regarding the medication and possible sequelae. The answers were credited using a 5-points Likert scale, from 1 (*never*) to 5 (*always*). The results are presented in Table 8.

Table 8. The distribution of questions regarding the fear of contagion, hospitalization, and infection side-effects[1].

Items	1	2	3	4	5	M ± st
I am afraid I am getting infected with COVID-19 from the pregnant patients	8 (8.50%)	23 (24.50%)	32 (34.0%)	23 (24.50%)	8 (8.50%)	3.00 ± 1.08
I am afraid that I will transmit the disease to colleagues, and I will be accused of this and stigmatized/marginalized collectively.	15 (16.0%)	17 (18.10%)	30 (31.90%)	25 (26.60%)	7 (7.40%)	2.91 ± 1.17
I am afraid I will pass on the disease to family members.	2 (2.10%)	9 (9.60%)	25 (26.60%)	25 (26.60%)	33 (35.10%)	3.84 ± 1.09
I am afraid of anti-COVID-19 medication and its side effects.	9 (9.60%)	21 (22.30%)	18 (19.10%)	22 (23.40%)	24 (25.50%)	3.33 ± 1.33
I am afraid of the precarious hospital conditions I might have if I had tested positive for COVID-19.	4 (4.30%)	1 (1.10%)	13 (13.80%)	31 (33.0%)	45 (47.90%)	4.22 ± 0.98
I am afraid that, in case of infection, I will have to interrupt my professional activity in the state/private system for a longer period.	4 (4.30%)	8 (8.50%)	28 (29.80%)	26 (27.70%)	28 (29.80%)	3.70 ± 1.11
I am afraid that, in case of infection, there is a risk that I will be accused by patients of getting COVID-19 infection from me.	22 (23.40%)	24 (25.50%)	20 (21.30%)	19 (20.20%)	9 (9.60%)	2.67 ± 1.29
I am afraid that, in case of infection, there is a risk of death.	10 (10.60%)	27 (28.70%)	24 (25.50%)	15 (16.0%)	18 (19.10%)	3.04 ± 1.28
I am afraid that, in case of infection, there is a risk of lung pathology.	2 (2.10%)	12 (12.80%)	30 (31.90%)	25 (26.60%)	25 (26.60%)	3.63 ± 1.07

Table 8. Cont.

Items	1	2	3	4	5	M ± st
I am afraid that, in case of infection, there is a risk of extra pulmonary pathology.	2 (2.10%)	23 (24.50%)	27 (28.70%)	21 (22.30%)	21 (22.30%)	3.38 ± 1.14
I am afraid that, in case of infection, there is a risk of remote sequelae.	0	18 (19.10%)	30 (31.90%)	21 (22.30%)	25 (26.60%)	3.56 ± 1.08

[1] Number of answers (N) and percentage (%), means and standard deviations (M±).

Comparative analysis revealed that there were significant differences regarding gender, the presence of a chronic disease, marital status, and doctors who chose to stay away from family members when it came to fear of treatment for infection and its consequences. We identified that:

- women were more afraid of anti-COVID-19 medication and its secondary effects than men (M_{women} = 3.55, M_{men} = 2.83, t = −2.555, p = 0.013);
- doctors who were married were more afraid of interrupting their clinical activity in case of infection (t = −2.201, p = 0.03, M = 3.92) compared to single people (M = 3.43);
- doctors with no children (M = 4.17) presented a significantly higher level of fear of transmitting the infection (t = 1.757, p = 0.003) compared to doctors who were parents (M = 3.52).

Several comparative differences were identified between doctors who were diagnosed with a chronic disease compared to those who did not have a long-term disease in terms of:

- *fear of anti-Covid medication and its side effects* (t = −2.070, p = 0.05) in the sense that those with chronic diseases had a greater fear (M = 3.93) compared to those without chronic diseases (M = 3.23);
- *fear/risk of death* (t = −2.904, p = 0.005) in the sense that those with chronic diseases had a greater fear (M = 3.93) compared to those without chronic diseases (M = 2.89);
- *fear of lung disease* (t = −2.549, p = 0.012) in the sense that those with chronic diseases had a greater fear (M = 4.29) compared to those without chronic diseases (M = 3.51);
- *fear of extrapulmonary pathology* (t = −2.707, p = 0.013) in the sense that those with chronic diseases had a greater fear (M = 4) compared to those without chronic diseases (M = 3.28);
- *fear of distant sequelae* (t = −2.890, p = 0.01) in the sense that those with chronic diseases had a greater fear (M = 4.21) compared to those without chronic diseases (M = 3.45).

Additionally, considering the decision to leave home for short periods of time in order to protect their families, we identified that there were significant differences between:

- doctors who decided to protect their families by living elsewhere or restricting visits and therefore presented a greater fear of transmitting the disease to colleagues, and the fact that he/she would be accused of this and stigmatized/marginalized collectively. (M = 3.13, t = −2.366, p = 0.013) compared to those who did not take these measures (M = 2.50),
- those who protected their families by living elsewhere or restricting visits had a greater *fear of transmitting the disease to their family members* (M = 4.05, t = −2.498, p = 0.016) compared to those who did not take these measures (M = 3.44);
- doctors who protected their families by living elsewhere or restricting visits had a greater *fear of anti-Covid medication* (M = 3.55, t = −2.352, p = 0.021) compared to those who did not take these measures (M = 2.91)

4. Discussion

Few studies have focused on the impact of COVID-19 on the psychological, physical, and professional life of obstetrics and gynecology physicians. The present research showed that a lot of changes affected physicians' lives, on all levels. Their personal life had to adjust to the new rules of isolation, social distance, and self-care. The relationship with the family was disturbed due to concerns about not transmitting a possible infection. We identified that most doctors (87.23%) applied additional protective measures when getting home. More than half of the doctors (65.96%) declared that they had short periods in which they had not lived at home or had not visited their families in order to protect them from possible infection, and a large majority maintained that they applied additional protective measures when getting home. In a similar research on ob-gyn doctors in Turkey, Bahat et al. (2020) found that 74.4% of ob-gyn doctors stated that they were afraid of getting sick, 64.8% reported that they had fallen into despair at times because of the pandemic, 66.5% stated that their family lives had been affected, and 72.4% had started living separately from their families because of the pandemic [9].

Another identified problem was the permanent involvement into clinical practice. We identified that almost a quarter of the doctors had no free days during the first six months of the SARS-CoV-2 pandemic, and more than a half maintained that there was an increased level of job stress. Almost a quarter of them (majority women) declared that they had thoughts of changing their jobs. The use of pills to cope with stress and the intake of energy drinks was found to be frequent among the respondents (37.23% for energy drink intake, including caffeine), with women consuming more frequently than men and residents consuming more frequently compared to specialists or consultants.

Sleep disturbance, anxiety, and fear of contagion were also identified by a few studies conducted among doctors during the first six months of the pandemic period. In the study of Pappa et al. (2020), it was found that at least one in five healthcare professionals reported symptoms of depression and anxiety, and almost four in ten healthcare workers experienced sleeping difficulties and/or insomnia. [20] Additionally, the prevalence rate of anxiety and depression in female healthcare workers and nursing staff obtained a high scores for anxiety. Zhang et al. found that 36.1% of doctors suffered from insomnia symptoms during the beginning of the pandemics [21]. Doctors working in isolation units and worrying about being infected were more prone to experiencing sleep disturbance. We identified that sleeping problems were present in half of the respondents (80% were women and 54% were residents, which is in congruency with the presented results). Appetite loss was also identified among psychosomatic problems in a quarter of the respondents.

The results of our study proved that doctors were afraid of passing on the infection to their family members, of being hospitalized, or having possible long-term sequels. Talevi et al. [5] showed that most individuals experienced considerable psychological distress during the initial stage of the COVID-19 outbreak in terms of anxiety, depression, and post-traumatic symptoms, and that the symptoms' severity was evaluated as mild to moderate. Moreover, in the early days of the outbreak, a survey found that 53.8% of respondents rated the psychological impact of the outbreak as moderate or severe, 16.5% reported moderate to severe depressive symptoms, 28.8% reported moderate to severe anxiety symptoms, and 8.1% reported moderate to severe stress levels [6].

Medical practice had to adjust to new rules (institutional organization, doctor-patient relationships, ethical and legal rights, etc. We identified that doctors who were working with confirmed pregnant women preferred a caesarean delivery instead of a normal one, with the purpose of avoiding infection.

The insufficient equipment problem that doctors had to deal with in the beginning of the pandemic period was a strong source of stress. Medical staff had to be equipped with full-body protective equipment under the negative pressure of providing medical care for pregnant women during medical care or the delivery process. We identified that more than half of the doctors strongly agreed that the suits warmed them too much, and that the thermal discomfort decreased their resistance and concentration during surgery (52%), reduced the mobility and the accuracy of surgical or medical gestures (40%), and caused intraoperative visibility (47%).

To avoid being infected while removing the protective equipment, ob-gyn doctors cannot eat, drink, or use the bathroom for several hours. Dehydration and excessive sweating, cystitis, and a rash were identified by Marjanovic et al. (2006) on medical staff during the previous SARS pandemic [22]. Doctors working with confirmed patients were more prone to have sleep disturbance and high levels of stress.

Our study revealed that the doctors had difficulty in counselling pregnant women, especially patients who missed mandatory tests in the prenatal consultation, due to their fear of exposing themselves to possible infection during pregnancy. The results are in congruency with Mappa et al., who showed that the COVID-19 pandemic induced a doubling of the number of women who reached an abnormal level of anxiety [23]. The authors identified that pregnant women were fearful that COVID-19 could induce fetal structural anomalies (in 47% of investigated pregnant women), fetal growth restriction (in the case of 65% of patients), and preterm birth (in 51% of the women). Derya et al. [24] showed that the tele-education offered to the pregnant women on pregnancy and birth planning during COVID-19 decreased their prenatal distress and anxiety levels.

We identified that a quarter of doctors offered online consultations to their pregnant patients. The study of Derya et al. [24] proved that tele-medicine considerably improved patients' mental health during pregnancy. Using a control group, the authors showed that pregnant women who received counselling scored lower for anxiety, fear of giving birth, and worries of bearing a physically or mentally handicapped child.

We identified that there was a permanent concern regarding pandemic-associated malpractice cases. Being afraid of the risk of malpractice—misdiagnosis (51.06%) and the lack of legal or professional regulation (43.61%)—were among the most challenging problems during the beginning of the pandemic. Similar results were obtained by other studies with higher rates; in a study conducted on ob-gyn doctors in Turkey, it was found that 82.6% of doctors declared that they were worried about malpractice during the pandemic period [9].

Our study showed that three quarters of the doctors (73.40%) declared that the pandemic had changed their view of the rules of the profession. The results proved that clinical activity changed after the COVID-19 pandemic compared to the period before the pandemic; most doctors (89.36%) believed that the pandemic had changed their view of patient interactions and led them to apply new rules and to be more cautious. The results are congruent with those obtained by Bahat el al. [9], who showed that many ob-gyn doctors (81.5%) believed that their workload increased significantly compared to the period before the pandemic. Additionally, the doctors declared that they were concerned about their private office work being interrupted in the case of infection. The results are similar to those identified in a study conducted at the beginning of the SARScoV2 pandemic in the United States. A few weeks into the pandemic, the Medical Group Management Association found that COVID-19 was having a negative financial effect on 97% of the 724 medical practices [25].

We identified that the older the doctor, the more a caesarean section was preferred in pregnant women suspected or confirmed with COVID-19, due to the patients' stress related to the birth. Additionally, we found that doctors who were working with confirmed pregnant women preferred caesarean section. The results are congruent with those identified by Bahat et al. [9], who identified that less than a half of ob-gyn reported that they did opt for more caesarean deliveries despite their fear of exposure.

4.1. Strength and Limitations of the Study

The most important strength of the research is due to the fact that this is the first study on obstetrics and gynecology doctors working under the pressure of SARS-CoV-2 infection in Europe. Secondly, the study provides a large amount of information relating to psychological and somatic health, clinical practice, behaviors to diminish the risk of infection, new daily habits practice in order to diminish the risk of self-infection and infecting the members of the family, and new institutional rules and methods to deal with daily and job-related stress.

The first limitation of the study is represented by the limited territorial research. The respondents were selected from a single university city center, both maternity hospitals being university centers. Because of this limitation, the results cannot be generalized for all obstetrics and gynecology physicians. Secondly, we must take into consideration the fact that, in Romania, ob-gyn doctors provide medical support in both types of delivery (C-section or normal delivery), so greater risks and concerns regarding infection and job stress could be generalized only for Romanian doctors. Thirdly, the study was conducted after the first six months of the COVID-19 pandemic, so the results reflected the practice of preventive measures applied during this period, congruent with the guidelines in the medical field, precisely because, in the very first months of the pandemic, there were insufficient scientific data concerning the transmission of the infection from mother to fetus/new-born.

4.2. Reflections and Planning

The present study shows that the COVID 19 pandemic had negative psycho-somatic effects and led to changes in lifestyle, interaction with family members and friends, the patient's medical approach, and the adoption of new practices among obstetrics and gynecology physicians. These results prove the need for the adoption of new strategies regarding both the doctors' health (psychological assistance to treat high levels of stress, overwork, burnout, depression, or fear of infection due to the long negative effect and the considerable period of the pandemic), identified, in general, among healthcare workers during this period [26] and patients' health, by adopting new protocol guidelines in the field of obstetrics and gynecology, focusing especially on female gender and resident doctors. Secondly, the need for new institutional rules to decrease the risk of infection has imposed new methods of communication (online meetings, tele-medicine, online education) that should be regulated to eliminate the risk for malpractice as much as possible [27]. The psychological assistance of healthcare workers (such as psychological counselling, cognitive-behavioral therapy, or Balint groups for doctors) must be a priority for medical institutions and health-policy makers, due do the fact that the pandemic seemed to be longer than expected and the negative impact on mental health could lead to chronic consequences.

5. Conclusions

Even if they were not in the front line fight against the COVID 19 pandemic, working under the stress that they could be at risk of infection, or infecting patients or family members, put a lot of pressure on obstetrics and gynecology doctors, which had a great impact on their physical and mental health. Understanding the challenges that ob-gyn doctors were facing, especially at the beginning of the pandemic, will help institutions to better provide psychological and organizational support, considering their gender, marital status, parental role, age, comorbidities, and type of institutions, and to highlight guidelines to help them cope better with pandemic challenges.

Author Contributions: Conceptualization, M.I., R.-V.S., and D.-G.S.; data curation, M.I., R.-V.S., A.C., and D.-G.S.; formal analysis, M.I. and C.S.; investigation, R.-V.S., A.C., and D.-G.S.; methodology, M.I. and C.S.; supervision, M.I. and D.-G.S.; writing—original draft, M.I., C.S., A.C., and D.-G.S.; writing—review and editing, M.I., D.-G.S., and C.S. All authors have read and agreed to the published version of the manuscript.

Funding: The publication of this manuscript was granted by COST Action CA18211: DEVoTION: Perinatal Mental Health and Birth-Related Trauma: Maximizing best practice and optimal outcomes (European Cooperation in Science and Technology).

Institutional Review Board Statement: The study was conducted according to the guidelines of the Declaration of Helsinki, and approved by the Ethical Committee of "Elena Doamna" University Hospital of Iasi, Romania, with the registration number No. 6843/26 August 2020.

Informed Consent Statement: Informed consent was obtained from all subjects involved in the study.

Data Availability Statement: The data presented in this study are available on request from the corresponding author.

Conflicts of Interest: The authors declare no conflict of interest. The funders had no role in the design of the study; in the collection, analyses, or interpretation of data; in the writing of the manuscript, or in the decision to publish the results.

References

1. Rasmussen, S.A.; Smulian, J.C.; Lednicky, J.A.; Wen, T.S.; Jamieson, D.J. Coronavirus Disease 2019 (COVID-19) and pregnancy: What obstetricians need to know. *Am. J. Obstet. Gynecol.* **2020**, *222*, 415–426. [CrossRef]
2. Hall, R.C.; Hall, R.C.; Chapman, M.J. The 1995 Kikwit Ebola outbreak: Lessons hospitals and physicians can apply to future viral epidemics. *Gen. Hosp. Psychiatry* **2008**, *30*, 446–452. [CrossRef] [PubMed]
3. Tucci, V.; Moukaddam, N.; Meadows, J.; Shah, S.; Galwankar, S.C.; Kapur, G.B. The Forgotten Plague: Psychiatric Manifestations of Ebola, Zika, and Emerging Infectious Diseases. *J. Glob. Infect. Dis.* **2017**, *9*, 151–156. [CrossRef] [PubMed]
4. Sim, K.; Huak Chan, Y.; Chong, P.N.; Chua, H.C.; Wen Soon, S. Psychosocial and coping responses within the community health care setting towards a national outbreak of an infectious disease. *J. Psychosom Res.* **2010**, *68*, 195–202. [CrossRef]
5. Talevi, D.; Socci, V.; Carai, M.; Carnaghi, G.; Faleri, S.; Trebbi, E.; di Bernardo, A.; Capelli, F.; Pacitti, F. Mental health outcomes of the CoViD-19 pandemic. *Riv. Psichiatr.* **2020**, *55*, 137–144.
6. Wang, C.; Pan, R.; Wan, X.; Tan, Y.; Xu, L.; Ho, C.S.; Ho, R.C. Immediate Psychological Responses and Associated Factors during the Initial Stage of the 2019 Coronavirus Disease (COVID-19) Epidemic among the General Population in China. *Int. J. Environ. Res. Public Health* **2020**, *17*, 1729. [CrossRef]
7. Kang, L.; Li, Y.; Hu, S.; Chen, M.; Yang, C.; Yang, B.X.; Wang, Y.; Hu, J.; Lai, J.; Ma, X.; et al. The mental health of medical workers in Wuhan, China dealing with the 2019 novel coronavirus. *Lancet Psychiatry* **2020**, *7*, e14. [CrossRef]
8. World Health Organization. WHO Director-General's Statement on IHR Emergency Committee on Novel Coronavirus (2019-nCoV); WHO: Geneva, Switzerland. Available online: https://www.who.int/dg/speeches/detail/who-director-general-s-statement-on-ihr-emergency-committee-on-novel-coronavirus-(2019-ncov) (accessed on 13 January 2021).
9. Yalçın Bahat, P.; Aldıkaçtıoğlu Talmaç, M.; Bestel, A.; Topbas Selcuki, N.F.; Karadeniz, O.; Polat, I. Evaluating the effects of the COVID-19 pandemic on the physical and mental well-being of obstetricians and gynecologists in Turkey. *Int J. Gynaecol. Obstet.* **2020**, 67–73. [CrossRef] [PubMed]
10. Iorga, M.; Socolov, V.; Muraru, D.; Dirtu, C.; Soponaru, C.; Ilea, C.; Socolov, D.G. Factors influencing burnout syndrome in obstetrics and gynecology physicians. *BioMed Res. Int.* **2017**. [CrossRef] [PubMed]
11. Na'ama, O.; Naimi, A.I.; Tulandi, T. Prevalence and predictors of burnout among obstetrics and gynecology residents in Canada. *Gynecol. Surg.* **2016**, *13*, 323–327. [CrossRef]
12. Ye, J.; Wang, H.; Wu, H.; Ye, L.; Li, Q.; Ma, X.Y.; Yu, X.; Zhang, H.; Luo, X. Burnout among obstetricians and paediatricians: A cross-sectional study from China. *BMJ Open* **2019**, *9*, e024205. [CrossRef] [PubMed]
13. Kannampallil, T.G.; Goss, C.W.; Evanoff, B.A.; Strickland, J.R.; McAlister, R.P.; Duncan, J. Exposure to COVID-19 patients increases physician trainee stress and burnout. *PLoS ONE* **2020**, *15*, e0237301. [CrossRef] [PubMed]
14. Chua, M.S.Q.; Lee, J.C.S.; Sulaiman, S.; Tan, H.K. From the frontline of COVID-19–how prepared are we as obstetricians? A commentary. *BJOG Int. J. Obstet. Gynaecol.* **2020**, *127*, 786–788. [CrossRef]
15. Vafaei, H.; Roozmeh, S.; Hessami, K.; Kasraeian, M.; Asadi, N.; Faraji, A.; Bazrafshan, K.; Saadati, N.; Aski, S.K.; Zarean, E.; et al. Obstetrics Healthcare Providers' Mental Health and Quality of Life During COVID-19 Pandemic: Multicenter Study from Eight Cities in Iran. *Psychol. Res. Behav. Manag.* **2020**, *13*, 563–571. [CrossRef]
16. Phelan, A.L.; Katz, R.; Gostin, L.O. The Novel Coronavirus Originating in Wuhan, China: Challenges for Global Health Governance. *JAMA* **2020**, *323*, 709–710. [CrossRef] [PubMed]
17. WHO. WHO Health Emergency Dashboard WHO (COVID-19) Homepage. 2020. Available online: https://covid19.who.int/ (accessed on 26 September 2020).
18. National Institute of Statistic. *Statistics NIo. Inhabitant population of Romania at 01.01.2020*; Romanian Statistical Review: Bucharest, Romania, 2020.
19. Statistics NIo. Coronavirus COVID-19 in Romania. 2020. Available online: https://covid19geo-spatialorg/ (accessed on 26 September 2020).
20. Pappa, S.; Ntella, V.; Giannakas, T.; Giannakoulis, V.G.; Papoutsi, E.; Katsaounou, P. Prevalence of depression, anxiety, and insomnia among healthcare workers during the COVID-19 pandemic: A systematic review and meta-analysis. *Brain Behav. Immun.* **2020**, *88*, 901–907. [CrossRef]
21. Zhang, C.; Yang, L.; Liu, S.; Ma, S.; Wang, Y.; Cai, Z.; Du, H.; Li, R.; Kang, L.; Su, M.; et al. Survey of insomnia and related social psychological factors among medical staff involved in the 2019 novel coronavirus disease outbreak. *Front. Psychiatry* **2020**, *11*, 306. [CrossRef]
22. Marjanovic, Z.; Greenglass, E.R.; Coffey, S. The relevance of psychosocial variables and working conditions in predicting nurses' coping strategies during the SARS crisis: An online questionnaire survey. *Int. J. Nurs. Stud.* **2007**, *44*, 991–998. [CrossRef]
23. Mappa, I.; Distefano, F.A.; Rizzo, G. Effects of coronavirus 19 pandemic on maternal anxiety during pregnancy: A prospective observational study. *J. Perinat. Med.* **2020**, *48*, 545–550. [CrossRef]

24. Derya, Y.A.; Altiparmak, S.; Emine, A.K.; GÖkbulut, N.; Yilmaz, A.N. Pregnancy and Birth Planning During COVID-19: The Effects of Tele-Education Offered to Pregnant Women on Prenatal Distress and Pregnancy-Related Anxiety. *Midwifery* **2020**, 102877. [CrossRef]
25. Rubin, R. COVID-19's crushing effects on medical practices, some of which might not survive. *JAMA* **2020**, *324*, 321–323. [CrossRef] [PubMed]
26. Gómez-Salgado, J.; Domínguez-Salas, S.; Romero-Martín, M.; Ortega-Moreno, M.; García-Iglesias, J.J.; Ruiz-Frutos, C. Sense of Coherence and Psychological Distress Among Healthcare Workers During the COVID-19 Pandemic in Spain. *Sustainability* **2020**, *12*, 6855. [CrossRef]
27. Marques, I.; Serrasqueiro, Z.; Nogueira, F. Managers' Competences in Private Hospitals for Investment Decisions during the COVID-19 Pandemic. *Sustainability* **2021**, *13*, 1757. [CrossRef]

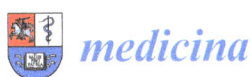

Article

Fear-Avoidance Behavior and Sickness Absence in Patients with Work-Related Musculoskeletal Disorders

Israel Macías-Toronjo [1], José L. Sánchez-Ramos [2], María J. Rojas-Ocaña [2,*] and Esperanza Begoña García-Navarro [3]

1. Department of Rehabilitation, Huelva Fremap Hospital, 21007 Huelva, Spain; israel.macias123@alu.uhu.es
2. Department of Nursing and Health Sciences, University of Huelva, 21007 Huelva, Spain; jsanchez@uhu.es
3. Research Group ESEIS, Social Studies and Social Intervention, Center for Research in Contemporary Thought and Innovation for Development, (COIDESO), Department of Nursing and Health Sciences, University of Huelva, 21007 Huelva, Spain; bego.garcia@denf.uhu.es
* Correspondence: mariaj.rojas@denf.uhu.es

Received: 30 October 2020; Accepted: 23 November 2020; Published: 26 November 2020

Abstract: (1) *Background and objectives*: The purpose of this work is to determine the association of fear-avoidance attitudes with sickness absence status, its duration and disability in a work accident context. (2) *Materials and Methods*: This is a descriptive observational design, conducting the study in two occupational insurance provider clinics with patients with nonspecific low back and neck pain during the study period. Clinical variables were the Fear Avoidance Questionnaire, Roland Morris Disability Questionnaire, Neck Disability Index, Numerical Pain Scale; sociodemographic variables were sex, age, occupational, educational level, sickness absence status, and duration in days of absence from work. Multiple logistic and linear regressions were used to explore the association between variables. (3) *Results*: Fear-avoidance behavior is related to sickness absence status (OR = 1.048, $p = 0.007$), and the physical activity dimension (OR = 1.098, $p = 0.013$) is more relevant than the work dimension (OR = 1.056, $p = 0.028$). The duration of sickness absence is related to higher values on the fear-avoidance behavior scale in its global dimension (b = 0.84, $p = 0.003$, r = 0.327), and the results of the physical activity dimension (B = 1.37, $p = 0.035$, r = 0.236) were more relevant than the work dimension (B = 1.21, $p = 0.003$, r = 0.324). Fear-avoidance behavior is related to disability in both dimensions (B = 0.912, $p < 0.001$, r = 0.505). (4) *Conclusions*: Fear-avoidance behaviors may influence the typification of sickness absence status, its duration both in its physical activity and work dimension, and its disability reported with higher values than in other healthcare contexts.

Keywords: avoidance learning; neck pain; workplace; employment; fear; exercise; attitude; accidents; disability

1. Introduction

Fear-avoidance behaviors are associated in an important way to the evolution and transition towards chronicity of musculoskeletal pain disorders [1,2]. The fear avoidance model focuses on patients' beliefs about disease, movement, and pain by creating myths related to erroneous thoughts about the nociceptive experience. According to this model, there would be an asynchrony between the natural pathological process and the clinical manifestation referred by the patient [3]. The pain referred would be exaggerated and not in accordance with the normal physiological process of the disorder. A central element of this model is the interpretation that the patient makes of an nociceptive experience as the origin of an important physical damage over which the patient has no control [3].

The avoidance and pain hypervigilance behaviors are based on catastrophic thoughts that activate limiting attitudes that, in turn, amplify the disability and pain [2]. As a result, catastrophic thoughts are related to fear of movement with worse results in terms of prognosis in therapeutic outcomes [4–6].

The working environment could be responsible for at least 37% of cases of low back pain (LBP) worldwide [7,8]. Workers exposed to forced postures, heavy lifting, or physically demanding jobs appear to be more likely to experience episodes of neck pain (NP) and LBP [9,10]. In addition, low levels of social coverage, job dissatisfaction, or stress levels caused by emergency situations could be associated with the development of musculoskeletal disorders [7,11].

High levels of fear-avoidance behaviors are associated with limitation of activity and greater levels of disability [12] and could condition recovery in processes of musculoskeletal disorders. In addition, fear-avoidance beliefs appear to be a predisposing factor towards long-term disorder processes, and their predictive value in acute problems is uncertain [13]. In this sense, the few studied which have focused on studying the association between fear-avoidance attitudes and time to return to work, in an occupational context, have questionable results [13–15], although the evaluation of this type of beliefs seems to have a positive result for determining the prognosis of patients with musculoskeletal disorders [14].

Different authors have insisted on the identification of psychosocial risk factors in the management of patients with musculoskeletal disorders [16–18]. Fear-avoidance behaviors and their influence on sickness absence and return to work have been scarcely studied in an occupational context. Musculoskeletal pain has been evaluated from the point of view of primary care within public health care [19–21], but more studies in an occupational health insurance provider context are necessary, taking into account that, in Spain, occupational disease is specifically managed by these institutions. In many European countries, these occupational health systems, similar to their Spanish counterparts, are responsible for managing occupational accidents [22], with a varied structure within the European Union [23]. Currently, Europe, Australia, Canada, USA, and others consider this system to be an essential part of the management of accidents and professional illness [23,24]. In Spain, occupational health insurance providers are non-profit organizations that manage health care and economic coverage in the process of an occupational accident or occupational disease. In this sense, these organizations have specific and earlier resources (specialized medicine, imaging tests, or rehabilitative treatment) as compared with public health services.

Considering that the presence of fear-avoidance attitudes may be associated with the evolution of low back and neck pain symptoms, the objective of this work was to determine the relationship of these variables as predictors of sickness absence status and its duration in an occupational health insurance provider context. Therefore, the aim of this article is to describe the association between fear-avoidance behaviors as psychosocial factors in patients with occupational low back pain (LBP) and neck pain (NP) and their influence on absenteeism in an occupational health insurance provider context. This analysis is justified by the need to identify these non-strictly clinical variables for prevalent disorders such as low back and neck pain, in order that they can be observed and taken into account in guidelines and multidisciplinary therapeutic approaches at an occupational context.

2. Materials and Methods

2.1. Type of Study

This is a descriptive observational study conducted at the Clinical Health Service of an occupational insurance provider.

2.2. Subjects

All the subjects who presented to an occupational health clinic with a diagnosis of nonspecific low back and neck pain due to a work accident between 1 June 2018 and 31 December 2019 and met the inclusion criteria were included in this study. Nonspecific pain is considered to be pain that is not caused by fractures, direct trauma, or systemic disease and where there is no proven root compression amenable to surgical treatment [25]. A work-related accident is any bodily injury that the employed worker suffers during the time, or as a consequence, of work. The target population was the entire group of patients who met the inclusion criteria. All patients ($n = 129$) who met this inclusion criteria were consecutively included.

The following inclusion criteria were applied:

1. Work-related nonspecific LBP and NP attending to an occupational health clinic;
2. Age between 18–65 years old;
3. Understanding the language, informed and signed consent.

The following exclusion criteria were applied:

1. Back pain or neck pain related to infection, cancer, fracture, visceral disease, spondylarthrosis, extruded disc herniation, or cauda equina syndrome;
2. Previous treatment for spinal pain;
3. Previous surgical intervention, commuting accident, common illness, or occupational disease;
4. Cognitive impairment.

The injured patients were attended by the occupational insurance medical service the same day as the work accident and, after diagnosis and typification as a work accident, it was noted if the patients were on sick leave or if they could reconcile their disorders with work activity. At the end of their visit with the physician, each patient who met the eligibility criteria was informed of the study objectives and was asked to participate. All patients included in the study signed the relevant informed consent form. The participants knew that the information collected was confidential and anonymous.

On the first day of attendance, the participants were interviewed by the physiotherapist in charge and sociodemographic information was collected, the content of the questionnaires was explained, and the questionnaires were completed only once, prior to any other therapeutic intervention. The duration of sick leave was measured by the days off from the day of the accident at work until the patients returned to work. Any re-injury or setback of the same LBP and NP disorder after the six months after the day of return to work were considered to be part of the same process of sickness absence and therefore were recorded as the same sickness absence. Any change in the initial diagnosis of nonspecific low back or neck pain of any of the participants throughout the follow-up process would cause them to not meet the inclusion criteria and be excluded from it. The recruitment process is shown in Figure 1.

The study was authorized by the Fremap Mutual Ethics Committee (code number FREMAP-2200631-Z) and followed the ethical principles for medical research in human beings according to the Declaration of Helsinki and the protection of data and guarantees of digital rights according to organic law March 2018 of 5 December 2018.

2.3. Study Variables

2.3.1. Fear-Avoidance Questionnaire (FABQ)

Fear-avoidance behaviors about work are closely related to sickness absence in musculoskeletal disorders processes [26]. The questionnaire reflects how physical and work activity influence the nociceptive experience [27]. It consists of two parts, one on fear-avoidance beliefs during work activity (Cronbach's alpha = 0.88) and another on physical activity (Cronbach's alpha = 0.77). The FABQ contains 16 items, 5 for a physical activity subscale (with a maximum score of 24), and 11 for the work subscale (with a maximum score of 42). Each item is answered on a 7-point Likert scale where 0 is totally disagree and 6 totally agrees. The Spanish version of the FABQ has good comprehensibility, consistency, and reliability, with the full version being as valid as both subscales, as well as being easier to score and analyze, thus, facilitating its use in clinical practice [27]. In this study, the full scale (Cronbach's alpha = 0.84) and both dimensions were used separately.

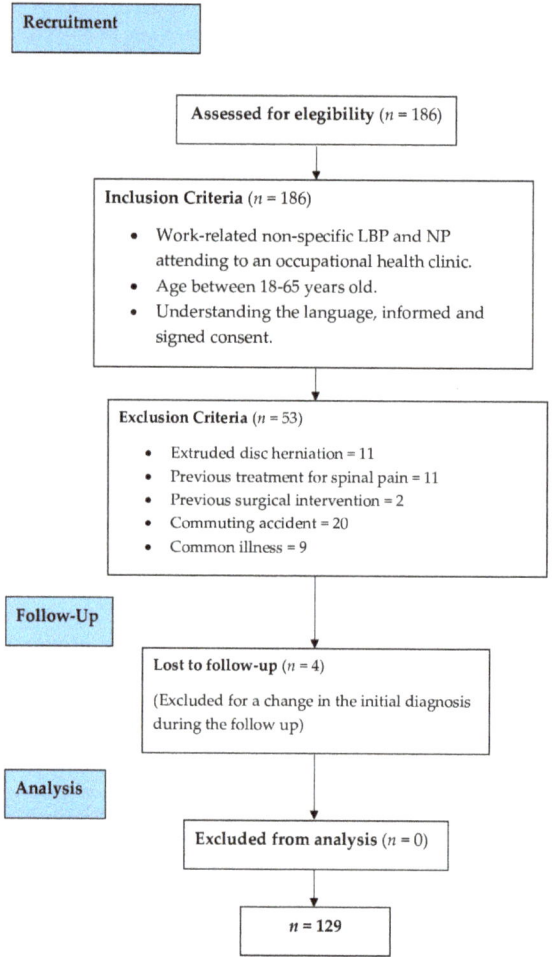

Figure 1. Recruitment process diagram.

2.3.2. Roland Morris Disability Questionnaire (RMQ)

Disability was measured using the Roland Morris Questionnaire instrument. It is one of the world's best validated and globally used scales to measure LBP disability. It consists of 24 items related specifically to daily physical activities likely to be affected by LBP scoring between 0 (no disability) and 24 (maximum disability). A reliable Spanish version has been validated to evaluate disability in patients with LBP [28], with an intraclass correlation of 0.87, good concurrent and construct validity, and a high internal consistency. Disability is expressed in absolute values.

2.3.3. Neck Disability Index Questionnaire (NDI)

Neck disability was measured with the Neck Disability Index Questionnaire. This 10-item questionnaire reflects limitations in activities of daily living of NP patients. It has 6 possible answers for each item scored from 0 to 5. It is a validated and reliable Spanish version to measure disability in patients with NP [29]. Neck pain disability is expressed in absolute values.

2.3.4. Numerical Pain Scale

The Numerical Pain Scale, an 11-item scale, in which 0 indicates an absence of pain while 10 represents the worst imaginable pain, was used to measure pain intensity [30].

2.3.5. Socio-Demographic Variables

Socio-demographic variables were collected on sex, age, occupational and educational level, as well as the following clinical variables: location, sickness absences status, and its duration.

For occupational level variable, the National Classification of Occupations 2011 (NCO-11) prepared by the Spanish National Statistics Institute (INE) was taken as a reference in the classification according to the level of skills. It consists of four skill levels [31]. The subjects were grouped into primary education, secondary education, pre-university education, and university education for the educational level variable.

2.4. Statistical Analysis

Firstly, a descriptive analysis of the variables studied was carried out. Means and standard deviations (SD) were incorporated for continuous variables and absolute and relative frequencies for categorical variables. To analyze the relationship between variables, a bivariate analysis of the variables associated with the sickness absence status, the duration of sickness absence and disability was carried out. The relationship of socio-demographic variables (sex, education, occupation, and location) with sickness absence status was checked using the Chi-square statistic, once the conditions of application were verified. The level of professional competence was recoded, grouping the only case of Level 4 with those of Level 3. The means of the clinical variables and age were compared using Student's t-test to see the differences between patients who were on sickness absence status and those who were not, after checking the absence of deviations by means of a detrended Q-Q plot and variance homogeneity. A linear regression model was used, controlling for occupation and educational level variables, to evaluate the association of fear-avoidance beliefs with the duration of sickness absence and the degree of disability. Multiple logistic regression was used, controlling for socio-demographic variables, to explore the association of the variables fear avoidance behaviors and pain intensity with the need for sickness absence. Using multiple linear regression, controlling for the socio-demographic variables, the association of the variables fear avoidance behaviors with the duration of sickness absence and the degree of disability was explored.

The Statistical Package for the Social Sciences (SPSS) software program was used for the statistical analysis in this work.

3. Results

This study included 129 subjects in which 71 were men (55%) and 58 women (45%) (CI 95% 0.52–2.17). Patients with low back pain were the majority ($n = 88$, 68.2%) versus neck pain ($n = 41$, 31.8%). Subjects on sickness absence ($n = 81$ vs. $n = 48$) status were the majority (62.8% vs. 37.2%) (CI 95% 0.23–1.05). The mean values of the age variable were 40.1 (standard deviation = 9.43) years. Mean duration of sickness absence was 23.74 (SD = 30.27) days. The levels of disability were higher in the group with low back pain (46.64%) than in the group of patients with neck pain (42.67%). The average of the Fear-Avoidance Behavior Questionnaire in its global dimension was 45.09 (SD = 13.15), in the physical activity dimension it was 18.03 (SD = 5.93), and in its work dimension it was 27.05 (9.15). The Numeric Pain Scale mean score was 7.02 (1.83).

3.1. Sickness Absence

The relationship between presenting fear-avoidance behavior and sickness absence is described in Table 1. Subjects on sickness absence presented a higher mean score on the fear-avoidance behavior scale (46.63 (11.80)) than those not on sickness absence (39.10 (13.24)) ($p < 0.001$). Subjects on sickness absence presented a higher mean score on the fear-avoidance scale for work (29.19 (8.13)) and physical activity (19.44 (5.21)) than those not on sickness absence status (23.46 (9.71)) (16.65 (6.35)) ($p < 0.001$). In the results presented, fear-avoidance behavior is related to sickness absence in its global version (OR = 1.05, p = 0.007), the relationship with the physical activity dimension (OR = 1.10, p = 0.013) was higher than with the work dimension (OR = 1.06, p = 0.028) (Table 2).

Table 1. Mean values for the different clinical variables as a function of the presence (yes) or absence (no) of sickness absence.

Sickness Absence	Yes			No			‡ p
	n	Mean	SD	n	Mean	SD	
Fear-avoidance behavior	81	48.63	11.80	48	39.10	13.24	<0.0001
Fear-avoidance Work	81	29.19	8.13	48	23.46	9.71	<0.0001
Fear-avoidance physical activity	81	19.44	5.21	48	15.65	6.35	<0.0001
Intensity of pain	81	7.23	1.55	48	6.69	2.19	0.101

‡ t-Student.

Table 2. Multiple logistic regression model. Influence of fear-avoidance behavior on the sickness absence variable, controlled by education and occupation.

1. Multiple logistic regression model: influence of fear-avoidance attitudes on sickness absence, controlled by education and occupation.

Sickness absence	p	Odds Ratio	CI 95% Odds Ratio
Fear avoidance	0.007	1.05	[1.01–1.08]
Education	0.090		
Primary/University	0.591	2.12	[0.14–32.59]
Secondary/University	0.905	0.85	[0.05–13.21]
Pre-University/University	0.862	1.26	[0.10–16.51]
Occupation	0.299		
Level 1/Level 3	0.291	3.86	[0.31–47.52]
Level 2/Level 3	0.844	1.32	[0.08–22.04]

2. Multiple logistic regression model: influence of fear-avoidance physical activity behavior on sickness absence, controlled by education and occupation

Sickness absence	p	Odds Ratio	CI 95% Odds Ratio
Fear avoidance PA *	0.013	1.10	[1.02–1.18]
Education	0.275		
Primary/University	0.638	1.91	[0.13–27.96]
Secondary/University	0.836	0.75	[0.05–11.22]
Pre-University/University	0.940	1.10	[0.09–13.97]
Occupation	0.208		
Level 1/Level 3	0.193	5.18	[0.43–61.57]
Level 2/Level 3	0.730	1.64	[0.10–26.90]

3. Multiple logistic regression model: influence of fear-avoidance work behavior on sickness absence, controlled by education and occupation.

Sickness absence	p	Odds Ratio	CI 95% Odds Ratio
Fear-avoidance work	0.028	1.06	[1.01–1.11]
Education	0.290		
Primary/University	0.534	2.35	[0.16–34.97]
Secondary/University	0.977	0.96	[0.06–14.46]
Pre-University/University	0.841	1.30	[0.10–16.67]
Occupation	0.280		
Level 1/Level 3	0.269	4.08	[0.34–49.60]
Level 2/Level 3	0.807	1.42	[0.09–23.32]

* Fear-avoidance physical activity.

3.2. Duration of Sickness Absence

No relationship between socio-demographic variables and the duration of sickness absence was found. Regarding the clinical variables, the duration of work absence rises by 0.84 days for each unit of increase in the fear-avoidance behavior scale on its global dimension (B = 0.84, p = 0.003, r = 0.33), and the relationship with the physical activity dimension (B = 1.37, p = 0.035, r = 0.24) was superior as compared with the work dimension (B = 1.21, p = 0.003, r = 0.32) (Table 3).

Table 3. Multiple linear regression of the duration variable with clinical variables controlling for occupation and education variables.

Duration of Sickness Absence	b	95% CI (b)	r	p
Fear-avoidance behavior	0.84	[0.29–1.38]	0.33	0.003
Fear-avoidance work	1.21	[0.41–2.00]	0.32	0.003
Fear-avoidance physical activity	1.37	[0.10–2.64]	0.24	0.035
Pain intensity	2.78	[−1.58–7.15]	0.14	0.208

3.3. Disability

Regarding the association between fear-avoidance attitudes and disability, this variable increases 0.91 units for each point on the global fear-avoidance attitudes scale (B = 0.91, p < 0.001, r = 0.50), and the scale on physical activity was superior (B = 1.70, p < 0.001, r = 0.41) as compared with the work scale (B = 1.1, p < 0.001, r = 0.42). The relationship between pain intensity and disability shows statistical significance (B = 4.36, p < 0.001, r = 0.33). In multiple linear regression among fear-avoidance attitudes, intensity of pain, and disability, the scale of fear-avoidance attitudes remains stable in both groups of subjects for sickness absence status (B = 0.81, p < 0.001, r = 0.44) and in the group of subjects who remain active at work (B = 0.81, p < 0.001, r = 0.44) (Table 4).

Table 4. Multiple linear regression of the disability variable with clinical variables individually controlled by the confounding variables education and occupation (initial and final model).

(a) Multiple linear regression of the disability variable with clinical variables individually controlled by the confounding variables education and occupation (initial model).

Disability	B	CI 95% Odds Ratio	r	p
Fear avoidance	0.91	[0.61–1.22]	0.50	<0.0001
Fear-avoidance work	1.10	[0.65–1.55]	0.42	<0.0001
Fear-avoidance physical activity	1.66	[0.99–2.34]	0.41	<0.0001
Pain intensity	4.36	[2.18–6.54]	0.33	<0.0001

(b) Multiple linear regression of the disability variable with clinical variables individually controlled by the confounding variables education and occupation (final model).

Disability	B	CI 95% Odds Ratio	r	p
Fear avoidance	0.81	[0.51–1.11]	0.44	<0.0001
Pain intensity	3.19	[1.17–5.22]	0.24	0.002

(c) Multiple linear regression of the disability variable with clinical variables in the context of sickness absence (final model).

Disability	B	CI 95% Odds Ratio	r	p
Fear avoidance	0.88	[0.50–1.26]	0.44	<0.0001
Pain intensity	4.63	[1.76–7.51]	0.30	0.002

4. Discussion

4.1. Sickness Absence and Duration of Absence

The results presented indicate an association of fear-avoidance behavior with sickness absence status and with the time to return to work in patients with work-related LBP and NP. This association is reflected both in attitudes related to physical activity and in those related to the work dimension. In this analysis, education and occupation variables have been considered to be confounding variables, and therefore controlled in the statistical process.

The ability of the fear-avoidance questionnaire to predict sickness absence status and time to return to work has previously been shown to be questionable [32]. However, other authors have pointed out that high levels of fear-avoidance attitudes in the work dimension were related to long term sickness absence and no improvement in disability and pain in patients with LBP [33]. The results presented, in this study, are based on data collected at the beginning of the sickness absence process and on the follow-up of the duration of the absence. In this sense, these authors worked with a sample of chronic patients, while the results obtained in this project were collected from a follow-up of acute, subacute, or chronic patients until the day of return to work. Therefore, the control of the subjects in the sample presented in this work was done from the first day of the work accident, which would make the follow up of the measure stricter without any time period from the accident until the patient started to be controlled.

In the analysis presented in this project, the two dimensions are related to both the sickness absence status and the duration of sickness absence, with the physical activity dimension having a stronger association. Grotle et al., in a follow-up study at 3, 6, 9, and 12 months, reported that chronic pain patients presented significantly higher values of fear-avoidance behaviors in the work dimension than those in acute pain [34]. In this regard, these authors [34] described that the results of the fear-avoidance questionnaire in the physical activity dimension gave higher initial results that were reduced during the first month of follow-up, which could explain why the patients in the sample presented higher levels of fear-avoidance attitudes in the physical activity dimension than in the work dimension. IN addition, it is the occupational health insurance provider that, in addition to managing health care, manages the economic compensations derived from sickness absence. In a sample of subjects in which occupational primary sector and nonpermanent jobs prevail, the answers referring to their own capacity to work or when they would expect to return to work included in the questionnaire in its work dimension, could be biased by an economic issue. Thus, the question referring to the economic compensation received for being in a sickness absence status (item eight in the questionnaire on fear-avoidance behavior) was, on many occasions, a reason for consultation by the workers on the obligatory nature of the response. In the same line, the fear-avoidance behavior questionnaire has been debated by some authors as a one-dimensional instrument capable of measuring fears and avoidance attitudes towards pain [35]. These authors proposed, in a detailed analysis of each of the items in the questionnaire, that it indicated more expectations for returning to work than actual fears and avoidance attitudes towards patient work activity. This, together with the bias proposed in the context of sickness absence/economic compensation, could question the use of this work dimension of the questionnaire in an occupational health insurance provider context. In any case, the data on both sickness absence status and its duration are related to both dimensions of fear-avoidance behavior, although in an occupational context, a greater association with the work dimension could be expected.

Storm et al. related high scores in their work dimension to the ability to work in a short four-week longitudinal study and considered it to be an important tool when assessing work capacity in patients with back pain [36]. Along the same lines, Jay et al., in a study that investigated the relationship among fear-avoidance variables with the time to return to work in patients with musculoskeletal disorders (lumbar, cervical/shoulder, and arm/hand pain), indicated that these psychosocial variables were related to absenteeism from work [37], something in line with the results presented in this work. In our case, the sample consisted exclusively of subjects who had suffered a work-related accident, while the sample of the authors mentioned above were on subjects on work and non-work-related sickness absence in a mixed population sample. In this sense, this work is novel by the fact that it relates work-related sickness absence with this type of attitude.

The values of the fear-avoidance behavior obtained are similar to other studies both in acute [38,39] and in chronic pain patients [40]. These data are also consistent with other observational studies in the same line [19,33,41,42], giving meaning to the fear avoidance model, according to which the perception of pain in the short term could lead to movement avoidance behavior, reinforcing this attitude in the long term and providing negative characteristics to movement after a work accident [42].

Both dimensions of the fear-avoidance behavior scale are related to the duration of sickness absence with a higher relevance than in other studies [33]. Thus, Kovacs et al., in a primary care study in the Spanish Health System, although they did not report a relationship between fear-avoidance behavior and disability, they did find a relationship between the duration of sickness absence in patients with low back pain during the year following the injury in the context of chronic pain [19]. In general, fear-avoidance behavior values are higher in workers who remain sedentary than in those who perform some activity [19,43], which is in line with the results of this work on a global scale and in both dimensions separately but, in this case, in a much more intense association [40]. The results obtained could be influenced by such an early intervention and this, in turn, could be related to the fact that the observed association between fear-avoidance behaviors and sickness absence and their duration was so strong. Be that as it may, the work environment seems to mediate this association in some way.

4.2. Disability

The results presented show a strong association between fear-avoidance behavior, in both dimensions, and declared disability in first attendance. In this same sense, Trinderup et al. related this type of attitude towards pain and disability in patients with chronic LBP [33]. In cross-sectional studies, this association with fear-avoidance behavior has been confirmed to be the main predictor of LBP disability in a study carried out in a primary care system [44]. In Spain, the influence of fear-avoidance behavior on disability in primary care has been previously studied, showing no association [19], or being clinically irrelevant [21]. Our study, in multivariate analysis, with the control of confounding variables (education and occupation) and including the intensity of pain declared in first assistance, does show a correlation between fear-avoidance behavior and pain intensity with disability both in patients on sickness absence as in the work active patients. Again, contrary to what might be expected, attitudes related to physical activity are more related to disability than occupational ones, and items related to return to work and economic compensations could influence the results at this level.

In the same line of the presented results, intensity of pain has also been pointed out as a predictor of disability in prospective studies [45] and likewise, the information collected was done the same day of the accident. This early intervention could determine the high levels of pain reported.

Thus, the reported disability would be related, according to our results, to fear-avoidance behavior and the amount of pain declared regardless of the work status of the subjects.

In this study, the subjects were recruited on the day of the work accident and followed up until the day of return to work. In this sense, the obtained results and interpretations could be influenced by this very early recruitment. Regarding the limitations of this work, other aspects of a psychological nature such as anxiety and depression have also been shown to intervene in patients' return to work [46–48]. In this work, this specific aspect has not been controlled and could be a confounding factor to our results. Furthermore, the methodological design used would not allow us to establish causal relationships among the variables studied. Although the follow-up was carried out until the day of return to work, we would recommend longitudinal studies with larger sample sizes and more heterogeneous work groups.

5. Conclusions

Both dimensions of the fear-avoidance behavior questionnaire are related in a work-related health insurance provider context to the sickness absence status, its duration, and disability reported with higher values than in other health areas, and fear-avoidance behavior is lower in subjects who remain active at work.

Fear-avoidance behavior must be taken into account for the assessment and follow-up of these patients with the aim of reducing the time to return to work, work absenteeism, and achieving better results in clinical interventions.

Author Contributions: I.M.-T. conceived of the idea project; I.M.-T. and E.B.G.-N. contributed to the design and implementation of the research; I.M.-T. and J.L.S.-R. verified the analytical methods and did the statistical work; J.L.S.-R., M.J.R.-O., and E.B.G.-N. supervised the findings of this work. All authors have read and agreed to the published version of the manuscript.

Funding: This research received no external funding.

Conflicts of Interest: Authors declare no conflict of interest.

References

1. Luque-Suarez, A.; Martinez-Calderon, J.; Falla, D. Role of kinesiophobia on pain, disability and quality of life in people suffering from chronic musculoskeletal pain: A systematic review. *Br. J. Sports Med.* **2019**, *53*, 554–559. [CrossRef]
2. Zale, E.L.; Lange, K.L.; Fields, S.A.; Ditre, J.W. The Relation Between Pain-Related Fear and Disability: A Meta-Analysis. *J. Pain* **2013**, *14*, 1019–1030. [CrossRef]
3. Crombez, G.; Eccleston, C.; Van Damme, S.; Vlaeyen, J.W.; Karoly, P. Fear-Avoidance Model of Chronic Pain. *Clin. J. Pain* **2012**, *28*, 475–483. [CrossRef]
4. Niederstrasser, N.G.; Meulders, A.; Meulders, M.; Slepian, P.M.; Vlaeyen, J.W.; Sullivan, M.J. Pain Catastrophizing and Fear of Pain Predict the Experience of Pain in Body Parts Not Targeted by a Delayed-Onset Muscle Soreness Procedure. *J. Pain* **2015**, *16*, 1065–1076. [CrossRef]
5. Westman, A.E.; Boersma, K.; Leppert, J.; Linton, S.J. Fear-Avoidance Beliefs, Catastrophizing, and Distress. *Clin. J. Pain* **2011**, *27*, 567–577. [CrossRef] [PubMed]
6. Parr, J.J.; Borsa, P.A.; Fillingim, R.B.; Tillman, M.D.; Manini, T.M.; Gregory, C.M.; George, S.Z. Pain-Related Fear and Catastrophizing Predict Pain Intensity and Disability Independently Using an Induced Muscle Injury Model. *J. Pain* **2012**, *13*, 370–378. [CrossRef] [PubMed]
7. Schaafsma, F.G.; Anema, J.R.; Van Der Beek, A.J. Back pain: Prevention and management in the workplace. *Best Pr. Res. Clin. Rheumatol.* **2015**, *29*, 483–494. [CrossRef] [PubMed]
8. Punnett, L.; Prüss-Ütün, A.; Nelson, D.I.; Fingerhut, M.A.; Leigh, J.; Tak, S.; Phillips, S. Estimating the global burden of low back pain attributable to combined occupational exposures. *Am. J. Ind. Med.* **2005**, *48*, 459–469. [CrossRef]
9. Shankar, S.; Shanmugam, M.; Srinivasan, J. Workplace factors and prevalence of low back pain among male commercial kitchen workers. *J. Back Musculoskelet Rehabil.* **2015**, *28*, 481–488. [CrossRef]
10. Keown, G.A.; Tuchin, P.A. Workplace Factors Associated With Neck Pain Experienced by Computer Users: A Systematic Review. *J. Manip. Physiol. Ther.* **2018**, *41*, 508–529. [CrossRef]
11. Moretti, A.; Menna, F.; Aulicino, M.; Paoletta, M.; Liguori, S.; Iolascon, G. Characterization of Home Working Population during COVID-19 Emergency: A Cross-Sectional Analysis. *Int. J. Environ. Res. Public Health* **2020**, *17*, 6284. [CrossRef] [PubMed]
12. Vlaeyen, J.W.; Linton, S.J. Fear-avoidance and its consequences in chronic musculoskeletal pain: A state of the art. *Pain* **2000**, *85*, 317–332. [CrossRef]
13. Iles, R.A.; Davidson, M.; Taylor, N.F. Psychosocial predictors of failure to return to work in non-chronic non-specific low back pain: A systematic review. *Occup. Environ. Med.* **2007**, *65*, 507–517. [CrossRef] [PubMed]
14. Sieben-Wertz, J.; Portegijs, P.J.; Vlaeyen, J.W.; Knottnerus, J.A. Pain-related fear at the start of a new low back pain episode. *Eur. J. Pain* **2005**, *9*, 635. [CrossRef]

15. Pincus, T.; Vogel, S.; Burton, A.K.; Santos, R.; Field, A.P. Fear avoidance and prognosis in back pain: A systematic review and synthesis of current evidence. *Arthritis Rheum.* **2006**, *54*, 3999–4010. [CrossRef]
16. Haldeman, S.; Johnson, C.D.; Chou, R.; Nordin, M.; Côté, P.; Hurwitz, E.L.; Green, B.N.; Cedraschi, C.; Acaroglu, E.; Kopansky-Giles, D.; et al. The Global Spine Care Initiative: Care pathway for people with spine-related concerns. *Eur. Spine J.* **2018**, *27*, 901–914. [CrossRef]
17. Pincus, T.; Smeets, R.J.E.M.; Simmonds, M.J.; Sullivan, M.J.L. The Fear Avoidance Model Disentangled: Improving the Clinical Utility of the Fear Avoidance Model. *Clin. J. Pain* **2010**, *26*, 739–746. [CrossRef]
18. Oliveira, C.B.; Maher, C.G.; Pinto, R.Z.; Traeger, A.C.; Lin, C.-W.C.; Chenot, J.-F.; Van Tulder, M.; Koes, B. Clinical practice guidelines for the management of non-specific low back pain in primary care: An updated overview. *Eur. Spine J.* **2018**, *27*, 2791–2803. [CrossRef]
19. Kovacs, F.; Muriel, A.; Sánchez, M.D.C.; Medina, J.M.; Royuela, A. Fear Avoidance Beliefs Influence Duration of Sick Leave in Spanish Low Back Pain Patients. *Spine* **2007**, *32*, 1761–1766. [CrossRef]
20. Ramírez-Maestre, C.; Esteve, R.; Ruiz-Párraga, G.; Gómez-Pérez, L.; López-Martínez, A.E. The Key Role of Pain Catastrophizing in the Disability of Patients with Acute Back Pain. *Int. J. Behav. Med.* **2016**, *24*, 239–248. [CrossRef]
21. Kovacs, F.; Muriel, A.; Abriaira, V.; Medina, J.M.; Sanchez, M.D.C.; Olabe, J. The Influence of Fear Avoidance Beliefs on Disability and Quality of Life is Sparse in Spanish Low Back Pain Patients. *Spine* **2005**, *30*, E676–E682. [CrossRef] [PubMed]
22. Lappalainen, L.; Liira, J.; Lamminpää, A.; Rokkanen, T. Work disability negotiations: Supervisors' view of work disability and collaboration with occupational health services. *Disabil. Rehabil.* **2018**, *41*, 2015–2025. [CrossRef] [PubMed]
23. Manzanera, R.; Mira, J.J.; Plana, M.; Moya, D.; Guilabert, M.; Ortner, J. Patient Safety Culture in Mutual Insurance Companies in Spain. *J. Patient Saf.* **2017**. [CrossRef] [PubMed]
24. International Comparison of Occupational Accident Insurance System—OSHWiki. Available online: https://oshwiki.eu/wiki/International_comparison_of_occupational_accident_insurance_system (accessed on 26 March 2020).
25. Spanish Working Group of the European Programme Cost B13. Clinical Practice Guide for Non-Specific Low Back Pain. 2018. Available online: https://www.REIDE.org (accessed on 17 September 2018).
26. Waddell, G.; Newton, M.; Henderson, I.; Somerville, D.; Main, C.J. A Fear-Avoidance Beliefs Questionnaire (FABQ) and the role of fear-avoidance beliefs in chronic low back pain and disability. *Pain* **1993**, *52*, 157–168. [CrossRef]
27. Kovacs, F.M.; Muriel, A.; Medina, J.M.; Abraira, V.; Sánchez, M.D.C.; Jaúregui, J.O. Psychometric Characteristics of the Spanish Version of the FAB Questionnaire. *Spine* **2006**, *31*, 104–110. [CrossRef] [PubMed]
28. Francisco, M.; Kovacs, F.M.; Llobera, J.; Gil Del Real, M.T.; Abraira, V.; Gestoso, M.; Fernández, C. Validation of the Spanish Version of the Roland-Morris Questionnaire. *Spine* **2002**, *27*, 538–542. [CrossRef]
29. Kovacs, F.M.; Bagó, J.; Royuela, A.; Seco-Calvo, J.; Giménez, S.; Muriel, A.; Abraira, V.; Martín, J.L.; Peña, J.L.; Gestoso, M.; et al. Psychometric characteristics of the Spanish version of instruments to measure neck pain disability. *BMC Musculoskelet. Disord.* **2008**, *9*, 42. [CrossRef]
30. Williamson, A.; Hoggart, B. Pain: A Review of Three Commonly Used Pain Rating Scales. *J. Clin. Nurs.* **2005**, *14*, 798–804. [CrossRef]
31. INEbase/Clasificaciones Estadísticas/Clasificaciones Nacionales/Clasificación Nacional de Ocupaciones. CNO/Últimos Datos. Available online: https://www.ine.es/dyngs/INEbase/es/operacion.htm?c=Estadistica_C&cid=1254736177033&menu=ultiDatos&idp=1254735976614 (accessed on 30 October 2020).
32. Holden, J.; Davidson, M.; Tam, J. Can the Fear-Avoidance Beliefs Questionnaire predict work status in people with work-related musculoskeltal disorders? *J. Back Musculoskelet. Rehabil.* **2010**, *23*, 201–208. [CrossRef]
33. Trinderup, J.S.; Fisker, A.; Juhl, C.; Petersen, T. Fear avoidance beliefs as a predictor for long-term sick leave, disability and pain in patients with chronic low back pain. *BMC Musculoskelet. Disord.* **2018**, *19*, 1–8. [CrossRef]
34. Grotle, M.; Vøllestad, N.K.; Brox, J.I. Clinical Course and Impact of Fear-Avoidance Beliefs in Low Back Pain. *Spine* **2006**, *31*, 1038–1046. [CrossRef] [PubMed]
35. Aasdahl, L.; Marchand, G.H.; Østgård, S.G.; Myhre, K.; Fimland, M.S.; Røe, C. The Fear Avoidance Beliefs Questionnaire (FABQ) Does it Really Measure Fear Beliefs? *Spine* **2020**, *45*, 134–140. [CrossRef] [PubMed]

36. Storm, V. Bewegungsangstkognitionen, schmerzbezogene Selbstwirksamkeitserwartung und subjektive Arbeitsfähigkeit bei Personen mit Rückenschmerz. *Der Schmerz* **2019**, *33*, 312–319. [CrossRef] [PubMed]
37. Jay, K.; Thorsen, S.V.; Sundstrup, E.; Aiguadé, R.; Casaña, J.; Calatayud, J.; Andersen, J.L. Fear Avoidance Beliefs and Risk of Long-Term Sickness Absence: Prospective Cohort Study among Workers with Musculoskeletal Pain. *Pain Res. Treat.* **2018**, *2018*, 1–6. [CrossRef]
38. Marchand, G.H.; Myhre, K.; Leivseth, G.; Sandvik, L.; Lau, B.; Bautz-Holter, E.; Røe, C. Change in pain, disability and influence of fear-avoidance in a work-focused intervention on neck and back pain: A randomized controlled trial. *BMC Musculoskelet. Disord.* **2015**, *16*, 1–11. [CrossRef]
39. Myhre, K.; Røe, C.; Marchand, G.H.; Keller, A.; Bautz-Holter, E.; Leivseth, G.; Sandvik, L.; Lau, B. Fear–avoidance beliefs associated with perceived psychological and social factors at work among patients with neck and back pain: A cross-sectional multicentre study. *BMC Musculoskelet. Disord.* **2013**, *14*, 329. [CrossRef]
40. Diaz-Cerrillo, J.L.; Rondon-Ramos, A.; Clavero-Cano, S.; González, R.P.; Martinez-Calderon, J.; Luque-Suarez, A. Factores clínico-demográficos asociados al miedo-evitación en sujetos con lumbalgia crónica inespecífica en atención primaria: Análisis secundario de estudio de intervención. *Atención Primaria* **2019**, *51*, 3–10. [CrossRef]
41. Nava-Bringas, T.-I.; Macías-Hernández, S.I.; Ríos, J.R.V.; Coronado-Zarco, R.; Miranda-Duarte, A.; Cruz-Medina, E.; Arellano-Hernández, A. Fear-avoidance beliefs increase perception of pain and disability in Mexicans with chronic low back pain. *Rev. Bras. Reum. Engl. Ed.* **2017**, *57*, 306–310. [CrossRef]
42. Hiebert, R.; Campello, M.A.; Weiser, S.; Ziemke, G.W.; Fox, B.A.; Nordin, M. Predictors of short-term work-related disability among active duty US Navy personnel: A cohort study in patients with acute and subacute low back pain. *Spine J.* **2012**, *12*, 806–816. [CrossRef]
43. Fritz, J.M.; George, S.Z.; Delitto, A. The role of fear-avoidance beliefs in acute low back pain: Relationships with current and future disability and work status. *Pain* **2001**, *94*, 7–15. [CrossRef]
44. Igwesi-Chidobe, C.N.; Coker, B.; Onwasigwe, C.N.; O Sorinola, I.; Godfrey, E.L. Biopsychosocial factors associated with chronic low back pain disability in rural Nigeria: A population-based cross-sectional study. *BMJ Glob. Health* **2017**, *2*, e000284. [CrossRef] [PubMed]
45. Lardon, A.; Dubois, J.-D.; Cantin, V.; Piché, M.; Descarreaux, M. Predictors of disability and absenteeism in workers with non-specific low back pain: A longitudinal 15-month study. *Appl. Ergon.* **2018**, *68*, 176–185. [CrossRef] [PubMed]
46. Daubs, M.D.; Norvell, D.C.; McGuire, R.; Molinari, R.; Hermsmeyer, J.T.; Fourney, D.R.; Wolinsky, J.P.; Brodke, D. Fusion Versus Nonoperative Care for Chronic Low Back Pain. *Spine* **2011**, *36*, S96–S109. [CrossRef] [PubMed]
47. Finnes, A.; Enebrink, P.; Ghaderi, A.; Dahl, J.; Nager, A.; Öst, L.-G. Psychological treatments for return to work in individuals on sickness absence due to common mental disorders or musculoskeletal disorders: A systematic review and meta-analysis of randomized-controlled trials. *Int. Arch. Occup. Environ. Health* **2018**, *92*, 273–293. [CrossRef] [PubMed]
48. Hees, H.L.; Koeter, M.W.J.; Schene, A.H. Predictors of Long-Term Return to Work and Symptom Remission in Sick-Listed Patients with Major Depression. *J. Clin. Psychiatry* **2012**, *73*. [CrossRef]

Publisher's Note: MDPI stays neutral with regard to jurisdictional claims in published maps and institutional affiliations.

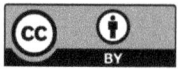

© 2020 by the authors. Licensee MDPI, Basel, Switzerland. This article is an open access article distributed under the terms and conditions of the Creative Commons Attribution (CC BY) license (http://creativecommons.org/licenses/by/4.0/).

MDPI
St. Alban-Anlage 66
4052 Basel
Switzerland
Tel. +41 61 683 77 34
Fax +41 61 302 89 18
www.mdpi.com

Medicina Editorial Office
E-mail: medicina@mdpi.com
www.mdpi.com/journal/medicina

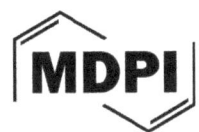